Maximise Your Fitness Potential

FOR ALL LEVELS

Wayne Lambert

Maximise Your Fitness Potential

By Wayne Lambert

Certified Personal Trainer, Nutrition Specialist and Master Life Coach

C.E.O & Founder – Whole Body Workshop & Weight Loss Dubai

Author of Visualise the new you, Psychology of weight loss, Exercise your whole body at home, Exercise therapy – progressive rehabilitation exercises and Why not stay fat?

ISBN 978-0-9561494-5-9

Important
The author assumes no responsibility for any consequence relating directly or indirectly to any action or inaction you take based on the information, services or other material contained or implied in this book.

There are no implied endorsements of any product mentioned herein.

I dedicate this, my favourite book to date to the 2 most beautiful princesses in my life, my wife Laila and my baby girl Eden Star.

I hope that 'Maximise Your Fitness Potential' provides you with everything that you desire related to health & fitness.

ACKNOWLEDGEMENTS

As always I would like to thank my family, relatives and close friends for their continued support. My gratitude for unconditional support in whatever I do goes to Laila who continues to inspire me on a daily basis. I thank all my good friends and fellow Royal Marine physical training instructors, who have all given me their professional opinion on my fitness books and who have continued to give me constructive criticism and comments in order for this edition to be the best it can possibly be. In particular I would like to thank Pete Jordan the current PT advisor to the United States Marine Corps for his feedback especially during the latter stages of writing. His advice and contribution as to what the avid reader will want to see within a fitness book was much appreciated. Pete has recently retired from competing in professional MMA (mixed martial arts) and is a training conditioning coach for many top level athletes in a variety of sports.

I must pay a special tribute to Saad Zaabi, a truly inspirational physical training instructor from the United Arab Emirates. Saad helped me a great deal when I put together my rehabilitation book, and he is featured in all of the photos, a book that covers how to rehabilitate yourself post injury, concentrating on specific exercises to strengthen weakened muscles.

My utmost gratitude again goes to Homrani Lotfi the Body Builder from Tunisia who is also in the first edition. Lotfi has been a good friend and colleague of mine for 6 years or so. Lotfi gave up his spare time to assist me with the completion of this book and he did so with commitment and desire. Lotfi owns his own gymnasium in Tunisia but currently works in Dubai physically training the UAE military. I wish him well with all his future conquests.

Apologies to anyone I may have forgotten to mention.

TABLE OF CONTENTS

INTRODUCTION

By opening 'Maximise Your Fitness Potential' you took your first step towards achieving your physical potential and training goals. This book is loaded with the most up to date training exercises and information based on the latest scientific research. Upon reading the text, you will know how to properly, safely and effectively perform 100's of exercises and you will be ready to begin a more functionally beneficial training program whatever your aim. The true importance of this book lies with the functional exercises found throughout. Performing the exercises in 'Maximise Your Fitness Potential' can provide significant aesthetic and functional strength benefits with an improvement in overall health and well-being as well as increased bone density, muscle, tendon and ligament strength, plus reducing the potential for injury in sports and every day activities. Strength training commonly uses a variety of exercises and types of equipment to target specific muscle groups and although strength training is primarily an anaerobic activity, some proponents have adapted it to provide the benefits of aerobic exercise through circuit training etc. A Fitness centre usually has a combination of free weights and machines but for those who choose the home based program you can utilise chairs, benches, balls and bands to name but a few pieces of equipment shown in the exercises within this book. Knowing what you want to achieve from the exercises you perform is a must before starting any kind of program. 'Maximise Your Fitness Potential' provides easy to follow exercise explanations to suit your individual needs. All exercises and activities are explained in detail so you know exactly what and where you are targeting. In all the programs the exercises we use adhere to our four rules of developing functional strength and fitness.

- Develop joint flexibility;
- Develop Tendon and ligament strength;
- Develop Core strength and stabilisers;
- Train movement's not just individual muscles.

'Maximise Your Fitness Potential' offers a variety of exercise choices and templates for your ease of planning, but ultimately it will be your fine tuning and choices that will determine your results. Our content has been specifically compiled for anyone of all levels, from beginner to advanced and even those who need that extra edge. We have catered for anyone who simply wants to advance their knowledge and/or fitness levels. We stress at all times that your number one criteria should be safety to you and others, this should include consulting medical advice prior to attempting any physical activity or changes in foods that you eat. It is also advised that you read all the exercise descriptions that explain about correct technique of each exercise. Wearing suitable clothing, breathing correctly and your everyday posture are all contributing factors to improving your knowledge about health and fitness.

Physiologically, training progressively increases your body's functional efficiency and in doing so your body adapts and you become stronger and fitter due to the demands placed on your body to improve its physical condition. Training requires many hours of work with exercises and routines repeated many times. Under these conditions, boredom and monotony can become barriers. 'Maximise Your Fitness Potential' overcomes these barriers by incorporating variety from the many exercises and program templates provided. This particular book has been specifically written to include the most relevant information but in it's simplest form, irrespective of the fact that it is an extremely overwhelming subject.

SPECIFICITY FOR YOU AS AN INDIVIDUAL

Time

Your time constraints will dictate what your program will include, and of course the length of your workout will have to be specific to your needs. If you believe that each workout should take 40 minutes then so be it and for some people this can be realistic, although certain sessions should take longer. The length of time of your program will depend on such criteria as the inclusion of a thorough warm up, the implementation of rest periods between sets and many other things which will be explained in detail later. There are many books available that attract individuals who want quick results due to busy lifestyles, and these books advertise shorter workouts, quicker and better results. The fact is that if you are proficient at exercising related to technique and safety etc and your time is limited then you can exercise in 2 minutes flat and feel better that you have done something – it is purely a psychological battle and if you have the time then you may as well use it in a safe and effective manner. For example if you are on vacation and your partner is in the shower and you feel the need to do some sit ups, push-ups and squats then you do this because time is limited, you are on holiday and you know you will feel better after doing (as good as) a whole body workout in a confined space, and in a minimum amount of time.

Avoiding the fitness performance plateau

Before long a familiar pattern often emerges with your level of fitness, and frequently your interest level with exercise wanes. Your performance plateaus and you start questioning the value of your workouts and you find yourself asking, where has your motivation gone? A fitness progress check often helps you overcome a plateau, both before you start your exercise programme and at regular intervals throughout the year. Checking your fitness progress will bring a whole range of benefits including:

- A motivational tool, as you see your performance improving;
- Information on how you've progressed since your last check up;

- Assessment of where your fitness levels currently are;
- The opportunity to alter your training programme.

A fitness progress check should really be carried out by professionals at a fitness centre irrespective of whether you plan to train at home or not, your aim at this stage is only to assess where you are at. When you commence an exercise program at home or join a gym you should complete a fitness check-up before you start which can serve two basic functions, a safety check before training and a baseline assessment of your fitness. It should be discussed with you concerning your needs, and if any, special considerations (injuries, limitations, adaptations, physician's directions, etc) that may limit your ability to train at full capacity. Checking that it is safe for you to exercise confirms your current fitness levels and any precautions that may be necessary for you to take prior to commencing your program. Your fitness check information should be recorded and completely confidential and will serve as a reference point both to base your training on and for future comparison. Once your baseline fitness levels have been established, you have something to measure future progress against. Additionally, your training program can now be designed to reflect both your goals and the specific areas you need to improve. All good fitness assessments should include a minimum of the following elements:

- Health questionnaire;
- Resting heart rate (RHR) & Blood pressure test (BP)
- Discussion about your fitness goals;
- Advanced fitness check;
- Flexibility tests.

The information from your fitness progress check then provides an instant comparison for your future progress, and at all times takes into consideration what exercises may fit your specific training needs. The following guidelines are a review of your conditioning principles:

Physical exam
Obtain a physical examination from your doctor so you will know if you have any limitations that affect your choice of exercise. Consider your training background before choosing any exercises. Beginners are often introduced to resistance training with machine or simple free weight movements, and machines although not necessarily safer, are easier to use because you do not have to supply a majority of the balance and coordination. As you begin to understand certain techniques related to body position and posture etc you can move to more complex free weight activities. You should consider the value of certain exercises in terms of movement specificity i.e. what your needs are

for your chosen activity or sport. The time it takes to learn a new exercise movement or how to use a certain cardiovascular machine you could be spending your time more wisely learning a more functional exercise for your specific needs.

Physiological & biomechanical analysis

Physiological analysis will allow you to devise a program that addresses the aspects of strength, muscular endurance, flexibility, conditioning, power, and speed required for success around your specific needs. A biomechanical analysis will allow you to choose training activities that assist you with your development in the specific manner, and also to determine the areas of critical stress within your chosen activities. You should have your strengths and weaknesses assessed as different activities, exercises and sports require various levels of fitness. Specific programs can be developed to address your needs, and your strengths and/or weaknesses. Many people have misconceptions as to which exercises are more important for them, and the importance of health and fitness in general. Choosing proper exercises and including them at the proper time during your training cycle is an art form.

Muscle balance

Imbalances – You need to keep in mind muscle balance between your opposite muscle groups when choosing your specific exercises i.e. if you have a weaker group of muscles on one side of your body compared with the other. Your exercise choice may need to include more exercises for those weaker muscles, in order to compensate for this imbalance. However you still need to spend time on all major muscle groups to insure overall development.

Individual body types

Within the human body there are many subtle differences and therefore strength and conditioning programs need to be designed so that your unique morphology and training background, as well as gender and age, are taken into consideration. Human beings display a wide variety of physiques and habits of physical activity. In order to respond to this diversity you need to be aware of, and open minded about your range of possible performance capabilities.

TESTING YOUR LEVEL OF FITNESS

Most fitness centres use testing procedures when you first apply to join, and these tests are designed to check your overall fitness levels and monitor your workout progress. A regular fitness test ensures you get the best results from your training, and to help you understand more about fitness testing we have explained it briefly for you below. These tests and the results gained from them should be used as a reference point in which you can look at over a period of time and see the areas where you are excelling the most, and in what areas you are lacking in. If you work out regularly, fitness tests are a great way to judge your progress, and these can be repeated and monitored every couple of months. Other specific tests include skin-fold and balance tests. Skin-fold tests are a good gauge of weight loss, as they tell you specifically if you have lost fat mass. Balance tests can be very critical for determining your physical capabilities, and if you excel on balance then you will have a better chance at performing your activity to optimum levels.

Endurance tests
These tests determine your current VO2 and Lactate thresholds as well as "maximum time to exhaustion" which for distance related events is invaluable. These normally include aerobic tests, a cycle test, a heart rate test, specific running tests and treadmill tests. Aerobic tests are a good assessment to perform if you've been working on your cardio. The cycle test determines your fitness and skill level very well. It is however extremely important to warm up and stretch your Quad (Quadriceps) muscles more so than normal on this particular test as these muscles are worked more predominately. The heart rate test allows you to see how well your endurance training is progressing and allows you to determine your ability to recover. Some of the most commonly used running tests are specific to measuring your maximum speed (VO2 max) i.e. for sprinters, or running tests that measure your aerobic endurance i.e. for distance athletes. The treadmill test assesses your pure level of fitness and of course minimizes external influences, such as wind resistance or uneven terrain etc. If you aren't an avid runner, walking tests are an alternative way of determining your aerobic abilities. You can perform walking tests going for speed, distance or incline gradient. All of these will challenge you physically and in turn enable you to see your progress.

Flexibility tests
These tests are used to ensure that if you already stretch, that it is paying off. It will certainly help to have these tests regularly to assess your risk of injury, these tests normally include flexion tests, sit & reach tests and static tests. By performing these flexion tests you are able to gauge how well you are able to move your hip joint

through a large range of motion. The sit and reach test is to determine your hamstring and trunk flexibility, and a modified test can be performed for those who have a limited range of motion. Static flexibility tests assess how large a range of motion you have when no movement is taking place i.e. how far past your toes you can reach or the distance your hip flexors can move.

Self fitness test
Certain tests can be conducted by you yourself as they do not require you to visit a fitness centre, and by conducting these tests you can also keep your results to compare over time. All you are required to do is as follows:

1. Perform each test in order;
2. Check your results and scores against the charts;
3. Write your results and scores within the charts;
4. Add up your scores, to acquire your total score.

In order for your results to be accurate, do not eat anything or drink alcohol or any type of caffeine at least 2 hours prior to the test. Do not exercise on the day of testing, and ensure that you complete only 1 test per day. Below is a self assessment chart for you to compare your results over time.

YOUR OWN PERSONAL FITNESS CHART				
TESTS	DATE:		DATE:	
MEASURE YOUR BODY				
Your weight				
Your waist				
Your chest				
Your hips				
Your thighs				
AEROBIC FITNESS	RESULTS	SCORE	RESULTS	SCORE
Resting Heart Rate (RHR)				
Step test				
FLEXIBILITY				
ABDOMINAL STRENGTH				
TOTAL SCORE				

Your measurements
To get a good indication of fat loss and gains in muscle you should measure your body size and compare these changes in measurements by regularly recording your progress.

Your waist - By keeping your stomach in a natural position, wrap the tape measure around your body, the tape should be level with your navel;

Your chest - Whilst standing naturally (relaxed) wrap the tape measure around your chest at nipple height, ensuring that the tape is at the same level around the back of your body;

Your hip - Wrap the tape and measure around the fullest part of your hips;

Your thigh - Wrap the tape and measure around the halfway point between the inside of your thigh and the top of your knee, ensuring that the tape is level all around.

Measuring your Resting Heart Rate (RHR)
Find your pulse on your wrist or neck and count the number of heart beats for 60secs.

YOUR OWN HEART RATE CHART					
Rating	**Score**	**Men**	**Women**	**Males under 15**	**Females under 15**
Good	2	Under 60	Under 65	Under 70	Under 75
OK	1	60-80	65-90	70-85	75-95
Poor	0	Above 80	Above 90	Above 85	Above 95

You should be aware that RHR alone is not an indication of your level of physical fitness, it is simply a clinical measurement, and must be considered alongside many other factors. However, a change in your average RHR may be an indication of an improvement or decrease in your level of fitness. A decrease in your RHR is usually attributed to an improvement in your cardiovascular fitness, and is more likely the result of an improvement in metabolic conditioning.

Measuring your aerobic fitness with a 3 minute step test
Your consistency during this test is of paramount importance i.e. complete this test the same way every single time that you do it. This test measures your cardiovascular endurance, and by working out regularly you will see your improvements over time.

All you are required to do is as follows:

1. Find a stable object that is approx. 40cm in height i.e. bench, platform or step, 30cm if your height is under 160cm;
2. Your aim is to step up fully onto the object, with the whole of your foot, then step back down onto the floor, change legs each time;
3. For 3 minutes you should maintain a steady speed throughout;
4. Immediately find your pulse on completion of the test. Calculate your heart rate (HR) per minute by counting the number of heart beats for 1 minute or 15 seconds and multiply by 4.

YOUR OWN (3 MINUTE) STEP TEST					
Rating	Score	Men	Women	Males under 15	Females under 15
Good	7	Below 110	Below 116	Below 120	Below 124
Above average	6	111-124	117-130	121-130	125-134
OK	4	125-140	131-146	131-150	135-154
Below average	2	141-155	147-160	151-160	155-164
Poor	1	Above 156	Above 161	Above 161	Above 165

Measuring your flexibility with the sit and reach test

This test should always be carried out on completion of the step up test and/or an adequate warm up, and is designed to measure the flexibility of your hamstrings and your lower back. You should have a tape measure set in the correct position, with the start of the tape level with your toes. All you are required to do is the following:

- Sit on the floor with your legs straight and your toes pointing upwards;
- With your legs remaining as straight as possible, slowly lean forwards from the trunk, reach forward as far as you can and hold for 2 seconds;
- Whether your fingertips touch your toes or not, measure the distance reached;
- The measurement is regarded as a minus score if you don't reach your toes, a zero if you touch them and a plus score if your fingertips pass your feet.

YOUR OWN FLEXIBILITY TEST (in cm)			
Rating	Score	Below 40 years of age	Above 40 years of age
Very good	3	15+	7+
Good	2	15 to 5	7 to 0
OK	1	5 to 0	0 to -5
Poor	0	0 and below	-5 and below

Measuring your abdominal strength with a 40 second test

Once you have mastered the technique and you are stronger, this test can be modified in 2 ways. 1. Measured over a longer period i.e. 90s or you can perform as many as you can until failure. Until this time, all you are required to do is as follows:

1. Place your feet on a chair whilst lying on your back, ensuring that your knees are bent at a 90 degree angle;
2. With your elbows pointing forwards, cross your arms across your chest;
3. Endeavour to touch your thighs with your elbows as you raise your shoulders from the floor, crunch forwards and then repeat the movement once your shoulders have returned back to the floor;
4. Your aim is to carry out the correct technique and complete as many as you can in 40 seconds.

YOUR OWN ABDOMINAL TEST				
Rating	**Score**	**Below 29 years of age**	**Between 30-39 years of age**	**Between 40-59 years of age**
Good	3	34 or more	30 or more	26 or more
OK	2	24-34	22-30	20-26
Poor	1	24 or below	22 or below	20 or below

Your total score

Add together your scores collated from your self fitness tests and find your rating of fitness as described below. The results are only a basic indicator of your overall fitness but can still be compared to tests that you complete in the future.

RATING OF YOUR FITNESS	YOUR TOTAL FITNESS SCORE
Very good	15-12
Good	12-9
OK	9-6
Poor	6-3
Very poor	3 or less

Other tests are explained in their respective chapters and sub-chapters such as:

- Sports specific tests;
- Explosive tests;
- Strength tests.

RECORDING YOUR EXERCISE PERFORMANCE

In this section you will discover how to record your exercise performance for the best results possible. Whether you require strength, weight loss, toning, an increase in size or simply to maintain your health 'Maximise Your Fitness Potential' provides you with exercises and activities for your individual requirements. The content from this book will enable you to get fit to mimic everyday activities and movements used commonly in everyday life and sport. "Functional strength" is the successful basis behind gaining real strength that has lasting benefits for everyone, no matter what your goal. As creatures of habit we tend to stick with what we like and enjoy, instead of trying out new ideas, only you know what activities you like doing, this is why we have supplied you with numerous alternative exercise choices for you to contemplate doing.

Critical to your success is to start an exercise and food journal to record your new habits and improvements. Recording these new habits helps you to notice trends in your performance, but more importantly you will notice differences between your actual performances and how you felt that you performed. Recording how you feel before, during and after exercise enables you to compare your 'feelings' over a set time. Journals give you the edge in order to begin a new life changing habit.

Tips for keeping your journal

There are many uses for keeping a journal to reach your health & fitness goals, irrespective of what you want to achieve. Use the fitness or diet components as a tool to help you reach your goals, but not to turn you into an obsessive compulsive, but keep it simple and easy so you stick with it. The purpose is to help you crystallize your thinking and to help you remain focused on your way to accomplishing your goal. If you keep a good fitness journal, you not only increase your chances of reaching your goal, you will in all likelihood decrease the time it takes for you to reach your goal. Sometimes journals are referred to as any of the following:

- Fitness diary;
- Exercise log;
- Diet log;
- Or a performance log, and others.

When you write down your fitness goals you dramatically increase the chances of accomplishing those goals, therefore your chances of success are higher. Several benefits of keeping a fitness journal include the following:

1. Helps you focus your mind on your fitness goals;
2. Helps you see your progress, which motivates you even more;
3. Helps you deal with the mental blocks that you might have about your diet plan, exercise program, or particular performance goals;
4. Helps you work through exercise burnout, and writing down what is keeping you from exercising. Following through with your fitness plan can help remove your obstacles.

No confusing charts or graphs are required as the only recommendation is that you divide your fitness journal into specific sections, such as:

Beginning of journal
At the start of the journal write down your written fitness goals so it is easy for you to review them often. This is the most important part of the journal.

Mid section of journal
Within your fitness journal keep a log of some of your diet plan progress, a log of your workouts, or a log of your training sessions, especially if you are training for a particular event, i.e. a strength competition or a marathon.

Weekly section
Throughout your fitness journal you should make weekly entries (daily entries for more intense training), however weekly entries should be suffice for most.

Psychological section
This section in your journal should be devoted to the mental part of your fitness goals, where you can work through the mental blocks that you are dealing with on the road to your fitness goals. This section can help you get more motivated, and it can also be a good place to record your credits for your rewards / incentive system.

Achievement section
Write down your diet / fitness accomplishments in your fitness journal, and make sure you have a separate section for this. Some examples of statements of accomplishment that you could record in your fitness journal include:

- If you found something difficult or if something in particular is really paying off;

- If you managed to lose a set amount of weight since you stopped eating a certain food type etc.

The process of writing down your accomplishments is a good idea because it helps to remind yourself that you are making progress and that the hard work is paying off. It is good for your self esteem and your level of motivation. It can also help if you are suffering from overtraining syndrome which is explained in more detail later in this book.

Remarks column
If you have a copy for each training day, you can simply make notes next to each exercise or training session for that particular day. These methods allow you to gauge your weekly progress i.e. if you are trying to lose weight and you are on a diet plan, you can make copies of your weekly diet plan for each day of the week. All seven days of the week could be on one diet plan sheet that is just copied each week. Writing down what you eat each day and perhaps even how many calories you eat. Putting pictures in your fitness journal that represent your fitness goals or even before and after photos, these will all help you. Only you will know which method is going to help you and this will be through trial and error. Some people are more visual, others are more auditory i.e. they would prefer to listen to motivational tapes which will help them accomplish their goals. Whichever method you choose, you will see the progress that you have made over time, and this will help motivate you. To monitor your training more efficiently, there are 2 other systems that you could use and these systems enable you to maintain

your motivation and record any changes related to adaptation and progression. These systems are:

1. The inbuilt computer monitoring system – where you are assigned your own personal key which contains all of your details. This key records everything that you do in your CV and strength sessions, on a continuous basis;

2. The program sheet – this system is particularly more useful for recording your strength training progress and is similar to the fitness journal method. As you work through your session you update the details yourself related to the CV equipment you use, the resistance, reps and sets etc you use.

Whichever system that you use to monitor your training, the value of a fitness check and recording system should not be underestimated. You should choose the most suitable system that fits for your training needs.

Recording your strength training performance
Strength training is explained in full detail in its own specific chapter, however it is extremely important for you to understand that recording your progress is as essential as actually doing the workout itself. Endeavour to record the following information in your fitness journal: Record the speed in which you perform each repetition i.e.

•   The average number of seconds you take to perform the contraction phase;
•   The average number of seconds you pause in the fully contracted position;
•   The average number of seconds you take to perform the negative phase.

If you use this standard protocol, you should be performing a 2 second contraction phase, a 1 second pause, and a 4 second negative phase. Within your fitness journal you can record it as 2/1/4 or however you choose. The amount of weight you use for a specific exercise, the number of repetitions you perform or the time the exercise is performed for, can all be recorded in the columns provided within your program. Using the remarks column for anything else is always beneficial, which may save you time later i.e. record the height of the seat on a particular machine or the height setting for the cables etc. When you record the amount of repetitions you perform, try and indicate if a particular number of repetitions were almost performed, or if the exercise was performed with poor form. In doing this you are indicating that the weight should not be increased for the next workout and you can use small arrows i.e. an arrow pointing up means that next time the repetitions can be increased and likewise an arrow pointing down means the opposite. Writing a plus sign (+) after the amount of repetitions you perform can indicate that the exact number of repetitions performed is unknown i.e. more than the number written. If you use a set of extension techniques such as forced reps or breakdowns (explained in detail later) you can also use the plus sign. For example: if you performed 8 repetitions and failed on the 9th, then your training partner helped you perform an additional 2 forced reps, you would record 8+2FR in the repetitions section of the performance box. If you do not complete a particular exercise you should still place something in the box i.e. an X but try not to leave the performance box empty for any exercise. If the exercise order is performed differently from what you have planned, you should re-number the exercise boxes to show the correct order of performance, especially if for example a particular shoulder exercise involves the triceps, then you may want to perform another muscle group first before you attempt a specific triceps exercise. However you choose to record your information is up to you, but it will never be a wasted effort. What you want to achieve can be recorded like the following example:

AIM	Muscle Endurance	A combination of Strength, Size & Endurance	Muscle Mass	Aerobic Fitness
HOW CAN YOU DO THIS?	Perform 13-20 reps	Perform 6-12 reps	Perform 1-5 reps	Perform 20+ reps

The majority of individuals who strength train perform 1-6 sets per exercise and 1-3 exercises per muscle group with adequate rest in between each set. Those who prefer circuit training have little or no rest between exercises. There are many different ways for you to strengthen your body and this is explained in more detail in the actual strength chapter.

Recording your cardiovascular training performance

Cardiovascular training is explained in full detail in its own specific chapter, as is heart rate training (HRT) however, it is extremely important for you to understand that **a** heart-rate monitor can record all of your cardiovascular training sessions and can be preset for specific training limits, both for heart rate and recovery time. On completion of your exercise, this information can then be viewed for comparison or downloaded onto a computer and directly compared with graphs and charts against your previous performances. The frequency for most common cardiovascular exercise programs is shown below, begin by recording these examples:

FREQUENCY	INTENSITY & TIME	TYPE	REMARKS
3-5 days per week	20-60mins (in target heart rate zone)	CARDIO On treadmill	Alternate days of more intense exercise with a day of rest or easy exercise

Target heart rate zones are explained in their relevant sub-chapter, but be aware that the timings do not include the warm up and cool down. When you begin to record information within your fitness program, the main components that you should record are duration and intensity i.e. how much you have increased your duration (with good posture and form) before you work on and record, how much you have increased the intensity of your workout. It is safe to increase the intensity by 10% per week i.e. once you are walking comfortably and with good posture and form for approx. 60 minutes at a time, then work on increasing the intensity by adding speed, hills, or intervals.

Exercise abbreviations

Certain words or abbreviations are used to define words linked with exercise, and you may come across them within a program that is given to you or you may find some throughout this book. If you are a complete beginner to exercise then you may not understand some of them, so we have listed a few basic examples for you.

WU – Warm up / CD – Cool down / MINS – Minutes / S – Seconds / MS – Main set
Two of the most common strength training related words you may come across are: Reps and Sets and they are explained below:

REP or Repetition - A repetition is one complete movement in the exercise, from the starting position to a position of maximum contraction and then back to the starting position. This ensures that you complete full range of movement (ROM).

SET - Several exercises intended to be done in a series, and the number of sets you perform depends on the following:

- Your training experience, the number of muscle groups trained per session;
- The size of the muscle group being trained.

Common muscle related terms

Abbreviation	Meaning
GLUTES	Gluteus muscles
HAMS	Hamstrings
BI'S	Biceps
TRI'S	Triceps
QUADS	Quadriceps
PECS	Pectorals (chest muscles)
DELTS	Deltoids (shoulder muscles)
LATS	Latissimus dorsi

Common movement related terms

Abbreviation	Meaning
ROM	Range Of Movement
EXT	Extension
FLX	Flexion
ABD	Abduction
ADD	Adduction
UG	Under-grasp (supinated) Grip
OG	Over-grasp (pronated) Grip
ROT	Rotation or Rotary (Single Joint)
CPD	Compound (Multi-Joint)
RT	Right
LT	Left

Common high intensity training protocols and techniques

Abbreviation	Meaning
BD	Breakdowns
FN	Forced Negatives
FR	Forced Reps
MC	Maximum Contraction
MR	Manually Resisted
NA	Negative Accentuated
NO	Negative Only
SC	Static Contraction
SH	Static Hold
SS	Super Set
HR / HRT	Heart Rate / Heart Rate Training
MHR	Maximum Heart Rate
RHR	Resting Heart Rate
LI	Lactate Threshold/Training
LI	Lactate Intervals

Common exercise start positions

Abbreviation	Meaning
Std	Seated
Stg	Standing
Ly	Lying
Kn	Kneeling

Common equipment terms

Abbreviation	Meaning
BB	Barbell
DB	Dumbbell
TB	Trap Bar (Shrug Bar)
EZ	EZ Bar
CM	Cable Machine
MB	Medicine ball
If thick bars are used then the diameter should be written i.e. before BB e.g. 2.5"BB.	

These lists are by no means exhaustive as there are literally hundreds more terms and abbreviations. Remember that you can create your own abbreviations too, and you will find that it will make life easier for you in the long run.

INJURY PREVENTION & REHABILITATION

Prehabilitation

Otherwise described as, preventative measures to avoid injuries.

The following information can be used by almost anyone but is more relevant to someone who works out regularly that is familiar with the joints and muscles of the human body. Included within this sub-chapter are ways in which you can self analyze and stretch and strengthen specific muscles that are prevalent to common imbalances within the human body related to misalignments and/or injuries. Many individuals have structural imbalances within their body, yet continue to increase their chances of injury by incorrectly strengthening those areas.

The following factors need to be considered:

1. Tight muscles - This can be due to factors such as insufficient stretching after exercise or being overweight etc. More often than not our muscles shorten as we age, but all of these reasons and more can actually knock the body off balance and cause injury;

2. Muscle soreness - This could be due to intense exercise, poor lifting and carrying technique or even leading a sedentary lifestyle related to poor posture and/or being overweight. Muscle soreness can differ from person to person although is especially common in the lower back region;

3. Lifestyle - Today's society and current lifestyle adaptations can also lead to poor circulation which can be due to factors such as lack of movement, poor diet, poor flexibility and breathing to name only a few;

4. Injuries - If you have had any injuries (past or present) this could have been caused by your other muscles over compensating. This is your body's way of realigning you to what feels like a normal posture.

Benefits of good posture:

- Pain relief throughout your body;
- Allows you to move efficiently;
- Improves muscle function and increases your range of motion;
- Takes pressure off of compressed organs;
- Improves your circulation;
- Creates a trimmer appearance;
- Radiates an attitude of confidence.

Self analysis:

Prior to commencing any fitness program you should always seek advice from a medical practitioner who can give you a medical examination to test your posture and body alignment. Likewise if you have been training for some time and you feel fit and healthy there is absolutely nothing wrong with assessing yourself for your own peace of mind. Genetically our bodies have a more dominant or stronger side, but to ensure that you are not going down a path that could potentially put your health & fitness back to the beginning or put you at risk to injury, try the following:

Posture	Stand upright in front of a full length mirror with your feet level and shoulder width apart. Maintain a good posture, ensuring your head and eyes are facing forwards, with relaxed shoulders. Your body image should be one of symmetry i.e. both your upper body and your lower body should be naturally aligned for e.g. your collar bones (or shoulders) should be level with each other and also your hips & knees too. Ideally it is better if someone else can observe these findings for you whilst you concentrate on your stance and posture.

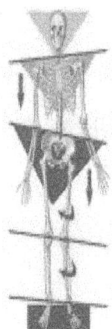

	From your above findings you should have some idea regarding whether you need to strengthen weak muscles and/or stretch tight ones. For e.g. If one collar bone (prominent landmark) is slightly lower than the other, then this will normally dictate that this side of your upper body is tight and you should therefore stretch the muscles on that side of your body. Likewise the side that is high i.e. shoulder/collar bone or hips/knees, then this side of muscles (upper or lower body) will more than likely be stretched/weaker and should be tightened/strengthened accordingly. This procedure is very specific but can be incorporated into your workout pro- gramme quite easily, especially during your periods of active rest.
Body alignment	

Your own specific injury prevention plan

Should your body be only slightly misaligned which incidentally is normal, yet you have no injuries and you feel fit and healthy then you can still add specific exercises to your workout to ensure that you prevent any occurrence of injury in the future. These types of exercises are very important, and even though they can be used as rehabilita- tion exercises (after an injury) it is ultimately just as important to include them into your fitness routine, especially in the beginning phase. A specific prehabilitation exer- cise program stemming from your findings should include stretching tight muscles and to strengthen weak muscles. Most injuries occur to ligaments, tendons and muscles, with only about 5% of sports injuries involving broken bones. Most frequent sports injuries are sprains (injuries to ligaments) and strains (injuries to muscles) caused when an abnormal stress is placed on tendons, joints, bones and muscle.

Ways to reduce injury:

1. Wear the right gear - wear comfortable clothing and appropriate footwear;
2. Increase flexibility - stretching exercises before and after exercise;
3. Strengthen muscles – adding resistance exercises to your workouts;
4. Use the proper technique- this should be reinforced during the initial stages;
5. Take breaks – certain rest periods can reduce injuries and prevent heat illness;
6. Stop your workout - if there is pain;
7. Avoid heat injury - By drinking plenty of fluids before, during and after exer- cise. Decrease or stop during high heat/humidity periods and prevent heat injury by wearing lighter clothing.

Things you must take into account

You should know that the way in which you walk can also affect your posture e.g. do you place your heel on the ground prior to rolling on the outside of your foot and propel your body forwards by pushing off the toe? Or do you breathe correctly? For example: do you fill each lung equally and if not this could also offset your posture. The most important factors we must not ignore are if there are any possible spinal discrepancies such as scoliosis, kyphosis or issues with your vertebral discs. Chiropractors, physiotherapists, manual therapists etc have many years of study in these areas should you require to be assessed further.

Reducing back problems and strengthening the core

Weak or poorly controlled core muscles have been associated with low back pain. The back muscles are responsible for movements such as extension and flexion of the spine and rotation of the trunk. Excessive or uneven shock on the spine may lead to back problems, and this may be exaggerated because weak core muscles lead to improper positioning or a forward tilt. In many exercises that use the back muscles, the abdominal muscles contract isometrically, stabilising the body. The stronger and more correctly balanced the core muscles are, the less the uneven strain on the spine. Abdominals get all the credit for protecting the back and being the foundation of strength, but they are only a small part of what makes up the core. Weak core muscles result in a loss of the appropriate lumbar curve and a swayback posture. While there are no doubt countless gimmicks on the market purporting to strengthen the core region most are useless in reality. There are however, several pieces of exercise equipment that are genuinely useful for strengthening the core region, and they include medicine balls, stability balls and balance boards, these are explained in more detail later. These simple pieces of equipment allow you to devise specific movements related to your fitness requirements. Medicine balls are particularly helpful for mimicking rotation movements that would be unpractical whilst using free weights. Of course even these pieces of equipment are not essential, but there are many exercises that use bodyweight or partner resistance that strengthen the core effectively. The use of free weights can be adapted accordingly to cater for the majority of required movements.

Exercise therapy

Best defined as the prescription of bodily movement to correct impairment, improve musculoskeletal function, or maintain a state of well-being. Exercise therapy varies from carefully selected activities restricted to specific muscles or parts of the body, to general and/or vigorous activities that can return an injured person back to their peak of physical condition. Exercise therapy seeks to accomplish the following goals:

- Enables ambulation;
- Release contracted muscles, tendons, and fascia;
- Mobilise joints;
- Improve circulation and improve respiratory capacity;
- Improve coordination;
- Reduce rigidity and improve balance;
- Promote relaxation;
- Improve muscle strength;
- Improve exercise performance and functional capacity i.e. endurance.

The final 2 goals mirror an individual's overall physical fitness, a state characterized by good muscle strength combined with good endurance. The final goal of rehabilitation is to achieve wherever possible an optimal level of physical fitness by the end of the exercise therapy regimen, irrespective of the initial types of exercise required to remedy an injured person's specific condition.

Rehabilitation & Fitness
Although most exercise therapy rehabilitation takes place in the gym, home exercises are also vital to ensure the success of a rehabilitation program. Retraining proprioception involves performing specific exercises with the eyes closed or on an unstable surface such as a 'wobble-board' so that you must rely more on your proprioception to perform the exercise. Hydrotherapy is also used in the treatment of sports injuries, as pool exercises are ideal for back pain, knee injuries, sprained ankle injuries, metatarsal fractures and broken leg injuries as they allow improved range of joint movement, muscle relaxation and maintenance of cardiovascular fitness. Hydrotherapy uses the buoyancy provided by wearing a buoyancy belt to allow the injured person to exercise in the pool without touching the bottom. This means that hydrotherapy exercises are non weight bearing and that there is no impact through the injured area, which assists healing and recovery. If you have been injured and are ready to start training again, the last thing in the world you want is for the injury to recur.

Equipment
Proprioception exercises using a wobble board or rocker board are perfect for improving joint stability and balance, and these exercises help to reduce the incidence of recurrent ankle sprains due to ankle instability. Resistance exercises to improve muscle strength and joint stability are another important aspect of rehabilitation. Resistance bands or thera-bands can be used to provide resistance to a muscle. These bands are commonly used in shoulder strengthening and ankle strengthening. They are particularly effective at strengthening the rotator cuff muscles following a shoulder dislocation or partial dislocation.

Resistance band colour grading

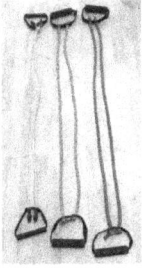

YELLOW = on left, a thinner tube of lighter resistance
GREEN = of medium resistance
RED   = on right, of heavier resistance

Other rehabilitation equipment can be used for home treatment as part of an exercise therapy program such as: Swiss balls, foam, physio balls, medicine balls, gym mats, Pilates and/or Yoga mats etc.

PLANNING YOUR WORKOUT

YOUR WORKOUT ROUTINE

A stale workout routine is like an old pair of shoes i.e. you know how they'll feel and you once loved using them, but you just don't want to go near them anymore. The fact is that we all need a little variety in our workouts, and an excessively repetitive workout program is one of the major causes of fitness burnout. Below are the 3 main variables you must consider when exercising your whole body and they are without doubt the 3 most important factors you need to focus on:

1. Your intensity i.e. how hard you train;
2. Your volume i.e. how much you should do;
3. Your frequency i.e. how often you should train.

In this advanced edition of our 'Whole Body Workshop' exercise books, we have included beginner to advanced techniques, exercises and types of training to assist you getting you past your plateaus and beyond. We have added workouts for gym users to include fitness machine workouts and specific programs for exercises with barbell and dumbbells. If you still exercise at home then you will gain all the knowledge you need by practicing before you go, should you decide to join a gym. The content of this book is your own personal library of knowledge to last you a lifetime. Each person is unique and therefore, whether you train alone, with a partner or in a group your own personal aim should remain the same. Some people need to be motivated by others and some can motivate themselves. The location where you train will also be specific to your goals i.e. do you need to join a gym, have you got your own equipment or do you want to continue to train in your own home. Your mind and your body combined will dictate your success whether it is daily, weekly, monthly or yearly, and this book assists you in understanding the importance of the working together of your mind and body, as one without the other is not an option for permanent success. We have included templates and specific programs for you; however before jumping ahead, you need to take certain considerations into account before commencing your workout. First and foremost you should select which program is best for you i.e. what is your aim?

a) To improve your flexibility?

b) To strengthen and tone your body?

c) To improve your muscle endurance, power or strength?

d) To improve your muscle mass?

e) To lose weight?

f) Anything else...?

Once you have decided on your aim, you can then move forwards with your plan, however certain considerations need to be taken into account before planning your own specific workout program. An individual training program could be specific to you and your needs, but may not be beneficial to someone else and vice-versa. Each day that you train can be affected by how you are feeling and/or what's going on around you, therefore you will have to be slightly flexible in your day to day planning. Having a program and a plan can and will undoubtedly motivate you to achieving great results. Being prepared is the key to success and if your aim is achievable, recordable, measurable and sustainable then you are on the right track for permanent results, whatever your aim. Below are some routine examples:

TRAINING DAYS (W)	MON	TUES	WEDS	THURS	FRI	SAT	SUN
2 days a wk	W	Off	Off	W	Off	Off	Off
3 days a wk	W	Off	W	Off	W	Off	Off
4 days a wk	W	Off	W	Off	W	Off	W
Every 3 days	W	Off	Off	W	Off	Off	W

Begin by asking yourself…When can you realistically train and for how often?

TRAINING DAYS (W)	MON	TUES	WEDS	THURS	FRI	SAT	SUN
__ days a wk							

Other circumstances will be important for you to consider, such as family, friends, workout timings and location… to name only a few. Your goals, level of motivation and the way you stick to your plan will be the deciding factors for your best results. Getting rid of negative thoughts, replacing them with positive ones, having realistic goals (food choices and exercise) and visualising what you want to look or feel like are all important factors too. The same goes for writing down why you want something, so long as you write it in the positive context i.e. I want to look toned so I can look good on the beach (instead of, so I don't look fat). Positivity will then embrace you and you will become more motivated through your new way of thinking.

Goal setting

When you don't have a specific goal, it is very difficult to keep exercising and to keep track of your progress to see how far you've come, but whatever it is that you desire it must be possible and reasonable. Begin by setting your goals and asking yourself these 5 questions:

26

1. What do you want to accomplish with your exercise program?
2. Is your goal realistic and attainable?
3. Do you know how to reach your goal?
4. When do you want to reach your goal?
5. How will you reward yourself when you reach your goal?

Reaching your goals

Many people are surprised at the daily effort it takes to reach their goals, once you know what you're doing and how you're doing it, you'll need some strategies for sticking with it:

- Schedule your workouts;
- Set weekly goals and reward yourself each time you succeed;
- Workout with friends or family for added motivation;
- Recommit to your goals every single day;
- Be prepared, always have your fitness bag with you;
- Take your lunch to work etc;
- Maintain your journal to stay on track and measure your progress;
- Regularly take your measurements.

Generally, if you can maintain an activity for 21-30 days you'll be more likely to stick with it. Better still, if you can maintain an activity for 60 days it will be harder to stop the habit than to continue.

Your strength training routine

Most people want to get great results in the shortest period of time but what they don't realise is that serious results require a systematic plan, as well as alot of hard work. To learn the core of a strength training routine requires you to know and understand the essential concepts of overload, progression, training volume and intensity. You must also understand the importance of correct training techniques before designing your own personal strength training program. You must begin by understanding the following:

1. How to select your exercises;
2. How to manipulate the weights used, sets, repetitions and rest periods;
3. How to increase your training intensity to achieve your specific goals.

Your cardiovascular training routine

As previously explained, setting your goals is your number one priority, because having your goals will help you to design your ultimate cardiovascular workout plan that will get you to where you want to be. Assessing your fitness level is a major priority but even if you don't complete the recommended assessments, you can try any cardio machine out for 10 minutes and assess how you feel after 10 minutes of medium intensity work. This is where you have to be honest with yourself, because if you're already breathing heavily then you will need to start your cardio workout plan with a very low intensity i.e. walking for an hour a day at least three times a week. If on the other hand you experience no problems at all, then of course you can incorporate jogging, cycling and other higher intensity exercises. You should never pass off seeking knowledge from personal trainers or advice from other professionals in the field of health and fitness. These people are highly specialized in their field and therefore professionally trained to create workout plans for people just like you, and ultimately to help people meet their personal fitness goals. To help you stick to your cardio workout plan it is advisable to join a gym, especially if you can afford the monthly membership. The motivation that you gain from being around like minded people is second to none. Boredom is one of the main reasons cardio workout plans fail, therefore you should try different classes to see which one you enjoy the most. Variation is also a key factor in preventing boredom, so why not try a martial arts class, aerobics or even spinning. You need to put your workout routine into your daily schedule i.e. same time, same place etc because setting aside a regular time for your cardio workout will not only create a schedule for you it will also help you to stick to your plan.

WARMING UP, COOLING DOWN & STRETCHING

General warm up

To prevent injuries and maximise the benefits of your workout, it is important to take the extra time to ease your body into the workout in a controlled manner. Most people know and understand the reasons why it is important to warm up, but very few even attempt or complete a warm up, and if they do is it sufficient enough? To reiterate the importance of warm ups, it is best to stress that your planned workout will be more successful and you will achieve more if your warm up is adequate for what you have planned. The intensity of your warm up preparation will also be dictated by the session that you have planned, and in basic terms your warm up should involve the mobility of your joints and the circulation of blood around your major muscles. There are many pre-workout (warm up) choices, but generally speaking your warm up should be easy and slow, yet progressive to fire up your muscles. If an injury prevents you from completing the warm up of choice, then try and utilise anything that does not incorporate weight bearing as this may cause pain, especially during the initial stages of the injury so as not to aggravate the injury. Your muscles, ligaments and tendons have to be warmed up so that they are less likely to be injured / re-injured. Your aim is to elevate your heart and respiratory rate, increase blood flow and increase muscle temperature to the specific area(s). If you are going to do upper body exercises, then start off at the top by gently moving your shoulders, prior to gently moving your head from side to side and up and down. Then work your way down to the shoulders again with gentle arm circling, forwards and back and side to side. Mobilise all the joints of the upper body as much as you can until your muscles feel warm and your joints move more freely prior to the stretch phase. If you are mobilizing your lower body prior to the stretching phase, move the hips, knees and ankles forwards and back and side to side to warm the muscles appropriately. If you can raise your the heels to your backside and knees to your chest then these are all different ways that you can raise your heart rate and prepare your muscles and joints for the stretching phase.

Stretching

This is a hotly debated area of muscle research and is constantly evolving. Clearly flexibility is important in order to achieve normal movement, but the question is... when a muscle is not flexible enough, does stretching actually help? The answer seems to be sometimes yes, sometimes no! The flexibility of a given muscle is determined by two main factors, the stiffness of the tissue within the muscle, and the background tone within the muscle. Tone can loosely be defined as the background activity in a muscle when it is at rest. Muscles which have excessively high tone are almost constantly 'on' even when at rest, usually because they are over-working to compensate for other muscles that aren't doing enough. Stretching of muscles with excessively high tone may produce gains in flexibility, but unless the muscle imbalances are addressed they are likely to 'tighten up' again relatively quickly as they continue to compensate for these other 'lazier' muscles. Stretching normally involves all areas of the body, although can be as specific to the workout that you have planned i.e. only stretching your lower body prior to going for a run.

Static stretching

This type of stretching should be used to gradually lengthen all the major muscle groups and associated tendons of the body, which increases your ROM. Both the opposing muscle group and the muscles to be stretched are relaxed, and at the point of increased tension the position is held or maintained to allow muscle lengthening.

Passive stretching

This type of stretching is very similar to static but involves another person or apparatus to help further stretch your muscles. If you use this type of stretching you must limit all bouncing and jerking movements. You should perform another warm up if you use passive stretching as a part of your warm up.

Dynamic stretching

This type of stretching uses a controlled, soft bounce or swinging motion to move a particular body part to the limit of its range of movement (ROM) Therefore dynamic stretching is seen more appropriate for warming up, however it should never become radical or uncontrolled.

Active stretching

This type of stretching involves using the strength of your opposing muscles to generate a stretch within the targeted muscle group, this helps to relax the stretched muscles.

PNF stretching – Proprioceptive Neuromuscular Facilitation is a more advanced form of flexibility training that involves the stretching and contraction of the muscle groups being targeted. Aswell as improving flexibility and ROM, it also improves muscular strength

For both the static and PNF methods, you should try to position the joints to enhance the desired flexibility, and then maintain the position for 6-12secs for 6-10 sets.

Breathing

The easiest way to remember how to breathe during a stretch is to exhale as you are moving into the stretch and inhale as you return to your original position. Breathing slowly and easily also helps to relax your muscles, which makes stretching easier and more beneficial. In our lifetime, the muscles shorten and become inflexible and even when we workout our muscles shorten due to them contracting in order to exert power. Short muscles limit our movement which can cause aches and pains, and therefore stretching is very important and is an essential part of any exercise routine. There are certain guidelines you should follow to ensure your stretches are effective:

- Go to the position where the stretch is felt and hold;
- Hold each position for 10–20secs;
- Your breath should be slow and deep, concentrating on relaxing;
- You should ensure good form and posture;
- You should always stretch warm muscles not cold;
- You should always avoid bouncing movements;
- You should always be patient.

Regular stretching will of course improve your flexibility, but more importantly though it will assist in improving your performance. You should endeavour to continuously think about your posture at all times i.e. the head, shoulders and hips need to be aligned at all times. A 2nd phase warm up should take place post stretching, this will lead you naturally into the main session you have planned which should ultimately be at a higher intensity gradually raising your heart rate and getting your muscles fully prepared.

Specifics for resistance training

Before beginning your strength session, you should complete some form of cardiovascular exercise at a light, comfortable intensity for about 5-10 minutes i.e. walking or cycling. If you are completing bodyweight exercises then an easier version of the exercise you have planned should be completed first i.e. perform an incline push up before you perform a declined push up and so on. If you are completing weight training exercises for specific muscle groups, then complete a warm up set with very light weights (approx. 50% of your target weight) for 12-20 repetitions i.e. if your first chest exercise is the bench press, then complete a warm up set of a lighter weight and then continue with your selected chest routine. When you have completed your chest workout and are ready to train the next muscle group, once again complete a warm up set, and then continue training that muscle group, and so on. A common mistake is to use too much weight during the warm up set, and the outcome consequently means you get tired too fast and don't have the energy necessary to push your muscles during the remaining sets. You can only build muscle by pushing your muscles past the point that they are used to lifting. If you don't have the energy to add sufficient weight to push your muscles, then you won't see any gains in muscle. You should spend time stretching each specific muscle you have trained in your strength program. You have to rest between your strength training sets anyway, so why not use this time more productively. After you have properly warmed up each muscle group, stretch between sets. Each set requires a resting period, usually between 30secs and 3mins (depending on what you are trying to achieve). Use this resting time wisely and stretch the specific muscle being trained. Remember to stretch only after the muscle has been properly warmed up and approx once every 2-3 sets per muscle group.

Specifics for cardiovascular training

A warm up of 5-10mins at low intensity will prepare your muscles for exercise and get your heart rate up. Start at an intensity of 50-60% of your maximum heart rate (i.e. effort) doing whatever activity will be your workout method. If you are walking or running, start by walking or running at an easy pace that puts you into this heart rate zone i.e. one where you can still carry on a full conversation. Once your muscles are warmed up you may benefit from flexibility stretches or drills specific for the muscle groups you will be using in the cardio workout. After you have completed your workout in your target heart rate zone, you should cool down with 5-10mins of lower intensity cardio. Aim for a heart rate of between 50-60% of maximum heart rate (i.e.

effort) for 5-10mins for your cool down. Traditionally, you would complete your workout with gentle stretching of the main muscles used in the workout i.e. legs and back for rowing etc.

You understand more about the importance of stretching before, during and after your workout, and you also know that stretching helps prevent injuries. The last thing you need is to have to stop training due to an injury. Maintaining the fitness level that you acquire over time is of the utmost importance. If you remember nothing else, remember to always include a warm up, stretch and a cool down to whatever you are doing (CV or strength) for maximum effectiveness and to prevent injuries.

Next you will have access to the most common stretches for each separate body part i.e. your back, chest, shoulders, triceps, biceps, legs and abdominals. Each stretch includes a detailed description.

COMMON BACK STRETCHES

Forward bend (supported)

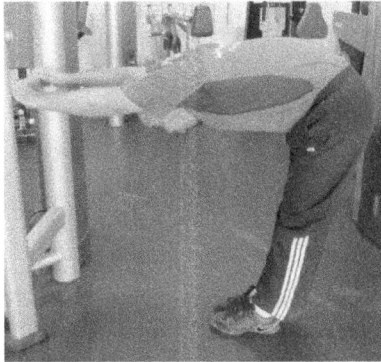

Choose a solid object that is around chest height and from the standing straight position ensure that your feet are flat on the floor and shoulder width apart. Place your hands on the object, bend your knees and under control lean forwards by bending at the waist. You should feel a stretch on the lower back as you hold the position, your breathing should be controlled at all times. Return slowly to the start position and repeat accordingly.

Forward bend (un-supported)

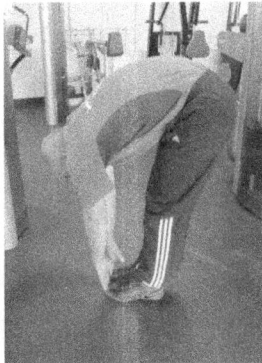

From the standing straight position ensure that your feet are flat on the floor and wide enough apart that you have enough balance. Bend your knees and under control lean forwards and attempt to touch your toes by bending at the waist. You should feel a stretch on the lower back and hamstrings (back of the legs) as you hold the position, your breathing should be controlled at all times. Make a mental note of how far you have reached down and attempt to get lower each time without straining yourself. Return slowly to the start position and repeat accordingly.

Forward bend (assisted)

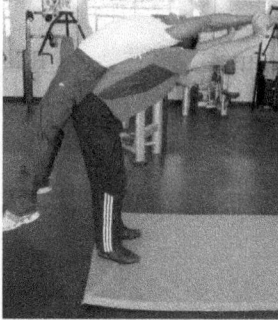

It is important to note that this stretch should be done with extreme care & caution! Choose a person that is fairly light and around the same height as you and from the standing straight position ensure that your feet are flat on the floor and shoulder width apart with your knees bent. Place your partner's hands in yours, bend your knees, tense your abdominals and under immense control lean forwards by bending at the waist. You should feel a stretch on the lower back as you hold the position, your breathing should be controlled at all times. Return slowly to the start position and repeat accordingly.

Tree hug

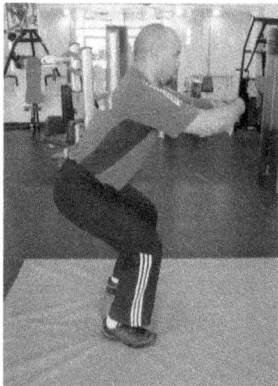

From the standing straight position ensure that your feet are flat on the floor and wide enough apart that you have enough balance. Bend your knees and under control lean forwards slightly and act as though you are hugging a large tree which will round off your back and give you a good stretch around the upper to mid section of the back. Hold your abdominals in whilst controlling your breathing at all times. Return slowly to the start position and repeat accordingly.

Twist & hold

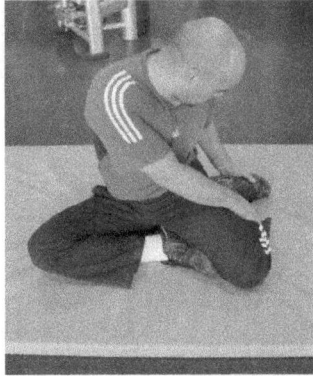

From the kneeling position twist to one side as far as you can go whilst breathing out without straining yourself. Breathe in as you return to the centre and repeat to the opposite side. This will stretch out your obliques at the side of your body but will also stretch out the lats and muscles positioned around the lower back. To make it easier you can try it whilst seated in a chair.

Pelvic tilt

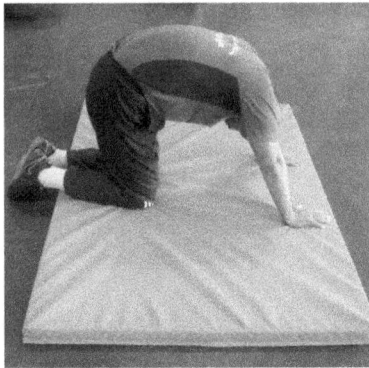

From the kneeling position ensure that your hands are level with your shoulders and your knees and hands are in line as much as possible. Your shoulders should be relaxed and your hips and shoulders initially should remain facing towards the ground along with your head and eyes. Initiate the movement from the abdominals and tilt your pelvis to the rear as you breathe out whilst pulling your head inwards. Slowly return to the start position whilst breathing in, repeat the movement in a controlled manner. Maintaining control throughout the movement is key whilst breathing correctly.

Knees to chest

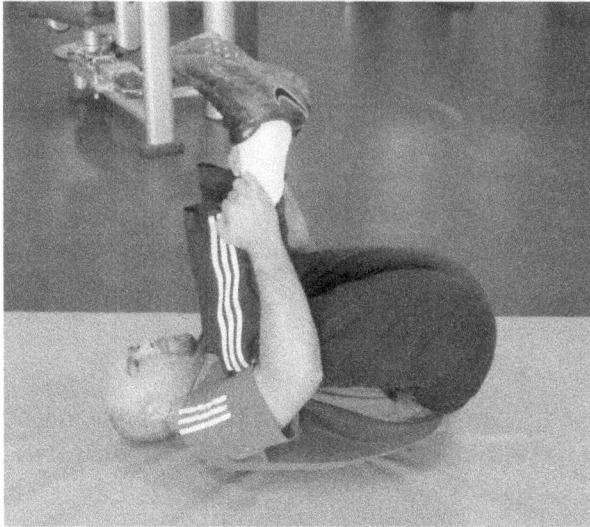

From the back lying position ensure that your hips and shoulders are facing upwards along with your head and eyes. Reach forwards to grasp the back of your legs and roll backwards until your back is flat on the floor. Maintain this hold as you feel the stretch which combines the hamstrings, glutes and lower back. Return to the start position and repeat.

COMMON CHEST STRETCHES

Hands to rear

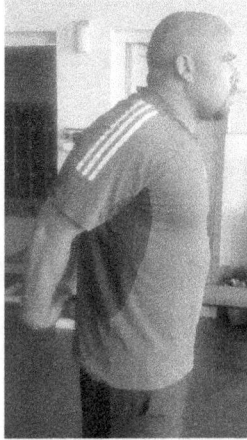

Stand upright with your hands clasped together behind your back, pull your arms as far from your body as possible whilst at the same time pulling your shoulders back and sticking your chest out. Your shoulders should be relaxed with minimum tension with your head and eyes facing forwards, breathe normally.

Wall Stretch 1

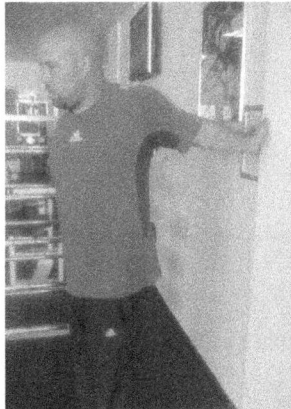

Stand upright and place one hand on a wall just below shoulder height, turn your body away from the wall whilst sticking your chest out. Your arm should be straight at all times with your shoulders relaxed, breathe normally.

Wall Stretches 2 & 3

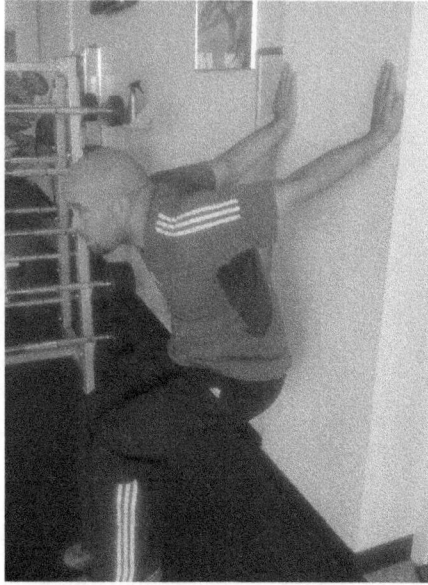

Initially, stand upright and place both hands on a wall just below shoulder height, bend at the waist as your body weight allows for the straight arms to apply maximum stretch on the chest. Your shoulders should be relaxed as you breathe normally.

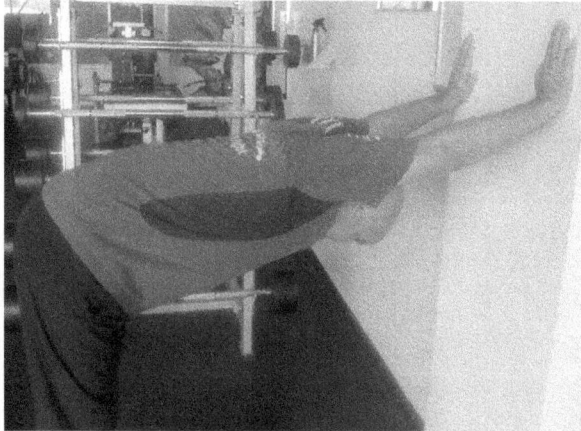

Arms above head (floor stretch)

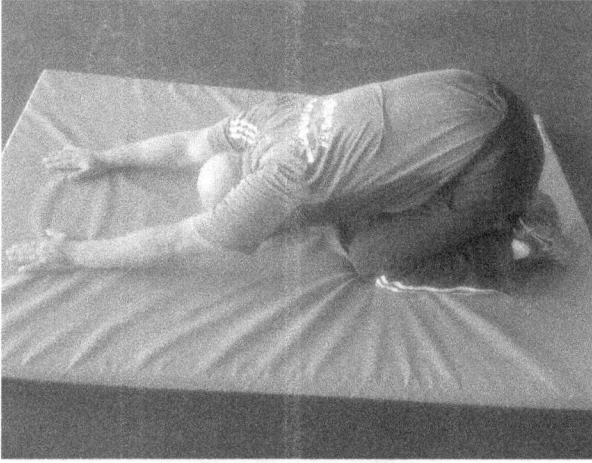

Kneel on all fours and lean forwards onto the mat with your arms outstretched in front of you; allow your bodyweight to apply a maximum stretch on the chest. Your shoulders should be relaxed as you breathe normally.

Arm out to side (floor stretch)

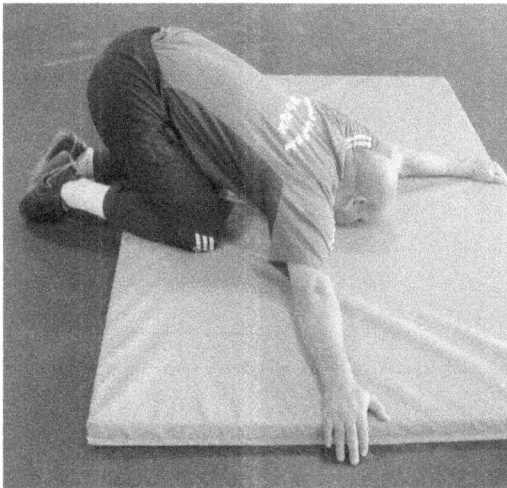

Kneel on all fours and lean forwards onto the mat with one arm outstretched to the side; allow your bodyweight to apply a maximum stretch on the chest. Your arm should be shoulder height and as relaxed as possible as you breathe normally.

COMMON SHOULDER STRETCHES

Most Common Deltoid Stretch

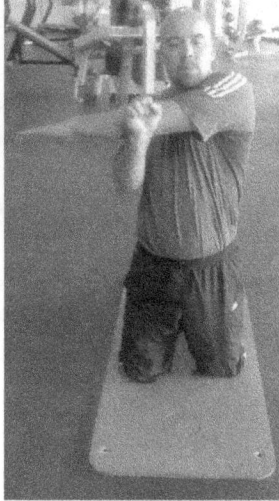

Kneel on all fours or stand upright and place your arm across your body whilst pulling it in with the opposite arm, this stretch can be increased further by another person assisting.
Breathe naturally

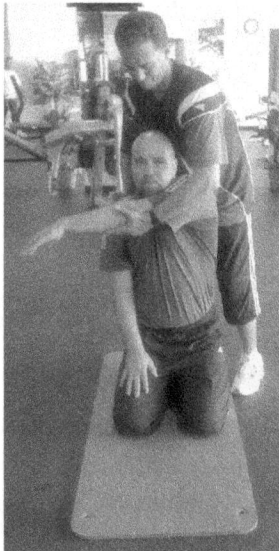

Anterior Deltoid Stretch

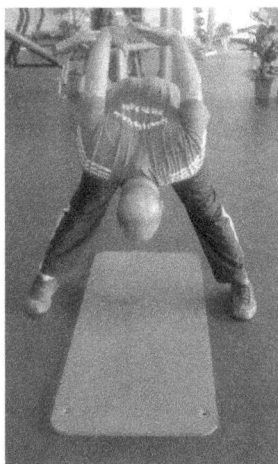

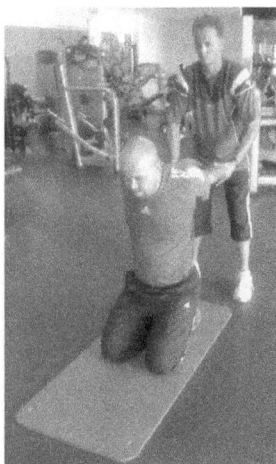

Kneel on all fours or stand upright and place your arms behind you whilst pushing them close together, this stretch can be increased further by bending forward or having another person assist you. Breathe naturally

Posterior Deltoid Stretch

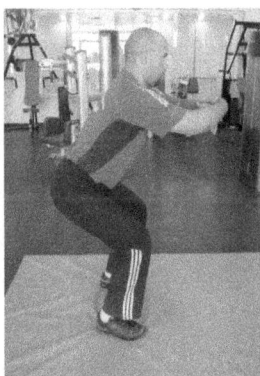

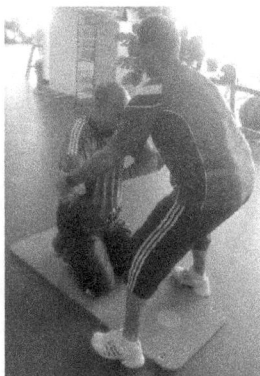

From the standing straight position ensure that your feet are flat on the floor and wide enough apart that you have enough balance. Bend your knees and under control lean forwards slightly and act as though you are hugging a large tree which will round off your back and give you a good stretch around the upper to mid section of the back. Hold your abdominals in whilst controlling your breathing at all times Return slowly to the start position and repeat accordingly. This stretch can be increased further by having another person assist you, whether you are standing or kneeling place your hands behind you whilst pushing your elbows to the front of you. Breathe naturally

Additional Deltoid Stretches (Both arms)

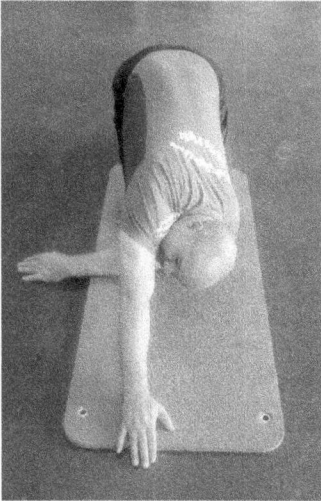

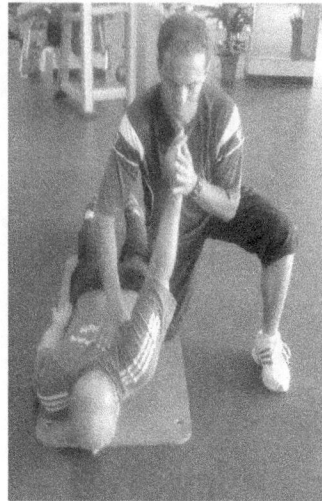

All of the stretches shown are a variation of all the stretches already covered, whether you are standing, kneeling, lying down, alone or assisted the principles still apply. So long as you hold the correct position, breathe naturally and maintain good posture and form to everything you do.

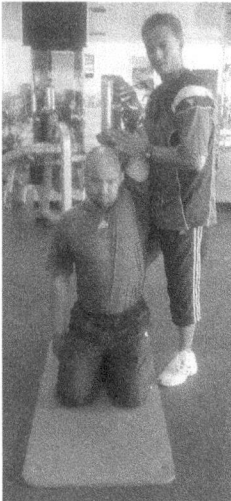

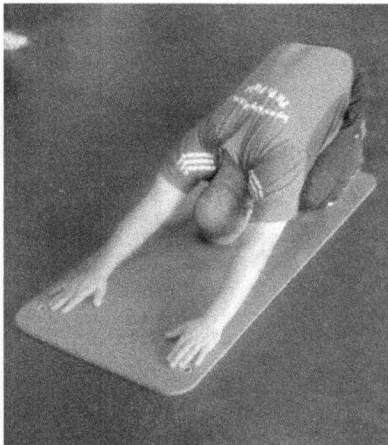

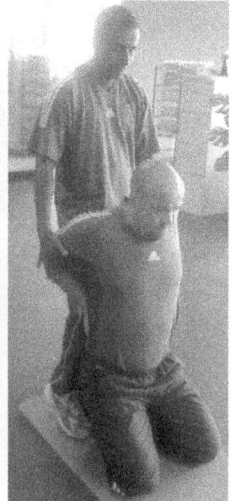

COMMON BICEP STRETCHES

Common Bicep stretch

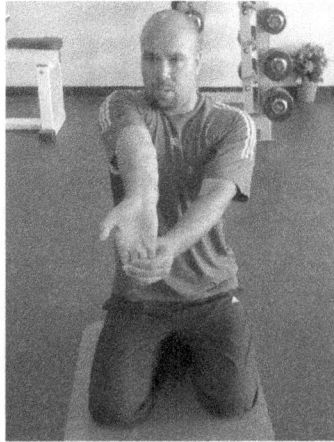

Pull your wrist backwards and away from your forearm whilst ensuring that your arm is straight, attempt to lock your elbow out in a safe manner.

Kneeling (all fours) stretch

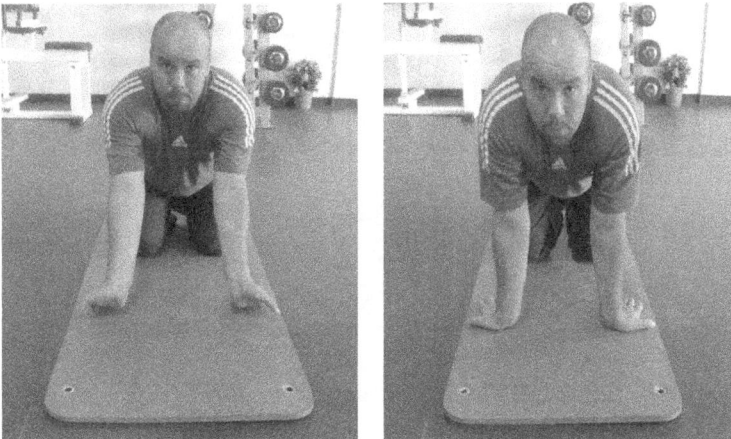

Kneel on the floor and place your arms out in front of you with the forearms facing away from you. Your hands should be facing towards you and you should ensure that your arms are straight, attempt to lock your elbow out in a safe manner. Roll your bodyweight forward of your hands to increase the stretch further but be careful as your wrists are delicate joints.

Arm out to side (floor stretch)

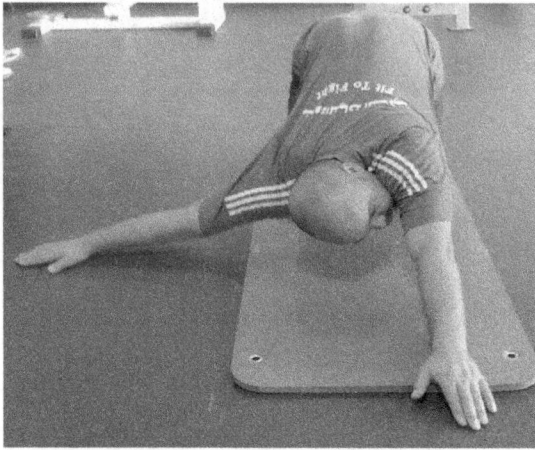

Kneel on all fours and lean forwards onto the mat with one arm outstretched to the side and one out to the front; allow your bodyweight to apply a maximum stretch on the bicep. Your arm should be shoulder height and straight but as relaxed as possible as you breathe normally.

Seated (arms to rear) stretch

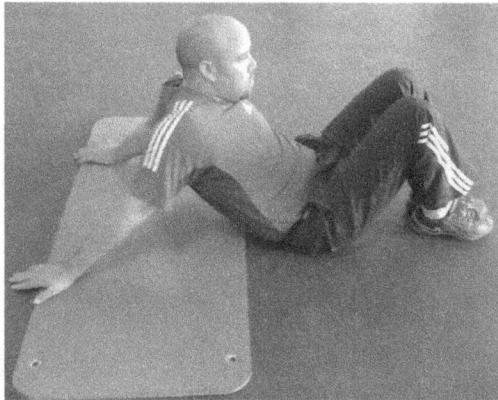

Sit on the floor with your arms behind you, your arms should be completely straight with your shoulders relaxed. Use your upper bodyweight to apply a greater stretch on the biceps and safely ensure that your wrists are bent with your hands facing away from your forearms at all times.

COMMON TRICEP STRETCHES

Most common triceps stretch

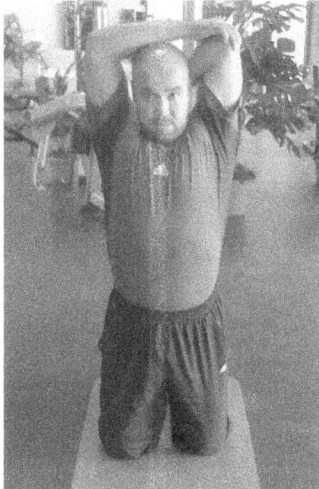

Start in the kneeling position with your hips, shoulders head and eyes inline and facing forwards. Place one arm behind your head and fully bend it at the elbow, attempt to place your hand as far down the centre of the back as possible. Increase the stretch by applying a resistance with the opposite arm, breathe normally

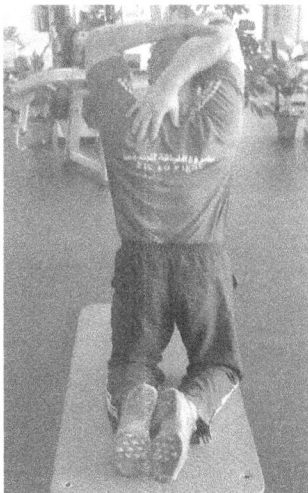

Assisted using a towel

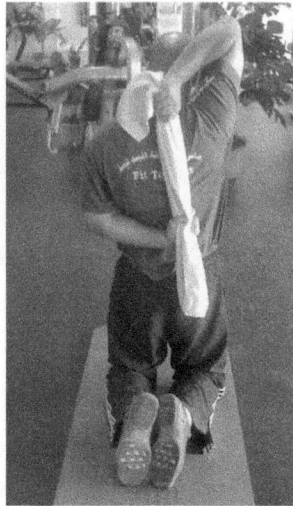

Start in the kneeling position with your hips, shoulders, head and eyes inline and facing forwards. Place a towel in one hand and place it behind your head, this arm should be fully bent at the elbow. With your opposite hand pull the towel down which should in turn increase the stretch of the arm you are stretching, breathe normally

Assisted using a bench

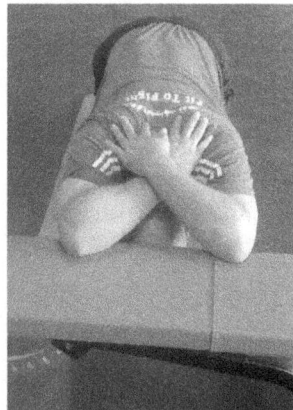

Start in the kneeling position, your hands crossed above your head and down the centre of your back, place your elbows on a flat sturdy surface. Use your bodyweight to move your hands as far down the centre of the back as possible. Increase the stretch by leaning more forward using your elbows down onto the bench, breathe normally

Assisted using a partner

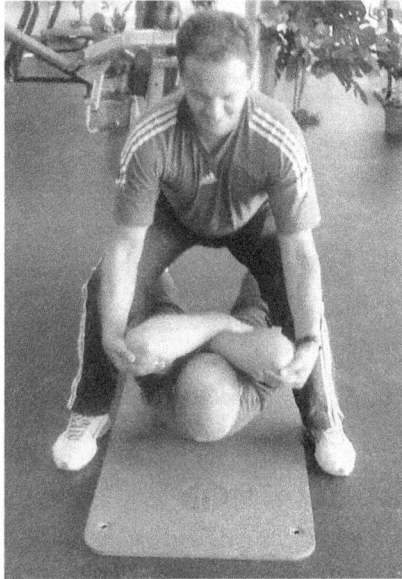

Start in the front lying position, your hands crossed above your head and down the centre of your back, your partner should hold your elbows pull you off the floor and attempt to move your hands as far down the centre of the back as possible by pushing your elbows down under control. Your partner should have a wide stance and keep his/her back straight, breathe normally.

Variations

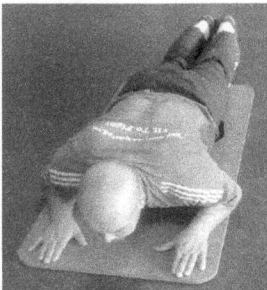

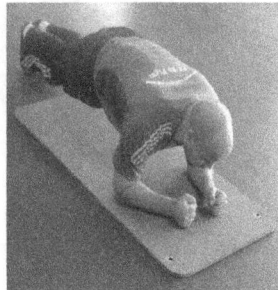

All of the triceps stretches require your arms to be fully bent at the elbow whether they are behind your head or in front of you. Utilising a partner (safely) can greatly increase your stretching abilities, holding a position (isometric – top right) can also provide a stretch so long as you maintain good form and good posture and breathe normally.

COMMON LEG STRETCHES

Hip flexors

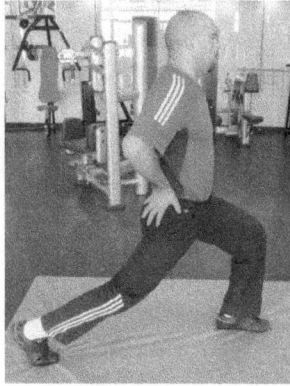

Stand upright with your feet flat on the floor, your head, eyes, hips and shoulders inline and facing forwards. Take a step backwards and endeavour to keep your body inline as mentioned above. To get a good stretch you must push your hips forwards whilst leaning backwards with the upper body, therefore stretching your hip flexors at the top of the upper thigh of each leg. Breathe under control and repeat with the opposite leg.

Glutes

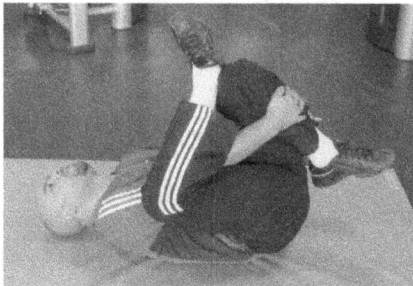

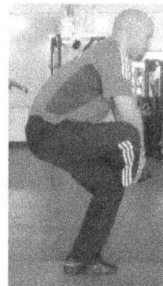

Lie on your back with your head, eyes, hips and shoulders inline and facing forwards. Place your hands around the sides of the leg that you are stretching, grasp your shin, pull the leg towards your chest and rock backwards. This stretch is for your glutes and you can do the same stretch standing up on one leg with the other leg crossed over the other in the same position as the picture although this requires more balance from the standing leg and you have to squat down to increase the stretch further. Breathe under control and repeat with the opposite leg.

Hamstrings

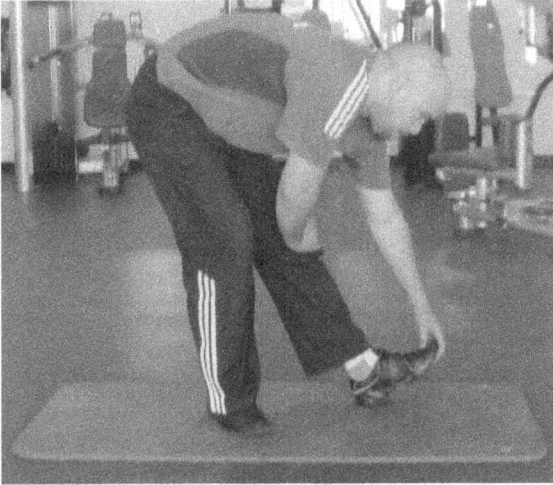

Stand upright with your feet flat on the floor and your head, eyes, hips and shoulders inline and facing forwards. Take a step forward with one leg and bend at the hips (forwards and down) towards your toe as far as you can safely go. To get a good stretch you can raise the toe off the ground. Breathe under control and repeat with the opposite leg.

Quadriceps

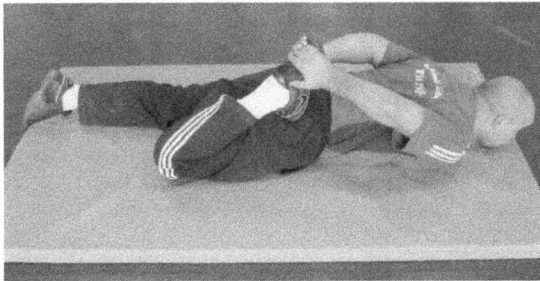

Lie on your front with your head, eyes, hips and shoulders inline and facing forwards. Bend one leg towards your backside and place your hands around the foot grasping it securely. This stretch is for your quadriceps and you can do the same stretch standing up on one leg with the other leg bent behind you in the same position as the picture although this requires more balance from the standing leg. To increase the stretch further you must push your hips forwards and pull the foot in more, you can also stretch both legs together. Breathe under control and repeat with the opposite leg.

49

Illio tibial band (ITB)

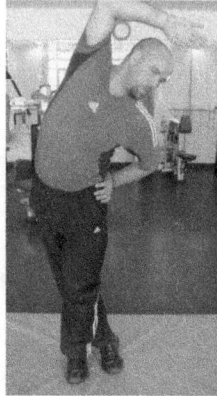

Stand upright with your feet flat on the floor and your head, eyes, hips and shoulders inline and facing forwards. Place one leg behind the other and lean with your upper body in the opposite direction i.e. If you place your right leg behind then you must lean left, pushing your hips right. To get a better stretch you can lean over further with your upper body. Breathe under control and repeat with the opposite leg.

Inner thigh

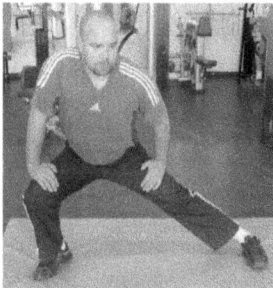 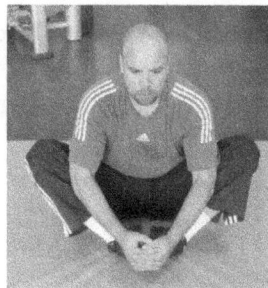

(A)   (B)

With your head, eyes, hips and shoulders inline and facing forwards, ensure that whichever stretch you are doing for the inner thigh that you adjust your bodyweight accordingly to get the maximum stretch from the relevant muscles. Breathe under control and repeat with the opposite leg. For stretch (A) the leg that you are stretching should be straight with your upper bodyweight forward of your hips whilst pushing the straight leg downwards. For stretch (B) the legs should be bent and the knees pushed outwards with the elbows ensuring that the feet are together and facing each other, again your upper bodyweight should be forward of your hips.

Calf

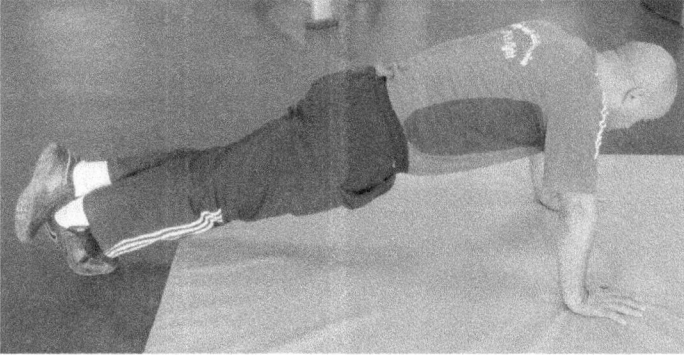

With both your hands and legs resting on the floor, ensure your head, eyes, hips and shoulders are inline and facing forwards. Place one leg on top of the other whilst pushing the heel of the leg that you are stretching as close to the floor as you can in a safe and controlled manner. Breathe under control and repeat with the opposite leg. You can achieve the same stretch in the standing position, just keep your heels lower than your toes.

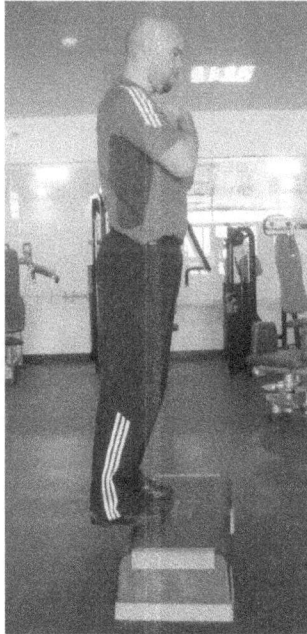

ABDOMINAL STRETCH

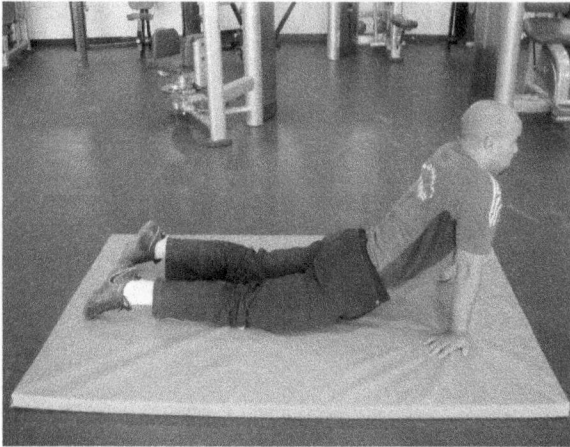

Lie on your front with your hips as close to the floor as possible, lift your upper body from the floor using your arms and push your hips into the floor. Breathe normally throughout the stretch without holding your breath. To stretch your oblique's, quite simply lie on a fit-ball (on your side) and lower your upper body below the height of your hips to ensure you get a good stretch, obviously ensure you are stable and your bottom leg is firmly on the ground.

Post exercise cool down

The reasons why you stretch after exercise are very different to warming up, but very necessary for a number of reasons. Any strenuous activity, particularly weight lifting, causes a small amount of damage to the muscle and associated soft tissues. These small rips and tears are what force the muscles to grow when they begin the process of repairing themselves. Damaged tissue is replaced by stronger tissue, which, for up to 48 hours after exercising, often causes soreness. This is called DOMS or Delayed Onset Muscle Soreness. The cool down will generally include longer stretches than the warm up because the muscles will be warmer post workout, although again this will depend on your planned activity i.e. for an athlete who competes in the 100m hurdles event they will need to complete a more ballistic warm up and stretch and will therefore require a much longer warm up phase but normally the cool down and post exercise stretches should be of a longer duration. Right after your workout your muscles are warm and elastic and the post workout stretching session affords you a second chance to increase your flexibility and range of motion, particularly around your joints.

It will be explained to you how to warm up, stretch and cool down specifically for resistance training and cardiovascular training within their respective chapters.

52

SPECIFIC GUIDELINES FOR PHYSICAL DEVELOPMENT

Cardiovascular development

Each time you complete a workout on a particular cardio machine or whilst walking, jogging, running outdoors etc you should endeavour to focus 100% on practicing perfect form. Many workouts are wasted when they aren't performed in the proper manner i.e. from the very beginning think about your body position on a machine, your posture and even the way you breathe. Especially with machines, some people allow the machine to dictate the workout whereas we should be in control at all times. By ensuring that you are performing each workout correctly with perfect form, you are truly maximizing your cardiovascular training routine.

Frequency - Beginning with only three days per week is fine, but your aim should be to set your sites on six days per week. We are not talking about a full 60 minutes of hard work because this can be progressed over time. To do something almost everyday of the week is more realistic for better results. Even if 1 of the days is walking around the neighbourhood for 10 minutes everyday, then so be it.

Intensity – If you can exercise your cardiovascular system on a daily basis, this is fantastic for your overall health, the difference being is to make it worthwhile and at the right intensity. Try HRT heart rate training and let your heart be your guide, as this is the most effective means of measuring intensity. Heart rate allows you to use other variables such as speed, incline, resistance, etc. HRT is explained in more detail later in this book. Your aim will always dictate the length of time you should spend exercising and of course your personal desires about your body will dictate the level of effort i.e. intensity you put into each workout. The intensity of how hard you push yourself during any type of exercise is usually measured on a scale of 1-10. With 10 being your maximum effort, and 1 being no effort at all, of course every person will differ in comparison. Remember, your aim will always dictate the length of time you should spend exercising and of course your personal desires about your body will dictate the level of effort i.e. intensity you put into each workout.

Time – Endeavour to lengthen your workouts over a period of time, and even if you only add 5 minutes or so to your daily routine until you reach your training duration goal, this will help substantially.

Type – Plan what type of exercises, activities or sports you want to be doing? It doesn't matter whether you run, walk, bike, swim, play racquetball, etc. As long as you are achieving an intensity and duration that are meaningful and you are doing this almost every day! If you only decide to commit to three days per week, for 45 minutes per session... it is very hard to add another day, so aim high from the very beginning with 6 short sessions per week and increase the length of each session slowly.

Strength development
Every time you complete an action i.e. every rep, every set, every movement, you should endeavour to focus 100% on practicing perfect form. Many repetitions of exercises are wasted when they aren't performed in the proper way. By ensuring that you are performing every move correctly with perfect form, you are truly maximizing your strength training routine.

Frequency - One day per week may help you maintain your current level of strength, but in most cases, it will not be enough to build muscle. Therefore you should aim to train each muscle group at least two times per week, and up to three if you have the time or are more advanced. To rest 1-2 days in between working the same muscle(s) is very important and gives them time to repair themselves from small tears that occur during strength training, and this is ultimately how you get stronger.

Intensity - The intensity is dictated by how much the resistance you lift challenges you, and it should be high enough so that when you approach your last repetition, you feel muscle exhaustion. Exhaustion means your muscle is so tired that you cannot do another full repetition in good form. Good form meaning, without any accessory movements or assistance from other muscle groups or put simply...no cheating. Many people tend to just lift the number of reps that they have subscribed to and stop, without even going to exhaustion. Training intensity serves as the major stimulus for muscle growth in your strength training routine. By increasing your training intensity, you provide a bigger stimulus for muscle growth. You can increase the intensity by increasing the amount of weight, amount of sets or repetitions, and the number of exercises, or reducing rest intervals between sets. As always the exact combination you choose depends on your overall goals.

Time - Number of reps and sets you should do i.e. progressing from the start position, through the action and back to the starting position counts as one repetition. Most workouts include lifting somewhere between 8 and 15 reps, which equals one set and includes 1-3 sets with rest in between each set. As long as you are working to the point of exhaustion, you can maintain and even build strength by doing only 1 set, but unless you are stuck for time, most beginners start with 2 sets of each exercise. Your resting periods should be between 30-90 seconds between sets, and you can use this time wisely to stretch the muscle you are working or to catch your breath and replenish yourself with water. The longer you rest, the more strength you will have to finish your next set just as strongly as the previous one, which will ultimately aid in your strength development.

Type - Perform exercises to target every major muscle group when strength training i.e. your arms (both biceps and triceps), shoulders, chest, back, core (abs, obliques and lower back), and legs (quads, hamstrings, glutes and calves). Make sure you work opposing muscles too, not just the ones you see when you look in the mirror. The opposing muscles should be worked alongside the muscles at the sides of your body i.e. your obliques, hips, abductors and adductors (outer and inner thigh). The idea being to achieve balance, and the same goes for the upper and lower body. Do not neglect one or the other just because one is more important to you. This creates imbalance and sets you up for injury and pain. Strength training can be performed using a variety of equipment such as resistance bands, stability ball, hand weights, machines, or body weight. We have included numerous examples of exercises and workouts for you to choose from within this book.

EXERCISE FOR SPORT

Specificity of training
Specificity refers to mechanical similarity between a training activity and a sport or event. The more similar the training activity is to the actual sport movement, the greater the likelihood of positive carryover to performance. Adaptations occur only in the muscles used in the exercise, and by training more specifically and efficiently for your sport is of paramount importance. As explained earlier you should not spend valued time on exercises unrelated to your specific needs. Some exercises will carryover and benefit a number of sports, just as some sports have similarities and similar movements. The better you can narrow this focus, the more specific and efficient your training will be.

Sports specific tests
To get a better idea of how well your training is going you can measure your performance by undertaking a sports test and this can be taken as part of your program assessment which will help you dramatically. Clearly you should look for a test within your specific sport for a variety of movements, since this will then allow you to develop a better well rounded fitness program. You should endeavour to perform a sports specific test as often as you possibly can, and as always these assessments will help you to monitor your performance following your training programs. Some of the most common sports specific tests have been highlighted overleaf:

Basketball tests – These are tests that assess your overall ability related to agility, dribbling and your shooting accuracy. These skills should be continuously practiced within your training program in order to see improvements on both the basketball tests and during your game.

Rowing tests - These will help you to determine your VO2 max levels as well as your muscular abilities, and they can be completed every 2-3 months, which is generally how much time it will take to notice a difference in your performance level.

Rugby tests - These tests allow you to assess a multitude of fitness factors, as rugby is a sport that calls upon aerobic fitness, strength and agility. Implementing a variety of these tests on a regular basis will assist you in reaching for optimum physical ability levels.

Track & field tests - These tests will assess a large range of skills and this is simply due to the fact that there are a large variety of events involved. These tests range from sprinting ability and jumping skills to throwing force power. By completing a combination of track & field tests such as these, you will get a good idea of your overall fitness level. Any runner, sprinter, long or high jumper or athlete who requires quick bursts of energy should be completing flexion tests on a regular basis. Depending on your sport some other tests may need to be completed, and they include:

TEST	REASON FOR THIS TYPE OF TEST
MUSCLE TESTING	Crucial for many athletes to understand fitness levels
SPEED TESTING	To determine how fast your body is capable of going, whilst using force as a determinant. You will be required to not only move fast but also be able to press some amount of weight over a type of movement
EXPLOSIVE TESTING	Your ability to generate a great deal of power over a short period of time, these tests are commonly used by sprinters, high jumpers, basketball players and football players. These tests assess how much force you can generate over a specified period of time
SPRINT TESTING	These tests are incredibly important for increasing your speed and take off time

The day before, and on the day of these tests, especially the sprint test, you must ensure that you include a good intake of carbohydrates within your diet. Weight measurement tests are just as important, because regular weight measurements can help keep you on track with your training. Whether it is a measure of loss or gain, you must achieve excellence by instilling the values of hard work, mental toughness and intensity. No one categorization system is regarded as set in stone, but the training program for each individual athlete is thought out and prepared thoroughly and systematically using good sound principles. If you are a serious athlete your needs as the individual performer must be analyzed in the context of the sport you are preparing for, and you should adhere to the following criteria:

- An analysis of the demands of the activity;
- Identification of which muscle groups are involved;
- Identification of the dominant muscle fibre recruitment;
- Prediction of which energy systems are dominant;
- Analysis of the duration of the effort.

Your main awareness should be related to the concept of periodization, and this can involve splitting your year up into convenient blocks of time, as shown below:

ANNUAL TRAINING PLAN					
PHASES	Preparatory		Competitive		Transition
SUB PHASES	General preparation	Specific preparation	Pre competition	Competitive	Transition

In most sports, the annual training cycle is conventionally divided into the 3 main phase as explained above. Each phase is composed of different cycles and each one has specific objectives which are derived from the general objectives of the annual plan. It may have any one of the following formats:

Macro-cycle
This format is defined as long term, usually a year, and this period can sometimes be longer, maybe up to 4 years depending on your aspirations.

Meso-cycle
This format is best defined as a middle term time span i.e. over a period of 3 months.

Micro-cycle
This format is best defined as short term which can be a week in length or even a month.

The nature of your training session and the major emphasis of your program may change according to these cycles, and there should be progression and development through the periods ultimately leading to a major objective or your peak performance.

Below is an example of a strength training program for a long jumper:

MONTH	DEC	JAN	FEB	MAR	APR
Macro cycle	1	2	3		4
Number of micro cycles	5	6	5		4
Objectives	Testing, Adaptation and prep of your body.	Maximum strength	Power and maintenance of max strength		Power and maintenance of max strength

Common sports such as hockey, netball, football or basketball have certain demands, and by identifying these demands you can break the sport down even more as with the example below:

TYPE	HOW TO ACHIEVE
Intermittent sprints	5secs - 1 min
Power bursts	1sec - 10secs
Prolonged high intensity	1 - 3mins
Steady state	General training and match play

Other demands include agility, specific and general strength and flexibility.
Practice time is also vital but these demands cannot all be met in one session or even in one week. Therefore the value and need for the concept of periodization can immediately be seen, whereby over time each and every one of these demands can be addressed in a progressive manner. Flexibility training and the skill practice would generally continue throughout the year except when complete rest is recommended i.e. during the holiday period.

Generally you should begin with the following:

1. **DEVELOPMENTAL PHASE -** a period of induction or acclimatization, followed by a period of base training as your program begins to develop.

Induction phase - A pre-developmental phase
Normally by this time most top level performers have just finished a period of rest lasting 2 - 4 weeks. Therefore this makes the induction phase the most important phase, although you must avoid launching straight back into full blown training. A period of readjustment is required, as is re-establishing a routine. What is often used during this phase is gentle aerobically biased training along with light strength training and flexi-

bility. The main aim is establishing the base, the solid and broad foundation upon which all performance should stem from.

Aerobically biased training

As with our example above regarding sports such as hockey, netball, football or basketball etc, base building becomes their central focus, even though they will not require the same base training as a marathon runner. An example of this would be:

FREQUENCY	REPS	SETS	TYPE	REMARKS
2 - 3 times per week	Moderate	20–40mins	Steady state running	Athletics track used

Strength development

Proceed with a low volume program on a wide range of exercises such as:

FREQUENCY	REPS	SETS	TYPE	REMARKS
2 times per week	12-16 reps	1 - 2 sets	Strength training	Split muscle groups

Good technique and form is as always of paramount importance, as is combining exercises which will be of direct relevance to your sport, for example:

- Lunges, squats, calf raises and bench press;
- Also involve exercises designed to provide a strong and stable base in potentially weak areas i.e. internal and external rotation, abduction and adduction; abdominal and low back exercises and extra work for the hamstrings.

Your strength work can also progress from low to more moderate loads as the period progresses, and your repetitions reduced to 8. Your weights should correspond to approx. 70% of your maximum potential, or so that your last 3 repetitions in a set feel very difficult. Your work volume can increase to 2 sets if required.

High intensity aerobic training

Introduce this training into your program as follows:

FREQUENCY	INTENSITY	TIME	TYPE	REMARKS
Once per week	Work periods of 1-3mins	6 x 1min- intervals	Interval training	Progress to 8, 10, then 12 x 1min

2. SPECIFIC PHASE - addresses the demands that make you really peak.

You should introduce shorter, more sprint based work in this phase i.e.

- Intermittent sprints 5secs - 1 min;
- Power bursts and agility, performed within circuit training (explained later)
- It may also be necessary to substitute one strength training session for one circuit training session in this phase so that specific movements can be included i.e. specific power or agility movements specific to your sport.

Your aerobically biased training should take the form of maintenance i.e. 1-2 sessions per week of high intensity sessions of 1 - 3mins each, supplemented by your power burst and intermittent sprint sessions.

This phase is very demanding, but your focus should most definitely be on good form and high quality exercises and drills. You will reap the benefits even at this phase especially if you have progressed accordingly. You may find that you prefer to do high intensity i.e. 1-3mins effort one week and intermittent sprints the next. This is completely your choice as differentiation for each individual is very important.
As with the first phase, your strength training must as always focus on good quality and should involve the following:

1 session per week of 10-12 reps to exhaustion, which maintains your strength developed over the previous phase, as this is only 1 session per week it should not interfere with your sprint or high intensity aerobically biased sessions.

TYPES OF TRAINING

SPORTS SPECIFIC TRAINING INTENSITIES

Most team sports are not characterized by continuous sub-maximal movement speeds, as these sports demand periods of high-intensity effort interspersed with maximal bursts of speed and periods of almost complete inactivity. A good example of this would be football i.e. a player may move at a moderate speed for several minutes while following the play and then the player may be forced to sprint at their maximal pace for the ball. After that, the player may have a stoppage in play for up to a minute or so due to various factors. Sport specific training, improves the following for the athlete:

1. Speed;
2. Lateral agility;
3. Strength;
4. Power;
5. Flexibility;
6. Endurance;
7. First step quickness;
8. Core stability.

Training drills that are devised to replicate movements from your given sport are referred to as 'sports specific' training drills or 'functional' training drills. This type of training involves exercises that consist of movements that are specific to your particular sport. Specifically targeting certain muscle groups during these training drill sessions may not actually change your performance under competitive circumstances or normal everyday function, and as yet there is no proof that this actually makes any difference. However if the playing conditions of your particular sport are replicated as much as possible within a training drill session, then this may be the only way that your performance benefits. Developing strength, co-ordination and agility during these training drill sessions by completing sports specific exercises will ultimately take up alot of your time. But ultimately the biggest question of all, is that if you learn to perform the exercises correctly within the training drill sessions, can the new skills learned be transferred back to your sport to improve your performance? The answer lies within the following criteria, and should you meet one or more of these criteria then it will make an actual exercise specific:

- The actual exercise must duplicate the exact movement witnessed in a certain segment of the sports skill;
- The exercise must involve the same type of muscular contraction as used in the skill execution;
- The exercise must have the same range of motion as the skill action itself.

63

Some experts may agree that the best sport specific exercise program, by definition, is by just playing the sport itself?

Aerobic dominant sports
By definition, aerobic training is any training in which oxygen is the muscles primary fuel source. Muscles derive most of their fuel from oxygen after approximately 2mins of continuous activity, for example: jogging or cycling etc at a moderate pace. In many sports, a high level of aerobic fitness is necessary for optimal performance because it promotes endurance and assists recovery in 'stop and start' type sports, such as ice hockey and football etc. To improve aerobic fitness, coaches have traditionally pre-scribed long and tedious sessions of continuous sub maximal exercise for athletes, regardless of their sport specific metabolic demands. Events such as running, cycling, swimming or even strength training that can help build your cardio-respiratory endur-ance are termed aerobic, and as mentioned should involve performing these activities continuously whilst meeting the following criteria:

FREQUENCY	INTENSITY	TIME	TYPE	REMARKS
No less than 3 times a week	70%-80% of max effort	15-20 mins	Aerobic fitness (endurance)	Train 4-6 days a week to achieve a higher level of endurance

FREQUENCY	INTENSITY	TIME	TYPE	REMARKS
No less than 3 times a week	30%-50% of max effort	15+ reps	Strength endurance	Field sports, rowing and martial arts.

Your heart has no idea what you are using your muscles for i.e. whether it is running, cycling, swimming or even strength training. Generally if your muscles are working harder, your cardiovascular system must also work harder to supply the working mus-cles with oxygen and remove the metabolic by-products of intense muscular work. For an activity to qualify as 'aerobic' or to be effective for cardiovascular conditioning it doesn't have to involve continuous or 'steady state' work of the muscles in the lower body, such as is the case in running or cycling. It is just as easy for you to achieve a significant degree of HR elevation by performing only moderate intensity activity using the lower body muscles. Most upper body exercises, however, do not involve enough muscle mass to place a significant demand on the cardiovascular system if only per-formed with a moderate degree of intensity.

Aerobically dominant sports specific training, should involve you working some significant part of your body at a high degree of intensity, and this means that there will still be a demand on the cardiovascular system. As long as you don't allow a significant degree of rest between exercises, the heart rate HR will remain elevated for the duration of the workout. Low intensity, long term activities:

| Distance cycling | Walking | Marathon running |

The activities above that are low in intensity and are performed over a long period of time all have a low absolute power output. This type of training relies more on the oxidative energy system (CHO / Glucose or Fat oxidation), and this type of system and method of training is inadequate for producing the required power output of the intermittent sports such as football, hockey and basketball etc. However, studies have suggested that anaerobic training can improve low intensity exercise endurance.

Training your energy systems for aerobic dominant sports
The table below illustrates the five intensity values for aerobic dominant sports:

INTENSITY NUMBER	TYPE	RHYTHM	HR/min	% of total volume
1	LA tolerance training	Maximum	180+	85-95
2	VO2 Max consumption	Very high	170-180	80-90
3	Anaerobic threshold	High	160-170	80
4	O2 threshold	Medium	150-160	70
5	O2 compensation	Low	130-150	40-60

Short, medium and long term muscular endurance
In order to hit the right muscular endurance range you must quite simply increase the reps and lower the weight so that you reach exhaustion around the 2-4min or 20min mark depending on what range you are aiming for.

TYPES OF M-END	MUSCULAR ENDURANCE SPORTS	INTENSITY
Short term muscular endurance (ME)	Wrestlers, Judo players and Rugby players etc	For a 2-4min period.
Medium term muscular endurance (ME)	Boxers, middle distance runners and swimmers, and even footballers due to rest in between bouts of exercise.	For up to 20min period
Long term muscular endurance (ME)	Marathon runners and triathletes etc	For longer periods

Acyclic and Cyclic muscular endurance

2 variants of circuit training sometimes called intensive/extensive with interval, which simply means:

TYPE	INTENSITY	% of LOAD	RHYTHM	REST
Acyclic muscular endurance	Intensive n.o of reps: (10-30 reps)	Dynamic loads of 50-80%	Slow	2-3 x more than work-out time
Cyclic muscular endurance	Extensive n.o: (30-50 reps per min)	Low loads of 20-50%	Med-slow	Shorter rest intervals

Anaerobic dominant sports

By definition anaerobic is any type of training in which creatine phosphate and glycogen are the muscles main fuel sources. This occurs during short, intense bursts of activity which normally lasts less than 2 minutes i.e.

Sprinting	Olympic Lifting	Jumping (long jump)	Throwing (Javelin)

Power sports - Anaerobic exercise, including interval training is highly effective for burning fat and at the same time building endurance for power sports. Anaerobic training is shorter than aerobic training in duration, as mentioned less than 2mins, in which oxygen is not a limiting factor in your performance, and requires energy from anaerobic sources. This energy source involves your body using phosphagen and lactic acid thus only enabling you to perform brief, near maximal muscular activity. The weekly frequency of your training remains the same i.e. 3 sessions, so your aerobic phase can still be covered during the other days. If only 2 or 3 weekly sessions are possible, then mixed programs can be adopted i.e. on completion of your anaerobic fitness, which is always done at the beginning of your session, add 15-20mins of aerobic fitness to balance the two phases i.e. anaerobic and aerobic.

Combination training

In order to enhance the capacity of your primary energy system, multiple energy systems should be trained together i.e. aerobic training can be added to the anaerobic training program. This enhances recovery from your anaerobic bouts of training. However, concern must be given to the relative amount of aerobic training being performed when prescribing aerobic exercise for the anaerobic athlete.

SPEED

The chart below represents the importance of the aerobic component in any program

TRAINING OBJECTIVE	ACTIVITY TYPE	PERCENTAGE
Improve endurance	Aerobic	Above 50%
	Anaerobic	Below 25%
	Compensatory	Remainder
Improve speed	Aerobic	Below 50%
	Anaerobic	Above 25%
	Compensatory	Remainder

Many elements influence speed development i.e. heredity, reaction time, ability to overcome external resistance, technique, concentration, willpower and muscle elasticity

Important

Training for your sport must not take you any longer than 1hr:30m otherwise the phase of catabolic processes is initiated, which is a phase in which your muscles self cannibalise. If you are a sports and endurance event athlete who performs in cycling, swimming or distance running etc, then you can improve your performance times by increasing your exercise intensity at which the anaerobic or lactate threshold occurs. Lactate threshold training is explained in more detail in the next sub-chapter. One of the important characteristics of your anaerobic fitness training is the use of general programs, during which almost all of your muscles are worked out in one training session. Any activity that lasts from 30secs to 2mins begins to rely on lactic acid (any activity that lasts more than 2mins actually becomes aerobic training). These energy systems are effectively developed using an interval training system (also explained in it's relevant sub-chapter) and although one energy system may be predominate for a given activity, all systems are in use to some degree during anaerobic, or interval training.

TRAINING IN THE ZONES OF INTENSITY

LACTATE THRESHOLD (LT)

Lactate Threshold (LT) training is best described as the exercise intensity at which blood lactate begins an abrupt increase above baseline concentration, after which diminished performance capacity is realised. Lactate Threshold (LT) training sessions also known as pace, tempo or aerobic/anaerobic training can either be continuous or intermittent in nature. Both training types require exercise intensity to be at, or slightly above your lactate threshold. To monitor your own heart rate is one of the most common ways to gauge your lactate threshold training intensity. Assuming that your lactate threshold will occur between 85-90% of your maximum heart rate is one of the simplest methods. You will learn more about this in the relevant sub-chapter related to HRT.

LT training sessions - To determine your work rate at its lactate threshold, your heart rate can be measured or equipment such as a power output meter can be used, as in the following example for a cyclist completing intervals and continuous type sessions:

FREQUENCY	INTENSITY	TIME	TYPE	REMARKS
2 per week	95-105% *LT 3-5 intervals	10m interval times	Interval LT training	2-3min rest intervals
2 per week	95-105% *LT	20-30mins	Continuous LT training	No rest

* LT = Training intensity at Lactate Threshold is measured via your heart rate or power output.

Training Effect

Training at intensities near, at or above the Lactate Threshold (LT) can "push your LT off the radar" i.e. greater exercise intensity is required to raise lactate levels to the LT. The accumulation of blood lactate remains a good indicator for subsequent exhaustion and can predict performance in many endurance events i.e. how it contributes to fatigue etc. Lactate threshold training can improve your performance times in endurance events such as distance running, cycling and swimming. Lactate threshold is often expressed as a percentage of VO2 max, for example if you reach VO2 max at a running speed of 15mph and lactate begins to accumulate at 10mph. Then you have a lactate threshold of approx. 67%, see other comparisons below:

VO2 max varies greatly between individuals and even between elite athletes that compete in the same sport. In comparison, the threshold of a world class endurance athlete can be up to 90% VO2 max compared to 50% in an untrained individual.

VO2 MAX TRAINING

VO2 max training is defined as the highest rate of oxygen consumption attainable during maximal or exhaustive exercise.

Other terms also used interchangeably with VO2 max are:

- Aerobic power;
- Aerobic capacity;
- Maximal oxygen uptake.

As your exercise intensity increases, so does your oxygen consumption but a point is reached where exercise intensity can continue to increase without the associated rise in oxygen consumption. VO2 max is usually expressed relative to bodyweight because oxygen and energy needs differ, relative to size. It can also be expressed relative to body surface area, and this may be more accurate when comparing children and oxygen uptake between sexes.

Your training & VO2 Max

In elite athletes, VO2 max is not a good predictor of performance. Perhaps more significant than VO2 max is the speed at which an athlete can run, bike or swim at VO2 max. You should think of VO2 max as your aerobic potential and the lactate threshold as the marker for how much of that potential you are tapping. Resistance training and intense anaerobic type training have very little effect on VO2 max, even when shorter rest periods are used between sets and exercises. There are many protocols used on treadmills, cycle ergometers etc where VO2 max can be determined, but more common is indirect testing as it requires little or no expensive equipment, none of these however are as accurate as direct testing. The best examples of these being:

- The bleep test;
- The 12 minute walk test;
- 1.5 mile run.

ANAEROBIC THRESHOLD (AT) TRAINING

Anaerobic threshold is an extremely reliable and powerful predictor of performance in aerobic exercise. In simple terms muscles can utilise glucose in 2 ways:

1. Aerobically i.e. with oxygen;
2. Anaerobically i.e. without oxygen.

Both of these systems generate a temporary energy store, which in turn produces mechanical work.

The anaerobic threshold zone – is approx. 80%-90% of your individual Max HR and this zone is reached by simply working harder, for example running faster. Training in this way you will get faster and fitter by increasing your heart rate as you crossover from aerobic to anaerobic training. At this point, your heart cannot pump enough blood and oxygen to supply the exercising muscles fully so they respond by continuing to contract anaerobically. This is the point where you can only stay in this high intensity zone for a limited amount of time, usually not more than an hour. The reason for this is because the muscle just cannot sustain working anaerobically without fatiguing. The working muscles protect themselves from overwork by not being able to maintain the intensity level.

The process is explained fully below:

- An all out sprint, i.e. high power output, uses the anaerobic system;
- Energy is quickly available, but anaerobic pathways are not very efficient;
- Short term energy stores rapidly deplete, lactic acid builds up, exercise stops;
- After a brief rest, the system is recharged and ready for the next sprint.

Anaerobic threshold (AT) varies, not only from person to person, but also within a given individual, sport to sport. Training your body to remove lactate better and applying the right types of workouts is the key to properly shape your AT. Individuals that are untrained tend to have a lower AT (approximately 55% of VO2 max) this can be compared to elite endurance athletes who generally have a higher AT (approx. 80 - 90% of VO2 max). These methods will be explained in greater detail within the next chapter.

Pushing your AT with specific workouts
Interval work consists of a repeated series of short, high intensity runs alternating with rest periods, and regardless of which distance you are training for i.e. 5k or a marathon distance, interval training will help you run faster. Intervals should be creative and fun but definitely not done every day, so long as you continually push yourself into a lactate burdened state your body will adapt, and you will become better at processing lactate. The only limitation with this system (phosphate) is in your body's ability to rebuild the stores to keep up to date with what's needed. In general terms, the fitter you are the quicker you can rebuild your energy (ATP) stores i.e. with shorter recovery periods. Until you are fit enough you will require longer recovery periods because you will not have the efficiency that a fitter individual will have. You can generally utilise all of your available energy (ATP) stores with 10-30 seconds of high intensity training, but they do replenish very quickly. The following table shows the replenishment periods:

70

% of ATP restored	Time after exercise (sec)
50%	30sec
75%	60sec
87%	90sec
90%	120sec
100%	180sec

By way of the above example, this explains why it is recommended that you wait a full 3 minute period of active recovery between your high intensity sets. This is so that your energy (ATP) stores are fully replenished. This is why individuals supplement their diet with creatine (creatine monohydrate) because it affects the phosphate system by adding more fuel into your system i.e. the creatine phosphate (CP) system. ATP-CP is broken down and regenerated, and when creatine is added you are in effect creating more energy for yourself, which ultimately leads to more growth.

AEROBIC THRESHOLD TRAINING

If you are an endurance athlete, aerobic system fitness is perhaps the single best way of determining your performance. The optimal way to train any physiological system is to create and frequently repeat a stress that precisely targets that system. When it comes to the aerobic system, that target is the aerobic threshold. When training at your aerobic threshold, all of the key aerobic systems are stressed, and that stress can be maintained for relatively long periods of time, just as you must be able to do in an endurance type race.

The aerobic zone – is approx. 70%-80% of your individual Max HR. As an athlete, your season in many ways must begin with the initial base period, as this is classed as the most important phase of the season. Great gains can be made during this time of the year, especially in 3 of the most important abilities in an athlete's fitness arsenal:

Endurance	Force	Speed skills

Many endurance athletes sell themselves short within this period by jumping ahead of themselves by completing anaerobic, race type workouts. This seasonal preparation could be used so much more productively, if only they took advantage of the gains that could be made by developing the above abilities i.e. endurance, force and speed skills.

Determining Intensity

There are several ways to know the level of intensity that targets the aerobic threshold, but it all depends on what technology you have available to you. The most common technology these days is quite simply your heart rate i.e. your pulse, and Heart Rate

71

Monitors (HRM'S) are explained in more detail within the next chapter. During exercise, your pulse will always be a good indicator of how your body is relating to the stress being applied by any of the following:

- Running;
- Cycling;
- Swimming;
- Cross country skiing etc

There seems to be a good correlation between aerobic threshold and anaerobic threshold i.e. if you know one, you can predict the other fairly closely with only 20 beats per minute apart. For example if an endurance trained athlete knows that their anaerobic threshold is 170bpm for their particular sport, then they will know that their aerobic threshold for that same sport will be approx. 150bpm. In knowing this information, you can quite simply wear a HRM and exercise steadily for long periods at 20bpm less than your anaerobic threshold.

To get an approx. measurement of your anaerobic threshold:

1. Conduct a 30min time trial;
2. At an all out race effort;
3. Use your HRM (split function) to find your average HR for the final 20mins of the effort.

Important

The main point to note is that, within the same athlete, both thresholds vary from sport to sport. Regarding your own zones of training, everyone is different and as long as you are not too far off the mark it will be ok, so remember that the % max is a guide only.

METHODS OF TRAINING IN DIFFERENT ZONES

Whatever your health and fitness desires, if you follow your goals and stick to a routine you will be well on your way to creating a healthier life for yourself. Your heart is a muscle, it can be strengthened, but if unused you can lose the hearts functional ability. Training in a zone is simply training within a range of heart beats which has powerful benefits. Training is your regime of exercising to achieve your specific goals. Heart rate (HR) is measured in beats per minute (bpm) and your resting heart rate (RHR) is the measurement when you are sitting, relaxed, sedentary. In general, the lower your resting heart rate, the better, and your resting heart rate should ideally be measured when you first wake in the morning before you get out of bed. Consequently your maximum heart rate (MHR) is the fastest your heart can beat for one minute. Some people use a mathematical formula to estimate MHR, although it has a lot of errors because it allows it to drop as you get older. Within most fitness clubs and gyms you will see the MHR charts which are generally genetically determined. You will find that according to those charts your MHR will simply not decrease, but if you maintain your fitness it shouldn't decrease unless you become de-conditioned. Using common mathematical formulas to estimate MHR are generally based on age and they don't really work well enough. Below is a formula found to be more accurate:

Age + Weight + Predicted Maximum Heart Rate

GENDER	STAGE 1	STAGE 2	STAGE 3
Males	210 minus 1/2 your age	minus 5% of your body weight	+ 4
Females	210 minus - 1/2 your age	minus 1% of your body weight	+ 0
You	210 minus - _____	minus _____ your body weight	+ _

An example for a 50 year old female, weighing 130Ibs would be: 210 – 25(yrs) minus 1.3 (w.t) + 0 (female) = MHR of 183bpm.

You can also ask anyone at your gym to explain the karvonen formula to you, which is just as accurate as the one above.

Important

Your MHR is altitude sensitive and increases as you go higher, the same as it would be if affected by drugs such as beta blocks and even antihistamines.

INTERVAL TRAINING

By definition is a short burst of intense activity alternated with shorter or longer periods of rest or light activity. The goal is normally to increase ones endurance or fat loss, but there are numerous ways in which to perform them. Interval training uses, as named, intervals that can consist of any of the following:

- Running;
- Swimming;
- Callisthenic exercises;
- Resistance training.

Work intervals, which also include rest intervals, vary depending on the mode of training, or need for example: work intervals of less than 30 seconds (phosphagen system), are typically performed with rest intervals of approximately three times this duration (1:3 ratio). Interval training utilises the body's two energy producing systems, the aerobic and the anaerobic.

The aerobic system is the system that allows you to walk or run for several miles, it uses oxygen to convert carbohydrates from various sources throughout your body into energy.

The anaerobic system on the other hand, draws energy from carbohydrates (in the form of glycogen) stored in the muscles for short bursts of activity such as sprinting, jumping or lifting heavy objects. This system does not require oxygen, nor does it provide enough energy for more than the briefest of activities. It's by-product (lactic acid), is responsible for that achy, burning sensation in your muscles that you may feel after. That said, interval training actually allows you to enjoy the benefits of anaerobic activities without having to endure those burning muscles. In its most basic form, interval or fartlek training might involve walking for two minutes, running for two (1:1 ratio) and alternating this pattern throughout the duration of a workout.

The concept of interval training is explained very briefly below:

➢ Sprint Intervals

The high intensity portions are called sprint intervals, and sprint intervals are measured either by time or distance. They can be as short as 15secs in activities like high intensity interval training (HIIT) or as long as 20mins for aerobic interval training. An example of a sprint interval would be running at full pace along a stretch of field for 30 seconds, another would be an indoor cyclist spending 15mins simulating a climb on the bike.

➤ Rest Intervals

The periods of recovery are called rest intervals. During a rest interval you should not stop the activity but generally exercise at a low intensity which allows the body to recover from the sprint interval. The length of these rest intervals are determined primarily by your fitness levels and the type of the sprint interval. The intervals themselves are very important and the idea is to ensure that your sprints are done at an optimal intensity, as without sufficient rest your interval training will resort back to an aerobic type of activity.

Intensity - As previously mentioned, the intensity of the sprint intervals is how hard you push yourself during the sprint. For e.g. the intensity is usually measured on a scale of 1 to 10:

1 = no effort whatsoever	10 = the maximum effort possible

This is clearly a personal scale and will depend on your own fitness level and the type of interval training that you are doing, so for example if you and another person were working on your speed work then, during your sprint phase which for e.g. could last for 15 seconds or so and your '10' is a flat out sprint by running as fast as you can, someone else who has not exercised in a while may decide to do intervals whilst walking and therefore after a 1 minute walk at a brisk pace may leave them completely out of breath, and this would be their 10. A '10' is merely the maximum amount of effort a person can safely expend for that particular interval.

Fartlek - (which means speed play) is a term which the Swedes came up with, that is not only an efficient training method, but it can help you avoid injuries that often accompany non-stop, repetitive activity, and provides the opportunity to increase your intensity without burning yourself out in a matter of minutes. Unlike traditional interval training, fartlek training does not involve specifically or accurately measured intervals. Instead, intervals are based according to the needs and perceptions of the participant. In other words, how you feel determines the length and speed of each interval. The intensity (or lack thereof) of each interval is up to you and how you feel dependant on what you are trying to achieve. The same is true for the length of each interval, for example: if it is your habit to walk two miles per day in 30 minutes, you can easily increase the intensity of your walk by increasing the pace every couple of minutes and then returning to your usual pace. A great method is to challenge yourself to run a particular distance, i.e. from the red car to the gates up ahead, and then walk from the gates to the next red car. When you first start fartlek training, each interval can be a negotiation with yourself depending on how strong or energetic you happen to feel during that particular workout. This helps to break up the boredom and drudgery that often comes from doing the same thing day after day. Consider the following four variables when designing an interval training program:

- Intensity (speed) of work interval;
- Duration (distance or time) of work interval;
- Duration of rest or recovery interval;
- Number of repetitions of each interval.

Lack of time is the number one excuse for people not exercising, and if they do eventually start exercising then a lack of results isn't far behind. Interval training is a great solution for many excuses and motivational problems. The most important principle of conditioning (sequencing) may be listening to your body, and just as with any other type of fitness, the intensity and duration of training must be increased gradually over time in a logical progression.

HEART RATE TRAINING (HRT)
Heart rate monitors (HRMs) allow you to feel in control of your training and most of the time they are an accurate guide of your cardio fitness. Generally they can prevent you from overtraining or under training by showing you that you need to work harder or easier dependant on your schedule. For many of you, HRMs will allow you to assess your progress in terms of numbers and charts etc instead of monitoring how you feel. Training at the proper intensity doing any type of activity is one of the key elements in improving your performance and staying injury free.

How does it work?
The chest strap of a heart rate monitor uses electrodes to monitor the electric volts that occur when your heart beats. The receiver detects this information from the electrodes via radio signal from the chest strap. The receiver then uses this information to determine your heart rate. A heart rate monitor receiver gives you a heart rate to compare to your targeted heart rate. Many HRMs will also take the information of your current heart rate and compare it to your programmed maximum heart rate to give you a percentage zone, and this number will allow you to know how hard you are working during your run.

How do you use it?

To use a HRM, you must first determine your maximum heart rate, then the HRM will generally do all the work for you. Finally, you can start tracking your information after each workout in order to see your progress over a period of time. Some HRMs will do the calculations for you and usually come with software that will track your progress for you. The vast majority of workouts should be performed at an easy to moderate intensity instead of thinking that harder is always better. Your first step however should be to rate your fitness level and second step to take your fitness test as you have already learned in the relevant chapter. Or you could take the following test which is a little more demanding. If you do not possess a HRM then you will have to calculate your own zones (as explained below) and after each run you can write your statistics in your workout journal.

One mile walk test

Find a 400m track, and walk four continuous evenly paced laps as fast as you can in your current condition. The first three laps will put you on a heart rate plateau where you hold a steady state ready for the fourth lap. Determine your average heart rate for this final lap. To predict your max heart rate MHR:

- Add 40bpm if you are in poor shape;
- Add 50bpm if you are in fair shape;
- Add 60bpm if you are in good shape.

How do you determine your proper training intensity?

When you train with a heart rate monitor it gives you immediate feedback related to your training effort. It is essential to develop a strong aerobic base which allows your body to efficiently metabolize stored body fat while sparing stored carbohydrate. It is very important to develop this aerobic base by exercising at an easy to moderate intensity, especially before commencing higher intensity sessions. Establishing heart rate training zones can be extremely confusing, but there are a number of formulas developed to estimate training zones based around your maximum heart rate. It is important to note that these formulas are only estimates and can be up to 30-40 beats off the mark for each individual.

Heart rate zones

Heart rate zones expressed as a percentage of your maximum heart rate (MHR), reflect your exercise intensity and the result benefit. Once you have established your MHR, the chart below shows you your specific zones, and they are each 10% of your MHR.

You can also fill in your own findings:

Percentage of your own Max Heart Rate MHR	Examples (bpm)	Enter your own heart rates here
50% of your Max Heart Rate =	e.g. 90 beats per min	
60% of your Max Heart Rate =	e.g. 108 beats per min	
70% of your Max Heart Rate =	e.g. 126 beats per min	
80% of your Max Heart Rate =	e.g. 144 beats per min	
90% of your Max Heart Rate =	e.g. 162 beats per min	
100% of your Max Heart Rate =	e.g. 180 beats per min	

To determine your own personal zone you just need to join together the percentages and put them in the chart below.

Your zone number	% of your own heart range	Enter your own heart rate range here for each zone
1	50%-60% - bpm	e.g. from chart above = 90 - 108bpm
2	60%-70% - bpm	
3	70%-80% - bpm	
4	80%-90% - bpm	
5	90%-100% - bpm	

Lactate threshold

If you can base these zones around your lactate threshold this will be a much more precise method for establishing your training zone. The burn that is felt in your muscles during hard efforts, this is lactic acid build up, and Lactate threshold is an exercise intensity in which your body can no longer clear this by-product as it begins to accumulate in your blood. To determine lactate threshold accurately, it has to be via laboratory testing or even field tests which can be performed alone to estimate lactate threshold heart rate, these tests are quite strenuous and you should first consult your physician. Field tests are a much more precise method than using the max heart rate formulas, but you will still need a heart rate monitor and preferably one that has a lap function. Be aware though that training heart rates can be very different for each sport, and you must ensure that you are well rested and hydrated prior to the tests. You should also plan a few days rest between both of these tests where possible. Due to the fact that Lactate threshold heart rate changes dramatically, your training zones should be re-tested regularly i.e. every 3–4 months. Prior to commencing the test, it goes without saying that you should warm up for 10 to 15 minutes first. The field test for an individual time trial of 30mins involves the following:

- Your effort should be maximum, but not so hard you slow down at the end;
- When you begin press the start button on the heart rate monitor;

- After the first 10mins, press the lap button and again at 30mins;
- Your average HR over the last 20mins is your lactate threshold estimate;
- On completion, you should cool down for 5-10mins.

Important point:
If there is no lap function on your heart rate monitor then you should:

1. Look at your watch every minute;
2. Make a mental note of your average HR over the last 20mins of the test.

Using the following chart, calculate your heart rate based upon the lactate threshold heart rate you established in your field test.

Zone Descriptions

Zones	Training Zones	% of Lactate Threshold	
		Lower	Upper
1	Active Recovery	<80%	
2	Endurance	80%	89%
3	Tempo	90%	93%
4	Sub threshold	94%	99%
5a	Supra threshold	100%	102%
5b	Aerobic Capacity	103%	105%
5c	Anaerobic Capacity	>105	

Zone 1 = Active recovery **Zone 2** = Aerobic threshold **Zone 3** = Tempo training **Zone 4** = Lactate threshold **Zone 5a** = Super-threshold training **Zone 5b** = Interval training **Zone 5c** = Anaerobic capacity training.

CIRCUIT TRAINING

By definition is one set each of several exercises done back to back, usually with little or no rest between sets, for example: a set of squats, followed by push ups, pull ups and step ups and then rest. That would be one circuit and then repeat. Circuit training is a workout routine that combines cardiovascular fitness and resistance training and is superb for general fitness and caters for a wide variety of fitness levels. A great time saver, it can be a refreshing and fun change from the more monotonous types of exercise. Circuit classes typically consist of the following:

CIRCUIT	INTENSITY	REST
10 exercise stations	60secs in sequence	30-60secs rest in between

A circuit can consist of 6 exercises (short circuit) 9 exercises (normal circuit) or 12 exercises (long circuit). The amount of exercise stations is based on your goals and/or pre-training levels. It is an efficient and challenging form of conditioning, which works well for developing strength, endurance (both aerobic and anaerobic), flexibility and coordination.

Sports conditioning circuits

A simple and effective way to train is to use a general sports conditioning circuit using a variety of fitness components with varying intensity organized to provide you with the best workout in the shortest time. This provides you with a time efficient way to train all of the fitness elements necessary for a well balanced team and/or individual sports conditioning workout. When developing a sports conditioning circuit a wide variety of exercises and equipment can be utilised.

Common equipment
- Cones, skipping ropes, resistance band tubing;
- Balance and coordination equipment i.e. boards, balls, mini trampolines etc
- Plyometric jump boxes, step platforms of various sizes;
- Assorted ball sizes, weighted (med) balls, slide boards, etc.

The versatility of a circuit has made it popular for everyone, not to mention for sportsmen and women who can use it during the closed season and early pre-season to help develop a solid base of fitness and prepare the body for more stressful subsequent training. Circuit training stations are generally sequenced in a way to alternate between muscle groups, which allows for adequate recovery. The rest interval between stations should be between 30-90secs and 1-3mins between circuits. A typical gym has several strength training machines and workstations, which enables the creation of several circuits. This benefit of variability challenges the skills of the participant and keeps them interested from session to session. By allowing only a short rest interval of 30-90secs between stations you gain cardiovascular fitness, along with the benefits gained from resistance type training for improving your strength endurance. Much of the equipment is relatively inexpensive and can include resistance bands, dumbbells, medicine balls, fit-balls and fitness machines, not to mention your own body weight (all of which and more are included within the functional resistance training chapter). A well designed circuit can help to correct the imbalances that occur in any sport played to a high level. Circuit training in itself is not a form of exercise, but the way in which an exercise session is structured. Routines can be developed from the exercises shown within this book, they can then be added to the exercise templates and used for strength development, for improving endurance or a combination of the two. A circuit can last for any length of time, generally between 10-30mins and the training demand is managed by indicating the time and/or number of reps. Heart rate (HR) could also be used to calculate when to rest.

POST TRAINING RECOVERY

In order for your body to fully recover and repair itself you need significant rest periods, especially days of rest between any of your sessions. Strength sessions specifically require substantial rest periods, where you are training similar body parts. In general, during a strength session it is advisable to rest between sets and between exercises. Regular performance evaluation assessments should be completed in order to identify overtraining before it occurs. A great indication that you are overtraining and not getting enough rest is if you notice that your results are considerably lower than last time.

Exercise recovery - For those who achieve higher intensities, a vital function of development for this method of training is the recovery phase i.e. resting and exercising simultaneously. Cross training whilst in each of these zones has their benefit, which means varying the demands on your body by completing activities such as walking 1 day cycling the next, and swimming another etc. Maintaining your own personal heart zone training journal and recording your training in various zones is the key to success. Adding this information to your journal will assist you in evaluating your total effort over a period of time. f you are training for muscular endurance (muscle definition) then you require a 48 hour recovery as this is how long it takes to fully restore your glycogen stores.

Delayed onset muscle soreness (DOMS) - This is the pain or discomfort that you may or may not have felt 24-72 hours post exercise, which generally subsides during a 2 - 3 day period. The precise cause of DOMS is still unknown, but can generally be caused by the breakdown of muscular fibres due to stress within specific resistance programs. Once this breakdown has occurred, the muscles then grow stronger and larger i.e. through hypertrophy. Some of the main causes of DOMS are:

- Downhill running;
- Many eccentric contractions;
- Overstretching.

Stretching before and after exercise has been suggested as a way of reducing DOMS, as have warming up before exercise, cooling down afterwards, and gently warming the area. Common treatment for DOMS is to do contrast bathing (showers) i.e. alternating between cold and hot water; as this may increase your circulation.

Overtraining syndrome - The name given to the collection of emotional, behavioural, and physical symptoms due to overtraining that has persisted for weeks or even months, and medically, the overtraining syndrome is classified as a neuro-endocrine disorder. Overtraining specifically can best be defined as the state where the athlete has been repeatedly stressed by training to the point where rest is no longer adequate to allow for recovery. In order to improve your performance you must work harder, but if your training is too hard this can break you and actually make you weaker and too tired to get the results that you desire. It is the concept and implementation of your rest periods that makes you stronger, and this adaptation is in response to maximal loading of the cardiovascular and muscular systems. These 2 systems build to greater levels to compensate for the stress that you have applied. These greater levels are only due to your recovery periods, which consequently place you at a higher level of performance. Regeneration cannot occur if a sufficient amount of rest is not included within your training program then, and the outcome is that your performance plateaus and in time declines. The most common symptom of overtraining is fatigue, as explained below:

Fatigue - Physical exercise, whether in training or actual sport participation, is never complete without an attempt to analyze fatigue. Any exercise at higher intensities will result in fatigue of the muscles and nervous system alike. Fatigue can also cause the human body to experience the following:

- A lack of co-ordination;
- Reduced ventilation;
- Poor transportation of oxygen and improper removal of waste products.

The majority of time, fatigue will only produce a lack of normal response, or a slowing down in the muscles alone, but it can also cause faintness, giddiness and often sickness.

Younger Athletes - A serious case of exhaustion is more often than not found in the younger athlete than in the experienced one, and this can be due to any one of the following reasons:

1. A lack of proper training and preparation;
2. Inadequate nutrition.

Very few cases of severe exhaustion have been noted with the experienced athlete, but some form of exhaustion is common to all games and sports and in particular cross country running, marathons and even boat racing. These findings have now led to the distribution of glucose drinks during most sports and especially during the majority of training regimes. In order to reduce the cases of fatigue, control is the key point to most training regimes, especially with younger athletes. Fatigue can be avoided somewhat by the provision of sound scientific training and conditioning, and of course an adequate diet i.e. carbohydrate reserves, vitamins and salt intake. Progression is also a big key factor to avoid burn out, involving a program that is gradually increased in intensity alongside natural stimulants as mentioned before such as creatine and glucose drinks to name only a few but never any enhancing drugs. To work towards a high oxygen intake and a low accumulation of acidity is extremely important, which in turn assists in creating efficiency in both heart and circulation. Fatigue also has other symptoms which are created from within, the only treatment being absolute rest. Other symptoms can include some of the following:

- Irritability;
- Decreased appetite;
- Insomnia;
- Acute sensitivity.

If you are training with a heart rate monitor you may notice that you cannot sustain your workout at its usual intensity, this can be due to regulation of glucose becoming altered. Generally speaking, your training journal is always the best method used for you to monitor your progress, and this will ultimately help you keep track of important data such as:

1. Distance you cover;
2. Your exercise intensity;
3. Your Resting Heart Rate;
4. Your weight;
5. Your general health;
6. How you feel during each workout;
7. Your levels of DOMS and fatigue.

Important
It is always better to be undertrained than over trained, with the key factor being rest which is the vital part of any training program.

STRENGTH TRAINING

DEVELOPING YOUR STRENGTH PROGRAM

Almost any form of exercise will stimulate some degree of strength and muscle development, however most people are not taught the principles essential for a safe and effective program. The following principles of strength training and exercise guidelines are extremely important for your safety and the effective planning of your strength training program. One repetition max (1RM) is explained in more detail in the next sub-chapter.

MUSCULAR STRENGTH - Muscular strength is the ability of the neuromuscular system to generate force. The magnitude of strength development is dependent on the prescription of the following:

- Muscle actions;
- Intensity;
- Volume;
- Exercise selection and order;
- Rest periods between sets;
- Frequency.

MUSCLE ACTION - Novice, intermediate, and advanced individuals, are recommended to include concentric, eccentric, and isometric muscle actions.

MUSCLE LOADING- Novice, intermediate, and advanced individuals, are recommended to train with the following loads:

NOVICE TO INTERMEDIATE	To maximise your muscular strength	ADVANCED
60-70% of 1 RM @ 8-12 repetitions	——————▶	Train at loads of 80-100% of your 1 RM

When you are training at a specific Rep Max load, it is recommended that you progress by using the following criteria:

INCREASE YOUR REP MAX		
Lower than 2-10% for small muscle mass exercises	Normally a 2-10% increase	Higher than 2-10% increase for large muscle mass exercises

You should aim to increase these set loads when you can perform the current workload for 1-2 reps beyond the target number, for more than one training session.

TRAINING VOLUME – The following progressions are recommended:

NOVICES	PROGRESSION TO INTERMEDIATE
1-3 sets per exercise	Use multiple sets with systematic variation of volume and intensity over time

To reiterate the importance of not overtraining consider the following:

1. A dramatic increase in volume is not recommended;
2. Not all exercises need to be performed with the same number of sets.

The emphasis of higher or lower volume is dictated by your overall aim i.e. your program priorities as well as what specific muscles you are training.

EXERCISE SELECTION - Novice, intermediate, and advanced individuals, are recommended to perform unilateral and bilateral single exercises in all resistance programs, and to maximise overall muscle strength, multiple joint exercises should be performed.

FREE WEIGHTS & MACHINES - Novice, intermediate, and advanced individuals, are recommended to perform a variety of free weight and fitness machine exercises within their program. However the emphasis should be placed on free weight exercises for the more advanced, and fitness machine exercises be used to compliment your specific program needs

EXERCISE ORDER - Novice, intermediate, and advanced individuals, are recommended to sequence the exercises for total body development i.e. all muscle groups trained.

METHODS FOR TOTAL BODY DEVELOPMENT		
METHOD	HOW?	REMARKS
Upper & lower body split	Train upper body musculature 1 day and train lower body musculature another day	Rotation of upper and lower body exercises. Perform larger muscle group exercises before smaller ones.
Muscle group split	Individual muscle groups trained during a workout	Perform multiple joint exercises before single joint exercises. Perform higher intensity exercises before lower-intensity exercises

REST PERIODS - Novice, intermediate, and advanced individuals, are recommended to include significant rest periods into their program for at least 2-3mins. This is especially important for all core exercises such as the squat and bench press, where heavier loads are used. A shorter rest period is required for all additional exercises i.e. assistance exercises which are used to compliment the core exercises, and a suffice length of time is 1-2min for these.

VELOCITY OF MUSCLE ACTION – The following velocities are recommended for each type:

UNTRAINED	INTERMEDIATE	ADVANCED
Slow and moderate velocities	Moderate velocity	From unintentionally slow to fast velocities.

The velocity you select should correspond to the intensity, and your intent should be to maximise the velocity of the concentric muscle action.

FREQUENCY OF MUSCLE ACTION - The following frequencies are recommended:

NOVICE	INTERMEDIATE	ADVANCED
Train the entire body 2-3 d/wk	Train the entire body 3-4 d/wk	Train 4-6 d/wk

More experienced strength trainers may benefit from using a higher frequency i.e. 2 workouts per day for 4-5 d/wk.

Improve your strength by performing the following:

METHOD	SETS	EXAMPLE
Perform more exercises per muscle group	Perform more sets of each exercise (a total of 18 sets)	If working chest, Perform 3 sets of bench press, 3 sets of dumbbell flyes and 3 sets of incline dumbbell press.

In this example, you would only train x1 other major muscle group, and if you are training only one or two muscle groups in a workout, you will be able to perform more sets than if you are planning to train 3 or 4. However if you plan to train more than 2 muscle groups, you would reduce the total number of sets per muscle group. In order to achieve sufficient stimulation, major muscle groups such as the legs and back generally require more sets i.e. 8-12 sets for the more advanced individuals.

SINGLE & MULTIPLE SETS

To achieve maximum stimulation you can choose to perform single sets or multiple sets. There are benefits to both types of training in this way but performing a single set of each exercise produces similar gains to performing several sets, so you don't necessarily need to perform multiple sets to achieve the greatest gains. Only beginners really benefit from a single set, however the discrepancy will always lie in the following:

- The quality of your reps;
- The distinction between your warm up set and your actual working sets.

So whether you achieve true failure on your first or tenth set it will all depend on the quality of your set i.e. how strict your form is, but your ultimate aim is to overload your muscles. Remember, the rest period you need to leave between your workouts depends on the intensity and duration of your workout, your training experience and your diet.

METHODS OF DEVELOPMENT

There are far too many different methods of developing your strength to list them all, from basic strength training, to training for combat athletes, utilising sand-bags, kettle-bells etc. But below we have listed some of the most common methods:

1. 1RM;
2. Power training;
3. Maximum strength training;
4. Hypertrophy;
5. Strength endurance;
6. Muscular size training;
7. Many more variations of the above.

As with most concepts related to fitness, before you commence any type of program it is recommended to first test yourself.

STRENGTH TESTS

What you ideally want from a strength test is to see a quantifiable measurement, especially at the start of your training. Strength testing on both your upper and lower body every few months is the best approach. A strength test allows you to see which muscle groups are progressing, and ultimately which are not.

Lower Body Tests - Including lower body tests into your strength test is an absolute must, especially if you want to get a full measure of your fitness level. The best lower body tests to perform will be ones that utilise many muscles at the same time i.e. compound movements for example the 1RM squat test.

Upper Body Tests - The 2 most common upper body tests to perform are the 1RM bench press, and the press up test. As above these are both compound movements, as they determine strength levels in a variety of muscle groups.

Push up test – Muscular endurance and muscular strength fall under the same heading of strength testing. Muscular endurance is the muscles ability to fight off fatigue for longer periods of time. Within the functional resistance training chapter you will find how to perform the push up. Should your strength or form need developing, you can see how you can modify this exercise to make it easier. Record the amount you can do in a set time (1-2mins) or to exhaustion and re-assess your progress every 4-8 weeks.

TYPE	Modified push up			Standard push up		
Number of push ups						

Core Tests - These tests determine the strength of your abdominal muscles and the muscles around your lumbar spine. Since core muscles should be activated and used in almost every activity you do, doing well on theses specific core tests will prove that you are more than capable on the other tests (explained in more detail in the Core training chapter)

1RM TESTING - Measuring your strength by performing specific exercises such as bench press, dead lift, squats and shoulder press, should be assessed by using the 1RM method of testing, which is the one most widely used to track your progress or gains in strength. 1RM stands for one repetition maximum, and is the maximum amount of weight that you can lift only once with perfect form. 1RM can be tested using any exercise but needs to be determined before you start an exercise program, when switching an exercise program, and/or when testing for results. Finding your 1RM for the bench press

- Warm-up for 5mins and complete a warm up set using a lighter weights;
- Choose a weight that you can lift approx. 6-12 times using perfect form.

You decide to lift a 30Ib DB (30 pound dumbbell) and find you can only lift it for a total of 7 reps i.e. until your muscles are completely fatigued.

%1RM	100	95	90	88	86	83	80	78	76	75	72	70
REPS	1	2	3	4	5	6	*7	8	9	10	11	12

*You can see that your ability to lift a weight 7 times until muscle fatigue is equal to 80% of your 1RM. Use a calculator to divide the weight you lifted by the percentage, and this gives you your 1RM for any exercise.

Weight you lifted	Repetitions you performed	% of your 1RM	Your 1RM (30Ib divided by .80%)
30Ib	7	80%	37.5Ib = your 1RM

Now record your results in the blank box above and then in your fitness journal and repeat every 3-4 weeks.

If you are a beginner stick with the basic 3 sets of 12 reps for each muscle group, which is 70% of your 1RM, but remember your muscles should be fatigued on the final rep. Lets just say that you know that your 1RM is 150Ibs for a specific exercise and you are following a workout program and it states 3x8 @ 75% i.e. 3 sets of 8 reps using 75% of your 1RM. Using the tables below and overleaf look over to the left hand column that is labelled 100% and scroll down to 150 pounds, glance over until it lines up with 75% and you'll see that you should be using 112 lbs for each set.....EASY!

100%	95%	92.5%	90%	87.5%	85%	82.5%	80%	77.5%	75%
1RM	2RM	3RM	4RM	5RM	6RM	7RM	8RM	9RM	10RM
155Ibs	147	143	139	135	131	127	124	120	116
150Ibs	142	138	135	131	127	123	120	116	112
145Ibs	137	134	130	126	123	119	116	112	108
140Ibs	133	129	126	122	119	115	112	108	105
135Ibs	128	124	121	118	114	111	108	104	101
130Ibs	123	120	117	113	110	107	104	100	97
125Ibs	118	115	112	19	106	103	100	96	93
120Ibs	114	111	108	105	102	99	96	93	90
115Ibs	109	106	103	100	97	94	92	89	86
110Ibs	104	101	99	96	93	90	88	85	82
105Ibs	99	97	94	91	89	86	84	81	78
100Ibs	95	92	90	87	85	82	80	77	75

72.5%	70%	67.5%	65%	62.5%	60%	57.5%	55%	52.5%	50%
11RM	12RM	13RM	14RM	15RM	16RM	17RM	18RM	19RM	20RM
112Ibs	108	104	100	96	93	89	85	81	77
108Ibs	105	101	97	93	90	86	82	78	75
105Ibs	101	97	94	90	87	83	79	76	72
101Ibs	98	94	91	87	84	80	77	73	70
97 Ibs	94	91	87	84	81	77	74	70	67
94 Ibs	91	87	84	81	78	74	71	68	65
90 Ibs	87	84	81	78	75	71	68	65	62
87 Ibs	84	81	78	75	72	69	66	63	60
83 Ibs	80	77	74	71	69	66	63	60	57
79 Ibs	77	74	71	68	66	63	60	57	55
76 Ibs	73	70	68	65	63	60	57	55	52
72 Ibs	70	67	65	62	60	57	55	52	50

Training Intensity - Training intensity serves as the major stimulus for muscle growth in your strength training routine, and by increasing your training intensity you are providing your body with a bigger stimulus for muscle growth. You can increase the intensity by increasing any of the following: the amount of weight, sets or repetitions, and/or the number of exercises. You will also increase the intensity by reducing the amount of rest intervals you have in between your sets. The exact combination you choose will depend on your training goals i.e. whether you want to improve your strength, power, size or your muscular endurance. Each of these are explained below in more detail, giving you specific guidelines for the number of sets, reps, weight, and rest intervals for your training program. Whether the program you design is specific for gaining strength, power, muscle size or muscular endurance, they each require a different way of training, as shown overleaf.

GUIDELINES FOR YOUR DIFFERENT TRAINING GOALS					
Training Goal	Number of sets/exercise	Number of reps	Weight (% 1RM)	Rest interval	*Training tempo
Max strength	2-6	Below 6	Above 85	2-5min	1:2
Power	3-5	1-8	70-85	2-5min	Explosive
Muscle size	3-6	6-12	67-85	30-90s	2:3
Muscular endurance	2-3	Above 12	Low Below 67	Below 30s	2:3

*The training tempo is best described as the number of counts for each concentric action i.e. lifting action, followed by the number of counts for the eccentric action i.e. lowering action. For example 2:3 = 2 counts concentric, 3 counts eccentric.

MAXIMUM STRENGTH TRAINING

Maximum strength is best developed using heavy weights and low repetition sets. Most maximum strength workouts are designed around the compound exercises such as squats, bench presses and shoulder presses. The consensus guideline is to perform 2-6 sets of 6 or fewer repetitions for the compound exercises. Only 1-3 sets are necessary for isolation exercises. Clearly you should select a weight that causes you to use maximum effort for that set - that is, reach the point of failure on the last repetition (between 85-100% 1RM). Your rest intervals between sets should be 3-4 minutes to allow sufficient recovery.

POWER TRAINING

Power training is simply defined as performing an exercise very quickly or explosively, and it can be developed by using any of the following:

TYPES	EXAMPLES
Plyometrics	Jumps and bounding exercises
Speed drills	40m sprints and shuttle runs
Strength training exercises	Cleans or any compound exercises

Power exercises are more suitable for those intermediate and advanced individuals who use power movements in their particular sport, as listed overleaf:

AIM	REPS	INTENSITY	POWER SPORTS	
To develop fast powerful movements	6-10	Medium to heavy loading (70-80% of max effort - 1RM)	Basketball, Football & sprinting	Most field athletic events (jumping and throwing events etc)

Technique and good form is essential for all individuals who perform power exercises, especially if you are a beginner, this is because total control of the weight must be adhered to throughout the whole movement, even when it is moved rapidly. The greatest power output is your main aim, and by using slightly lighter weights than maximal i.e. 70-85% 1RM allows you to perform the exercise with maximum speed, therefore almost doubling your output.

Power ratios

In the past, power ratios used to be anything up to 50%, the ratios are now between 50-70% and even higher on the percentage of 1RM. The only individuals that should really train at the upper weights are power/strength lifters and explosive/strength sports players i.e. American football players in the front line and forwards in rugby to mention only a few sports. The majority of the sporting world that repeat a movement more than twenty times throughout a game or bout should probably be performing lighter power weights, and maybe even Power Endurance i.e.

Training Goal	Number of sets/exercise	Number of reps	Weight (% 1RM)
Power Endurance	3 sets of Approx. 4-5 exercises per session	Up to 30reps	20-50% of 1RM

The intensity would be continued until speed or form starts to alter, and once 30reps is achieved with the same speed throughout each repetition, the weight should be increased.

MUSCLE SIZE TRAINING (hypertrophy)
Training for muscle size (hypertrophy) requires a higher training volume compared with pure strength and power training. With this type of program parallel increases should be expected in both muscle size and strength. Compound exercises should be performed i.e. squats, bench press, shoulder press, lat pull downs etc. Stimulating your larger muscle groups will assist in overall size development. In order to train with higher intensity split training systems should be used, especially for the more advanced individuals, who should perform 2-4 exercises per muscle group, incorporating 1-2 compound exercises.

MUSCULAR ENDURANCE TRAINING
Muscular endurance training is simply defined as the ability of a muscle or muscle group to sustain sub-maximal force over a period of time. Muscular endurance type training increases the aerobic capacity of your muscles rather than muscle size and strength. This type of training is developed by using lighter weights, a higher number of reps, and fewer sets per muscle group i.e.12 or more reps per set and 2 or 3 sets with minimal rest intervals between sets (approx. 30secs). Most circuit type weight training programs also promote your muscular endurance. The intensity of muscular endurance type training is very low with the overall volume being high. It is suitable for beginners and also for advanced trainers who want to improve this aspect of their fitness.

FUNCTIONAL RESISTANCE TRAINING

In this particular chapter it will be explained to you the different types of functional resistance training methods. Included are effective tools for building strength and muscle tone designed to work your target muscles in isolation and collectively, with or without the assistance of the surrounding muscles. Free weights and machines that provide the same equal resistance to a muscle allow you to target a particular muscle group and to engage other muscles that assist in the work. Once these assisting muscles are conditioned, they will help you to increase the weight you use in training the target muscles in order to stimulate the most growth in your muscle fibres. Your assisting muscles help to stabilise your body, support your limbs and help to maintain your posture during a lift, especially when lifting a set resistance i.e. whilst using free weights, as this may assist you with improving your coordination. You now have access to 100's of the most common exercises for all your major muscle groups.

BODYWEIGHT EXERCISES

Choosing the best exercise to achieve your specific needs can be difficult because everyone has various fitness levels and abilities when they begin a new program. Bodyweight exercises are an effective type of training because with each movement you tend to work multiple muscle groups, therefore making your body work hard which in turn increases your metabolism. Performing bodyweight exercises involves simple sequences of movements that not only strengthens and tones your body but also improves your endurance and stamina. Bodyweight exercises are generally faster to perform and more enjoyable than endless cardio workouts and better for your muscles and joints than heavy weight lifting sessions especially if you are a beginner to strength training. More importantly, bodyweight exercises are achievable by most people and they make a significant difference to your health and fitness. Most bodyweight exercise workouts can be completed in a shorter period of time and can quite literally be done anywhere. This type of training system can be performed 2-3 times per week for a period of 6 weeks, and you will see results so long as you progress the repetitions and sets accordingly. Your warm up should be intense enough for what you have planned and you should stretch according to your exercise choice. You should always write down your plan and specific routine within your journal, even down to your mood in a separate remarks column. Your introduction to bodyweight exercises should of course include achievable exercises until you are ready to progress to a more advanced selection. Correct technique of each exercise should be your most important aim in this phase in order to achieve perfect form. No gym membership, fitness equipment, or any monetary investment is required at all and may just be the answer you are looking for. Discover within this book, a series of bodyweight exercises that you can do on your own to condition and strengthen your body on your own, and for free. Workout templates specific to bodyweight exercises can be found at the rear of the book.

FIT-BALL EXERCISES
Detailed information can be found in the Core Training chapter.

RESISTANCE BANDS EXERCISES
Resistance bands are an extremely inexpensive way to get a whole body workout and can be used absolutely anywhere, they can be great for a Pilates routine or specific resistance workouts. You can avoid spending lots of money going to the gym as resistance bands alone can provide you with a complete upper and lower body workout, and they come in variable strengths for easy to advanced workouts. They can also be used one at a time or combined to add more resistance. Resistance bands and corresponding ankle straps can mount to your interior door or anywhere that is deemed secure, for safety reasons. They can also be used for rehabilitation purposes (as explained in the corresponding rehabilitation chapter) Workout templates specific to resistance band exercises can be found at the rear of the book.

FITNESS MACHINE EXERCISES
Unless you have a large area at home and money to spend on your own equipment, it is generally going to be easier to get a more complete workout at the gym. Apart from having a wider variety of equipment, you will also have continuous access to professional advice. Gym instructors & personal trainers can properly instruct you in the use of the available equipment. For many reasons it is the preferred option of many people to exercise at home instead of going to the gym.

The main reason allows people to get a very good physical workout at home, and some of the other reasons include the following:

1. The home gym option can be tailored to your specific fitness needs;
2. More privacy;
3. Over time, the home gym equipment will cost less than a gym membership;
4. Not having to exercise in front of strangers, fewer excuses allowed;
5. The timings are more of your choosing, with no travel time involved.

Almost 90 % of people who sign up for gym membership seldom use the membership to its full potential. Exercising in your home gym can assist with the lack of enthusiasm of going to the gym and you will be more likely to stick to your routine. With your home gym, you're already there in the zone, and whatever your reason for exercising i.e. you're trying to lose weight, gain muscle, maintain your health, or even to look good on holiday, it is a great feeling to be able to workout when it suits you.

These days, treadmills and other fitness equipment are generally more portable, and once it is paid for then there are no additional payments. The reality is that you will save money in the long run by purchasing your own home gym machines and you will save valuable time too. When the equipment is right in front of you then that becomes your motivation. If you have the space you can find adequate weight machines, free weights, aerobic equipment and much, much more to suit your needs and alot of them foldaway too. Workout templates specific to fitness equipment exercises can be found at the rear of the book.

BARBELL

By definition, a long bar you load plates onto. Most gyms have Olympic bars which weigh 45Ibs and feature rotating cylinders on each end. Barbells are used to lift very heavy weights on exercises that allow for it, such as the squat, dead-lift, bench press and shoulder press etc. Strength training with one barbell is better, especially if your local gym has no squat rack or bench, or only has smith machines. If you decide to workout at home and are low on budget or you lack the space, purchasing a barbell & a combination of weighted plates is a good option. Lifting heavy weights using specific exercises has its disadvantages such as:

1. **Squats** - without a power rack, you may have the problem of getting the bar on your back, front shoulders or overhead; depending on the squat variation.

However, you can often find a solution to overcome these problems i.e.

- Back Squat - Get the weight on your back using the Steinborn Lift, back squats allow you to lift the heaviest weights;
- Front Squat - power clean the weight onto your shoulders & squat, front squats are the best replacement for back squats;
- Overhead Squat - Snatch or clean & press the weight overhead, overhead squats are a full body exercise, which get you strong abs & healthy shoulders.

2. **Overhead Press** - Most power racks are not big enough to Overhead press inside them, especially if they don't have external safety pins. A solution for this would be to Power clean the weight onto your shoulders & press from there.

Lifting heavy weights using a barbell also has its advantages for e.g.

Dead-lift & Barbell Rows - Dead-lifts allow you to stress your body with heavy weights, and you don't need a power rack for Dead-lifts or Bent-over bar-bell rows. Barbell rows also work your back hard in absence of Pull ups.

Floor Press - If you don't have a Power rack of bench, the Floor press is a great alternative to the Bench press. The floor press speaks for itself, but works your triceps more, even though you are only doing the top part of the movement. If you are a beginner, a barbell will help you build muscle & strength, and once you get more experienced, space and/or money then you should endeavour to purchase a power rack. Workout templates specific to barbell exercises can be found at the rear of the book.

DUMBBELLS

By definition, the smaller, handheld weight bars. Dumbbells activate more of your core musculature than barbell training and they prevent your stronger side from doing the majority of the work. Dumbbells are preferable to machine weights because they allow you to focus on the correct form that is required for maximum results, and they provide you with excellent variety for your training programs. If you plan to workout at home and your budget is low then it is a good idea is to purchase 2 sets of dumbbells, i.e. Use the heavier set for exercises in which you can manage more weight like squats and lunges, and one set for exercises that work best with comparatively lighter weights like raises, rows, curls and similar joint taxing exercises. With dumbbells your weight selection is very important, and your approach is important in order to get the exercise technique and good form sorted prior to getting stronger and fitter. If you can afford them and you have the space, then you can buy a full rack of dumbbells or if your space is limited, then a set of adjustable dumbbells like Bowflex, Stamina and Bayou etc each have their own advantages. Another sound purchase is a bench with an adjustable back rest, and if you have this then you can perform all sorts of exercises like presses, rows, raises, curls and extensions etc, not forgetting all the bodyweight exercises you can perform using a bench such as dips and crunches etc. Workout templates specific to dumbbell exercises can be found at the rear of the book.

MOST COMMON BACK EXERCISES

USING YOUR OWN BODYWEIGHT

Seated back extension

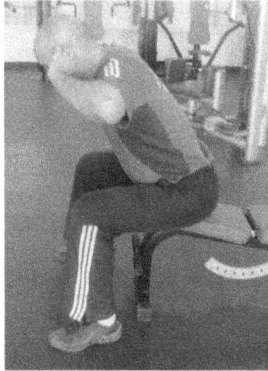

From the seated position ensure that your feet are flat on the floor and that your hips, shoulders, head and eyes are inline. Lean forwards under the control of your abdominals whilst breathing in, under control move your upper body backwards contracting the lower back muscles whilst breathing out. Repeat the movement in a controlled manner.

Standing back extension

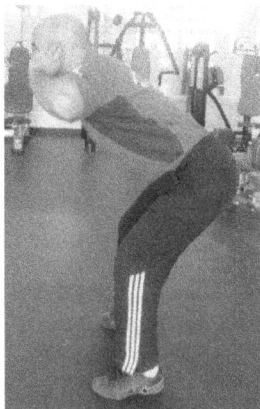

From the standing position ensure that your feet are shoulder width apart and flat on the floor and that your hips, shoulders, head and eyes are inline. Lean forwards under the control of your abdominals whilst breathing in, under control move your upper body backwards contracting the lower back muscles whilst breathing out. Repeat the movement in a controlled manner.

Alternate arm & leg raise 1

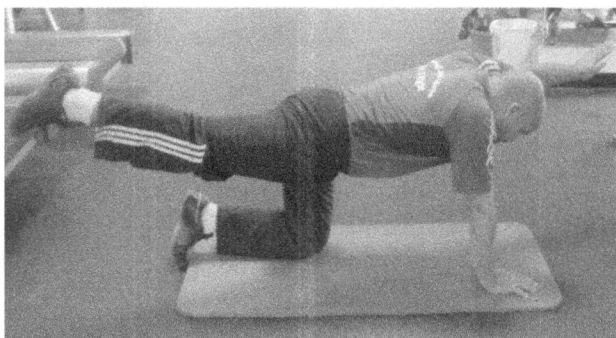

From the kneeling position ensure that your hands are level with your shoulders and your knees and hands are in line. Your shoulders should be relaxed and your hips and shoulders should remain facing towards the ground along with your head and eyes. Initiate the movement from the abdominals and raise one arm and the opposite leg simultaneously whilst looking forwards as you breathe out. Hold the position as if you are balancing something on your back and slowly return to the start position whilst breathing in. Repeat the movement with the opposite arm and leg in a controlled manner. If this is too difficult you can begin by moving one arm or one leg only and then progress accordingly. Maintaining control throughout the movement is key whilst breathing correctly.

Alternate arm & leg raise 2

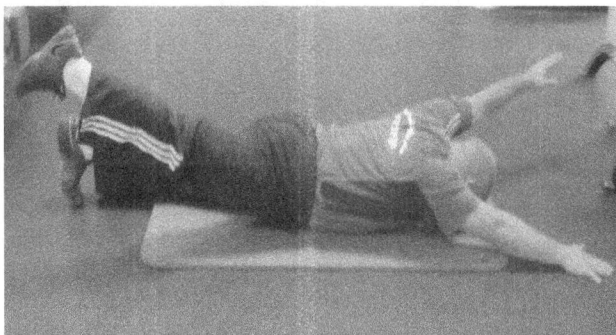

From the lying position ensure that your shoulders are relaxed and your hips and shoulders remain facing towards the ground along with your head and eyes. Initiate the movement from the abdominals and raise one arm and the opposite leg simultaneously whilst looking forwards as you breathe out. Hold the position as if you are balancing something on your back and slowly return to the start position whilst breathing in. Repeat the movement with the opposite arm and leg in a controlled manner. If this is too difficult you can begin by moving one arm or one leg only, then both arms only and then both legs only. You can then progress accordingly as explained above. Maintaining control throughout the movement is the key whilst breathing correctly.

Straight leg hold

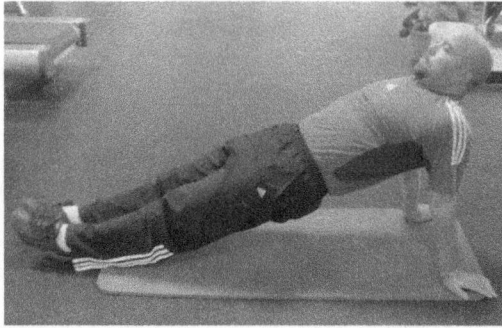

Start off by sitting on the floor with your legs outstretched, place your hands level with your shoulders and ensure and that your hips, shoulders, head and eyes are inline. Ensuring that your hands are flat on the floor, support your bodyweight as you raise your hips off the ground whilst breathing out. Hold the position as you contract both your abdominals and lower back, return to the start position under control whilst breathing in. Repeat the movement accordingly

Plank progressions

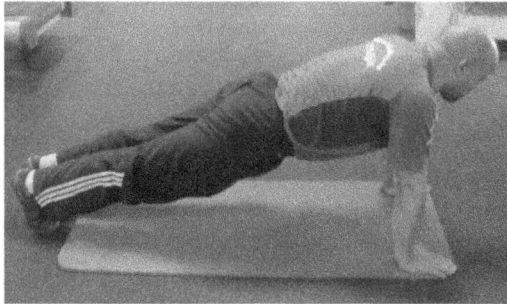

From the kneeling position ensure that your hands are level with your shoulders and your knees and hands are in line. Your shoulders should be relaxed and your hips and shoulders should remain facing towards the ground along with your head and eyes. Initiate the movement from the abdominals and move your legs to the rear whilst looking forwards as you breathe out. Hold the position as if you are balancing something on your back and breathe in and out in a controlled manner. Hold the position for as long as possible but you should aim to work towards 2 minutes. As you tire concentrate on your breathing whilst compressing your abdominals and lower back, tense your whole body (not shoulders) to assist you in keeping good form. If you need to rest, slowly return to the start position and repeat the movement in a controlled manner. If this is too difficult you can begin by placing your hands on a raised (secure) platform and do the same as above. You can make it more difficult by doing the same movement but on your forearms ensuring your elbows are level with your shoulders and also progress by placing your legs on a raised (secure) platform. Maintaining control throughout the movement is important whilst breathing correctly.

100

Hip raises

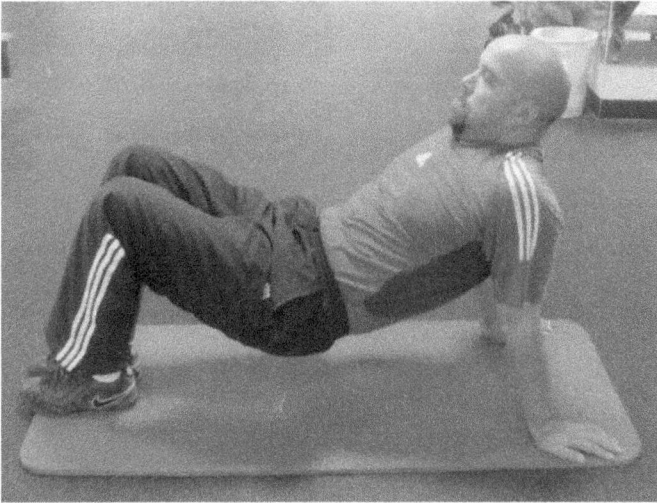

Start off by sitting on the floor with your knees bent and feet flat on the floor, place your hands level with your shoulders and ensure your hips and shoulders are facing forwards along with your head and eyes. Ensuring that your hands are flat on the floor, support your bodyweight as you raise your hips off the ground whilst breathing out. Hold the position as you contract your abdominals lower back and Glutes. Return to the start position under control whilst breathing in, repeat the movement accordingly.

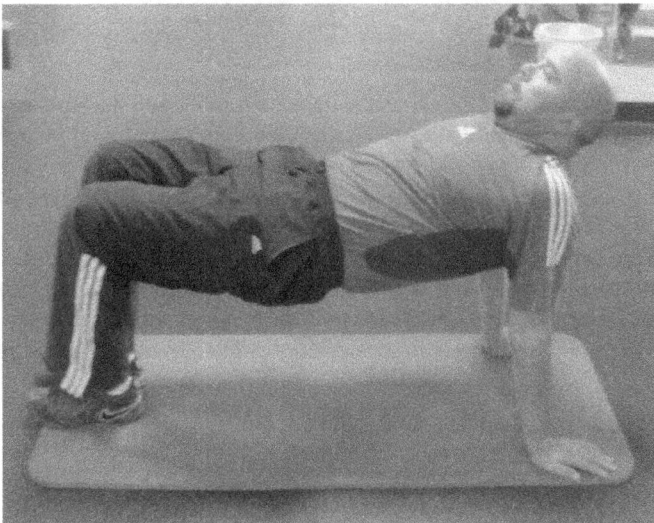

BACK EXERCISES USING RESISTANCE BANDS

Single arm row

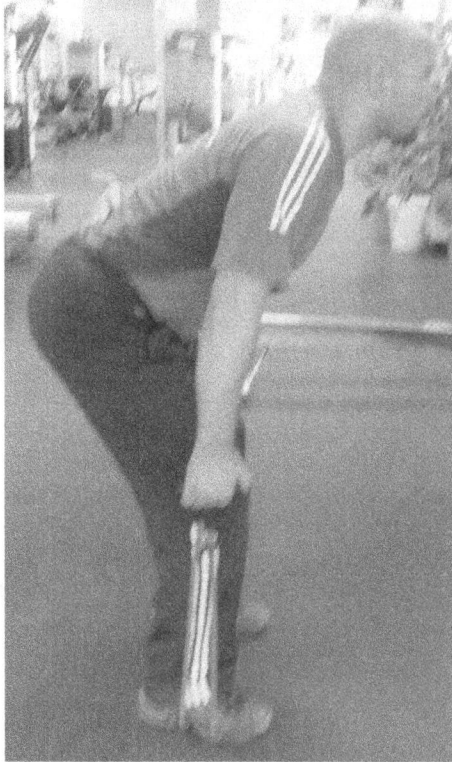

Firstly, choose a band that is the correct resistance for you and during the initial stages this will be a light weight until you master the technique. Stand with your feet flat on the floor and around shoulder width apart, stand on the band until there is enough tension for your back muscles to resist. Your hips, shoulders, head and eyes should be in line with a slight bend at the waist and knees. Start off with your arm straight whilst holding onto the band and pull it towards your waist whilst breathing out ensuring your elbow is close to the side of your body. Attempt to initiate the movement via your abdominals but use your back muscles to pull the band up with as little assistance from the biceps as possible. Return to the start position whilst breathing in and repeat accordingly.

Bent over row

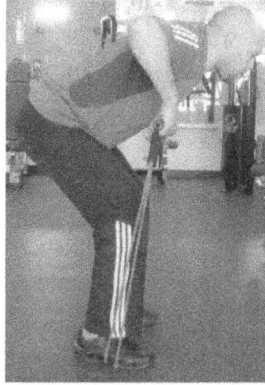

Firstly, choose a band that is the correct resistance for you and during the initial stages this will be a light weight until you master the technique. Stand with your feet flat on the floor and around shoulder width apart, stand on the band until there is enough tension for your back muscles to resist. Your hips, shoulders, head and eyes should be inline, with a slight bend at the waist and knees. Start off with your arms straight whilst holding onto the band and pull it towards your waist whilst breathing out ensuring your elbows are close to the side of your body. Attempt to initiate the movement via your abdominals but use your back muscles to pull the band up with as little assistance from the biceps as possible. Return to the start position whilst breathing in and repeat accordingly.

Seated row

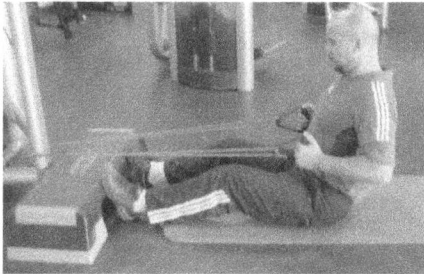

Firstly, choose a band that is the correct resistance for you and during the initial stages this will be a light weight until you master the technique. The band should be securely fitted around a solid object around waist height (whilst sitting). Sit with your legs outstretched on the floor and up against an object to ensure that there is a slight bend at your knees. The band should have enough tension for your back muscles to resist. Your hips, shoulders, head and eyes should be inline and you should start off leaning slightly forwards with your arms straight whilst holding onto the band and pull it towards your waist whilst breathing out ensuring your elbows are close to the side of your body. Attempt to initiate the movement via your abdominals but use your back muscles to pull the band towards you with as little assistance from the biceps as possible. Return to the start position whilst breathing in and repeat accordingly.

103

Lat pull down

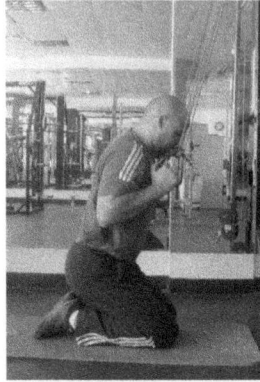

Firstly, choose a band that is the correct resistance for you and during the initial stages this will be a light weight until you master the technique. The band should be securely fitted around a solid object above head height. Kneel down on the floor and make sure the band has enough tension for your back muscles to resist. Your hips, shoulders, head and eyes should be inline and you should start off with the band above and in front of you. Your arms should start off straight whilst holding onto the band and then pull it towards your waist whilst breathing out ensuring your elbows are close to the side of your body. Attempt to initiate the movement via your abdominals but use your back muscles to pull the band towards you with as little assistance from the biceps as possible. Return to the start position whilst breathing in and repeat accordingly.

Reverse flyes

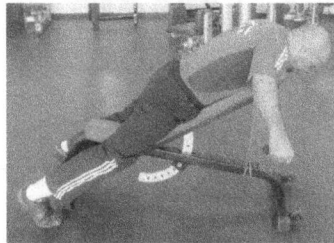

Firstly, choose a band that is the correct resistance for you and during the initial stages this will be a light weight until you master the technique. The band should be securely fitted around a solid object below you around chest height. Lean onto an inclined bench and make sure the band has enough tension for your back muscles to resist. Your hips, shoulders, head and eyes should be inline, and you should start off with your arms almost straight and towards the ground. Pull the band towards you whilst breathing out ensuring your elbows are slightly bent. Attempt to initiate the movement via your abdominals but use your upper back muscles to pull the band towards you as if you are bringing your shoulder blades together. There should be as little assistance from the shoulders as possible (no tension). Return to the start position whilst breathing in and repeat accordingly. This exercise can also be done standing

BACK EXERCISES USING A FIT-BALL

Single leg raise

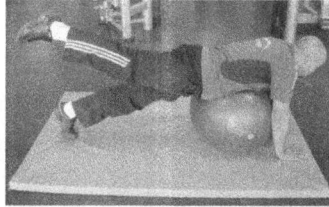

Lie on top of the ball with it positioned around the area of your chest; place your hands on the floor shoulder width apart. Extend your hip above waist height, ensuring at all times that you contract your abdominals whilst breathing out and keep your shoulders as relaxed as possible. Lower your leg to the start position whilst breathing in and repeat, change arms and legs accordingly. This exercise works your glutes in addition to your lower back muscles.

To increase the intensity:

- Do not rest the leg between repetitions;
- Use the same leg until fatigued;
- Hold the leg raised for 2-3 seconds;
- Insert a hold midway.

Alternate arm & leg raise

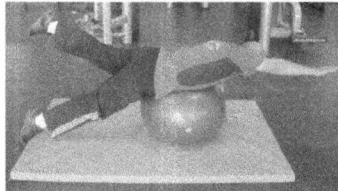

Lie on top of the ball with it positioned around the area of your chest; place your hands on the floor shoulder width apart. Extend one of your legs and the opposite arm above waist height, ensuring at all times that you contract your abdominals whilst breathing out and keep your shoulders as relaxed as possible. Lower your leg and arm to the start position whilst breathing in and repeat. Change arms and legs accordingly. This exercise works your glutes and rear deltoid in addition to your lower back   muscles.
To increase the intensity:

- Do not rest the leg and arm between repetitions;
- Use the same leg until fatigued;
- Hold the leg and arm raised for 2-3 seconds;
- Insert a hold midway.

Ball Pull with knees bent

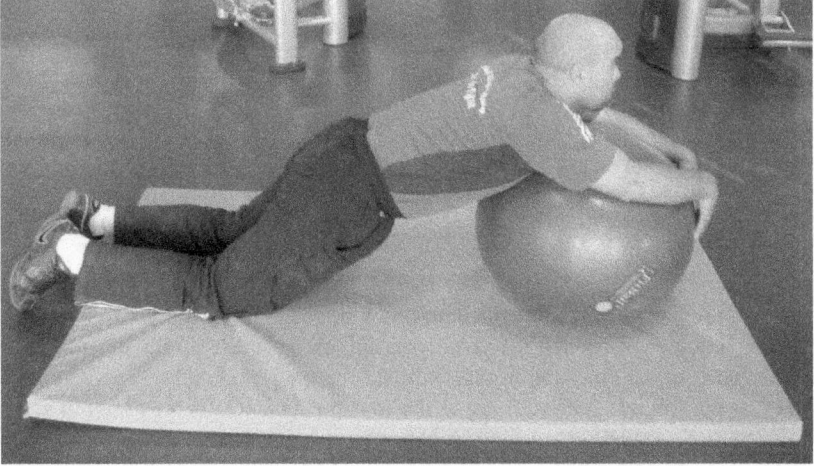

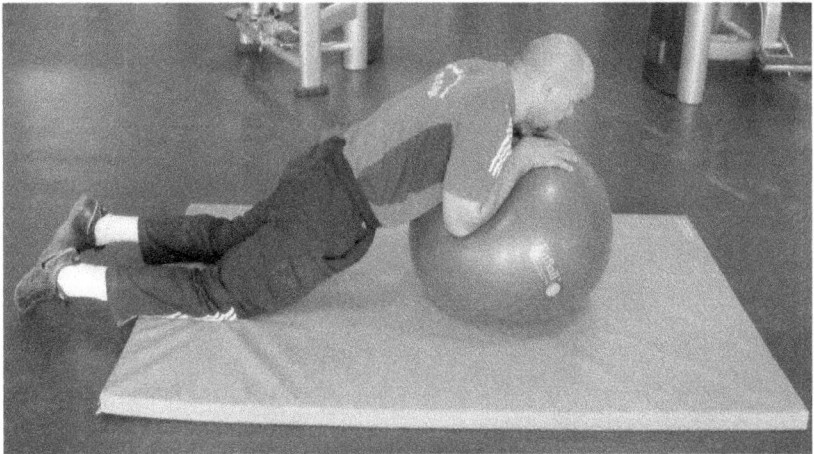

With your knees bent, lean onto the ball with your arms outstretched around it, Ensuring at all times that you contract your abdominals whilst breathing out and keep your shoulders as relaxed as possible. The emphasis should be on pulling the ball towards the body and holding for 2-3 seconds, push the ball back to the start position whilst breathing in and repeat.

Ball Pull with straight legs

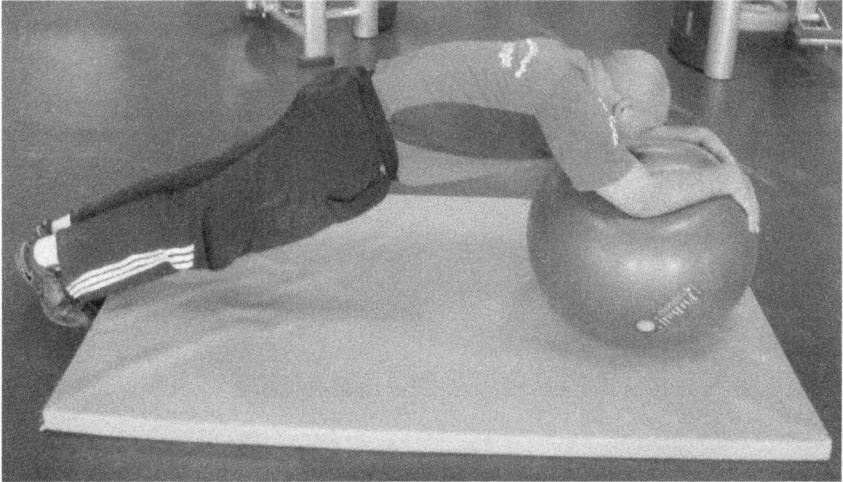

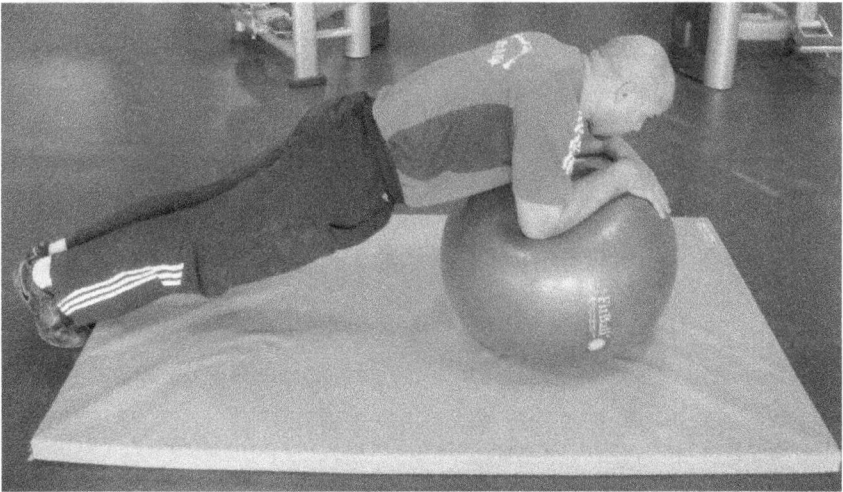

With your legs straight, lean onto the ball with your arms outstretched around it, Ensuring at all times that you contract your abdominals whilst breathing out and keep your shoulders as relaxed as possible. The emphasis should be on pulling the ball towards the body and holding for 2-3 seconds, push the ball back to the start position whilst breathing in and repeat.

Resistance band reverse flyes

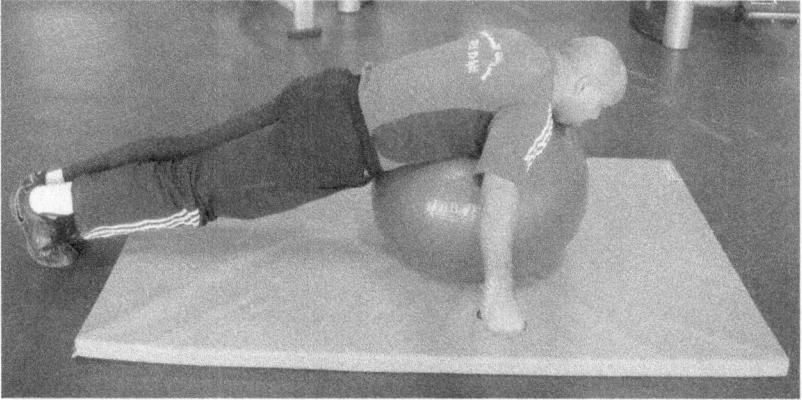

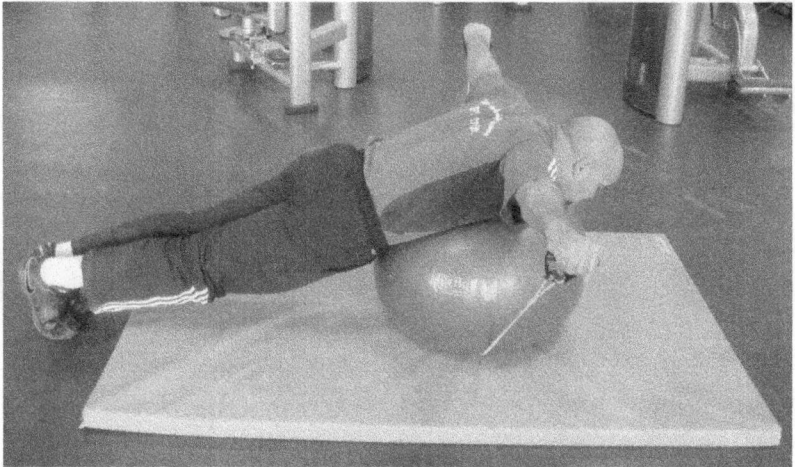

Making sure that the resistance band is not too heavy and positioned securely under-neath the centre of the fit-ball. Lie on top of the ball with it positioned around the area of your chest and grasp the band ensuring it is taught enough and that your arms are outstretched to the side with a slight bend at the elbow. Concentrate on bringing your shoulder blades together whilst breathing out and raising your arms above shoulder height. Ensure at all times that you contract your abdominals whilst breathing out and keep your shoulders as relaxed as possible. Lower the band back to the start position whilst breathing in and repeat.

Dumbbell reverse flyes

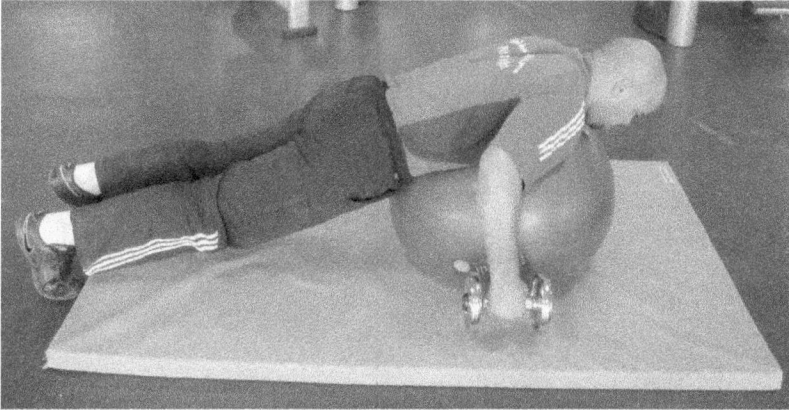

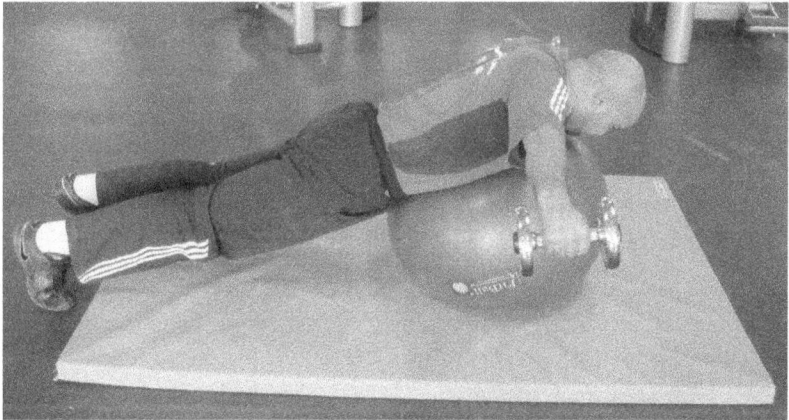

Making sure that the weights are not too heavy and they are positioned close to the centre of the fit-ball. Lie on top of the ball with it positioned around the area of your chest and grasp the dumbbells ensuring that your grip is tight enough and that your arms are outstretched to the side with a slight bend at the elbow. Concentrate on bringing your shoulder blades together whilst breathing out and raising your arms above shoulder height. Ensure at all times that you contract your abdominals whilst breathing out and keep your shoulders as relaxed as possible. Lower the weights back to the start position whilst breathing in and repeat.

Single arm Dumbbell row

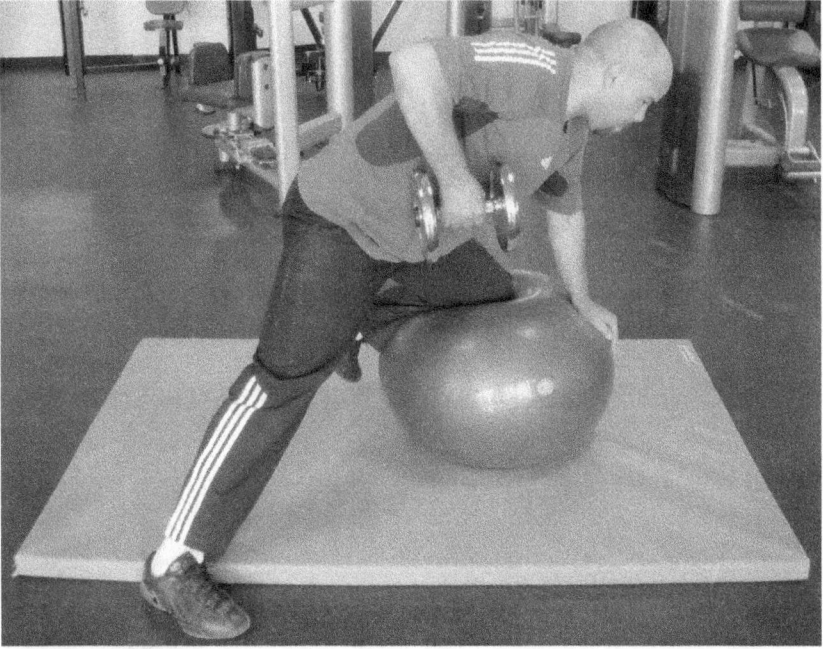

Making sure that the weight is not too heavy and that it is positioned close to the centre of the fit-ball. Kneel on top of the centre of the ball and grasp the dumbbell ensuring that your grip is tight enough and that your arm is straight. Concentrate on using your back muscles only whilst breathing out and bending your arm until the weight is close to the side of your body. Ensure at all times that you contract your abdominals whilst breathing out and keep your shoulders as relaxed as possible. Lower the weight under control whilst breathing in and repeat accordingly, change arms.

BACK EXERCISES USING FITNESS MACHINES

Lat pull down (wide arm)

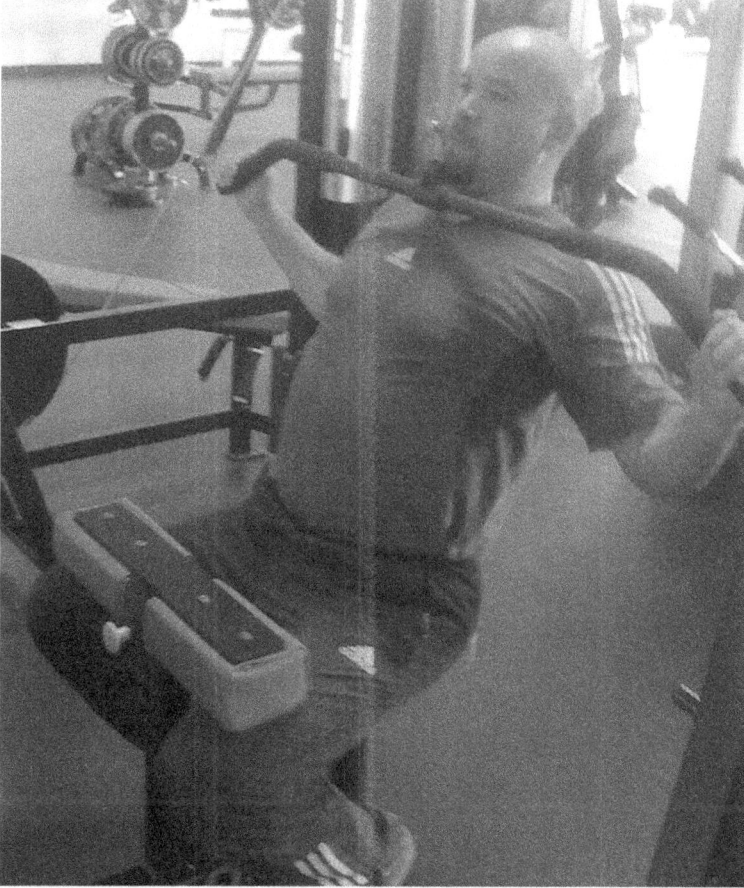

First of all, always select a safe weight that is achievable and this will generally be a lighter one until you have mastered the technique. Sit on the seat provided and ensure that the support is adjusted so that your upper thighs are secure. Your grip can vary from wide (as shown) or narrow grip, to under-grasp or over-grasp (as shown) and you can pull the bar down towards the chest (as shown) or behind the neck. You should initiate the movement by the abdominals and as you pull the bar down you should breathe out. Return to the start position whilst breathing in and repeat accordingly.

Standing pull downs 1

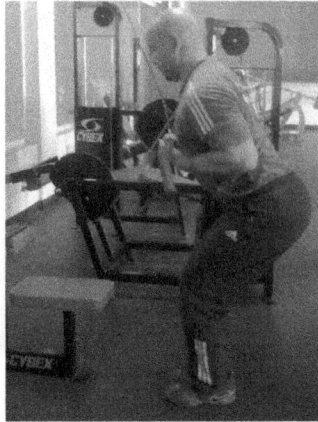

First of all, always select a safe weight that is achievable and this will generally be a lighter one until you have mastered the technique. Stand with your feet flat on the floor and knees bent. Your grip should be narrow and in an under-grasp position, pull the bar down towards your chest keeping your elbows close to the side of your body. You should attempt to isolate the back and allow minimum assistance from the biceps. You should initiate the movement by the abdominals and as you pull the bar down you should breathe out. Return to the start position whilst breathing in and repeat accordingly.

Standing pull downs 2

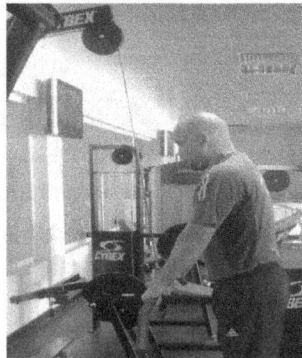

First of all, always select a safe weight that is achievable and this will generally be a lighter one until you have mastered the technique. Stand with your feet flat on the floor and knees bent. Your grip should be narrow and in an over-grasp position, pull the bar down towards your hips keeping your arms straight at all times. You should attempt to isolate the back and relax the shoulders at all times. You should initiate the movement by the abdominals and as you pull the bar down you should breathe out. Return to the start position whilst breathing in and repeat accordingly.

112

Pull ups (assisted)

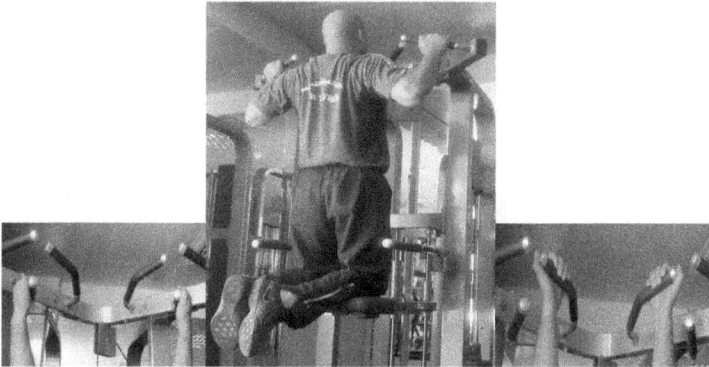

Select a weight that you would like to assist you, i.e. if you weigh 70 kg then you should not select anything higher than that as you will not be achieving anything. The aim is to master the technique first (with assistance) but to gain enough strength to be assisted as little as possible. Most people should be able (in time) to pull themselves up without assistance at all i.e. without this machine. You should start with your arms completely straight and as you breathe out raise up until your chin is level with your hands and breathe in as you lower down under control and repeat accordingly. Different grips can be used (as shown below)

Standing row

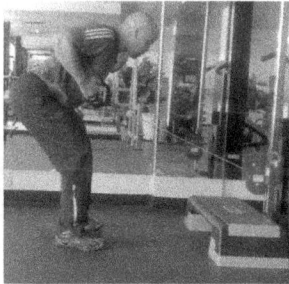

First of all, always select a safe weight that is achievable and this will generally be a lighter one until you have mastered the technique. Stand with your feet flat on the floor and knees bent, you should maintain good posture throughout the movement. You can use a bar or a rope for this exercise but cables are preferred and you should pull them towards your chest keeping your elbows close to the side of your body. You should attempt to isolate the back and allow minimum assistance from the biceps. You should initiate the movement by the abdominals and as you pull the cables you should breathe out. When you release the weight you should breathe in and straighten your arms. Repeat accordingly. This exercise can also be completed in the seated position using something like the step in the picture so that the legs start off in a bent position. The principles are exactly the same.

Seated row

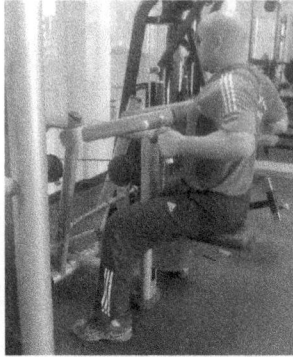

First of all, always select a safe weight that is achievable and this will generally be a lighter one until you have mastered the technique. Sit and adjust the pad in front of the chest so that you can grasp the bars with a slight bend at the elbow. You should maintain good posture throughout the movement as you pull the weight towards your chest keeping your elbows close to the side of your body. You should attempt to isolate the back by relaxing the shoulders and allow minimum assistance from the biceps. You should initiate the movement by the abdominals and as you pull the weight you should breathe out. When you release the weight you should breathe in and straighten your arms. Repeat accordingly.

Back extension

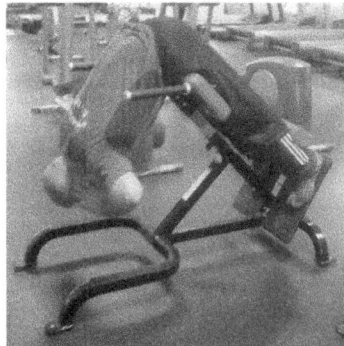

Adjust the equipment so that your feet are resting on the plates and your upper body can bend forwards comfortably. In the start position (as shown) it ensures that your hips and shoulders are facing downwards along with your head and eyes. Under control raise your upper body until it is level with your hips or slightly beyond if possible whilst contracting the lower back muscles and breathing out. Return to the start position under control whilst breathing in and repeat the movement in a controlled manner.

BACK EXERCISES USING A BARBELL

Back extension

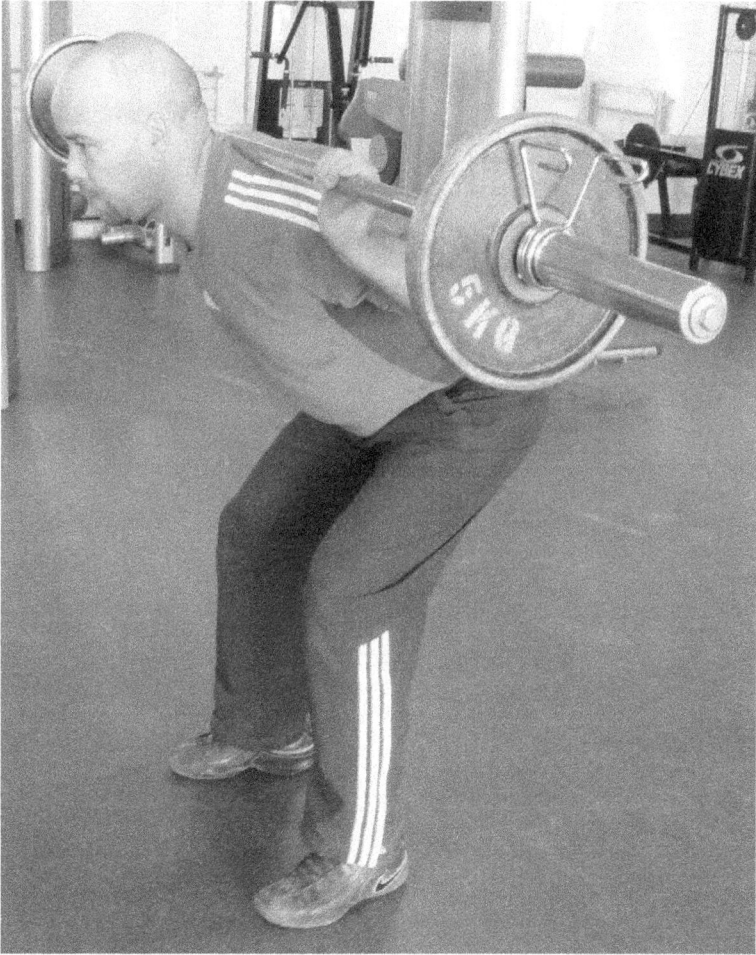

Select a weight that is low enough for you to master the technique first, place the bar on your shoulders and stand with your feet flat on the floor and wide enough to maintain good balance. Bend the knees and lean forward ensuring that your hips, shoulders, head and eyes are inline and facing forwards. Initiate the movement via the abdominals whilst using the lower back muscles to raise your body back to the upright position and beyond if possible, whilst breathing out. Breathe in as you return to the start position and repeat. All movements should be under control and safe!!

Dead lift

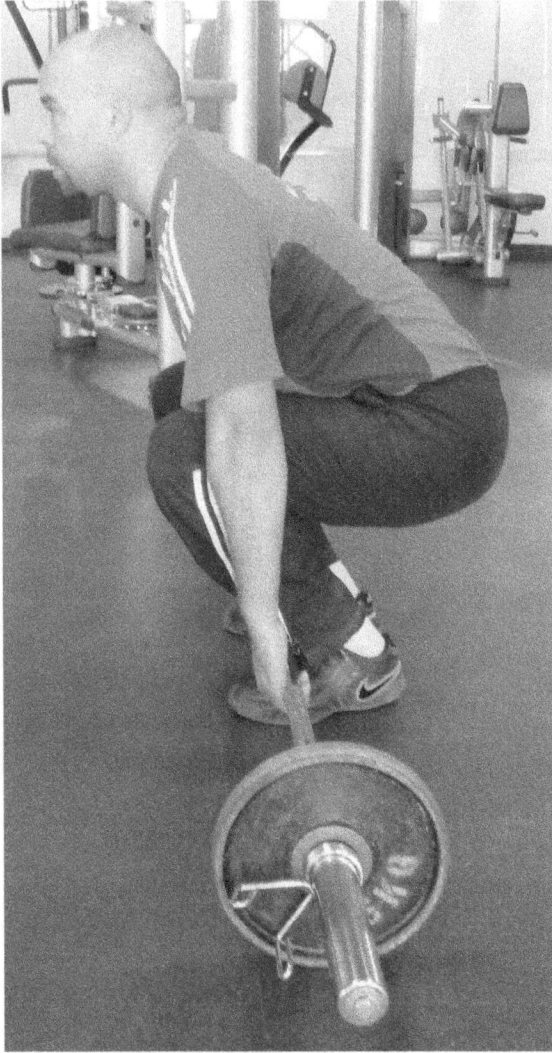

Select a weight that is low enough for you to master the technique first, stand with your feet flat on the floor and wide enough to maintain good balance. Bend the knees and lean forward and down to grasp the bar with a wide grip. Your arms should be straight ensuring that your hips, shoulders, head and eyes are inline and facing forwards. Initiate the movement via the abdominals whilst using the lower back muscles and legs to stand upright, whilst breathing out. Breathe in as you return to the start position and repeat. All movements should be under control and safe!!

Bar Pull with knees bent

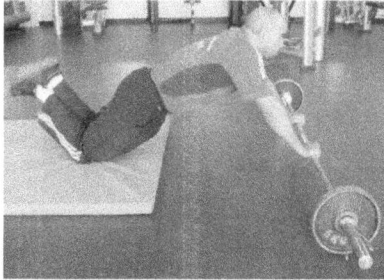

Select a weight that is low enough for you to master the technique first, kneel on the floor and lean onto the bar ensuring you have a good grip on the bar which should be in front of you. Your arms should be straight ensuring that your hips, shoulders, head and eyes are inline and facing forwards. Initiate the movement via the abdominals whilst using the lower back muscles and abdominals to pull the bar towards you, whilst breathing out. Breathe in as you return to the start position and repeat. The shoulders should be relaxed and offer no assistance to the exercise and you should endeavour to keep the lower body as still as you can. All movements should be under control and safe!! Of course a progression of this would be to have straight legs.

Bent over row 1

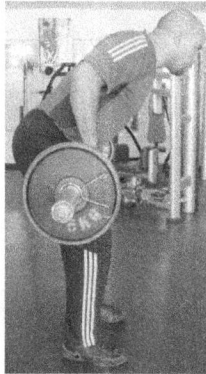

Select a weight that is low enough for you to master the technique first, stand with your feet flat on the floor and wide enough to maintain good balance. Bend the knees and lean forward and down to grasp the bar with a wide grip. Your arms should be straight ensuring that your hips, shoulders, head and eyes are inline and facing forwards. Initiate the movement via the abdominals whilst using the lower back muscles and straight arms to pull the bar away from the floor. Hold the start position using the strength of your abdominals and lower back. Pull the bar towards the body, whilst breathing out and ensure the elbows remain close to the side of the body. Breathe in as you return to the start position and repeat. All movements should be under control and safe!! You can vary the grip (over or under grasp)

117

Bent over row 2

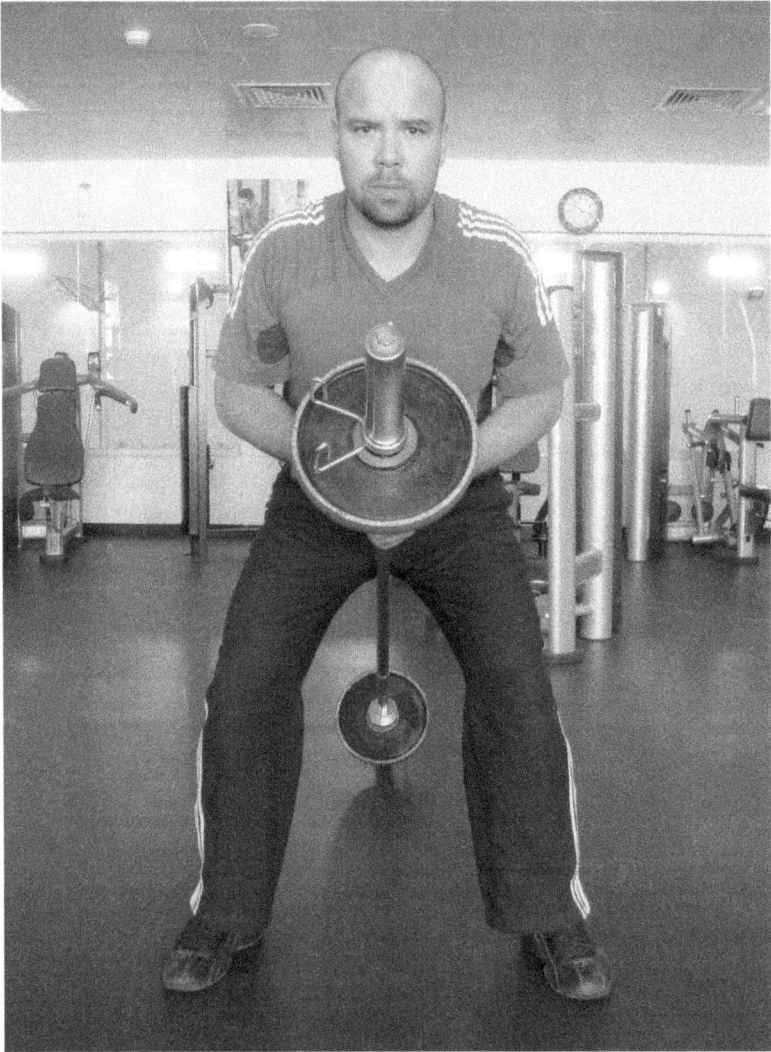

Select a weight that is low enough for you to master the technique first, stand with your feet flat on the floor and wide enough to maintain good balance. Bend the knees and lean forward and down to grasp the bar with a close grip. Your arms should be straight ensuring that your hips, shoulders, head and eyes are inline and facing forwards. Initiate the movement via the abdominals whilst using the lower back muscles and straight arms to pull the bar away from the floor. Hold the start position using the strength of your abdominals and lower back. Pull the bar towards the body, whilst breathing out and ensure the elbows remain close to the side of the body. Breathe in as you return to the start position and repeat. The shoulders should remain relaxed at all times and all movements should be under control and safe!!

BACK EXERCISES USING DUMBBELLS

Bent over row 1

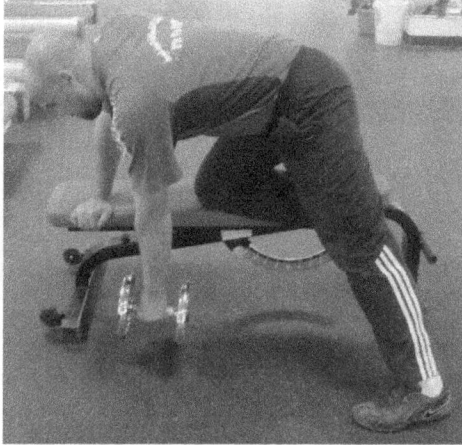

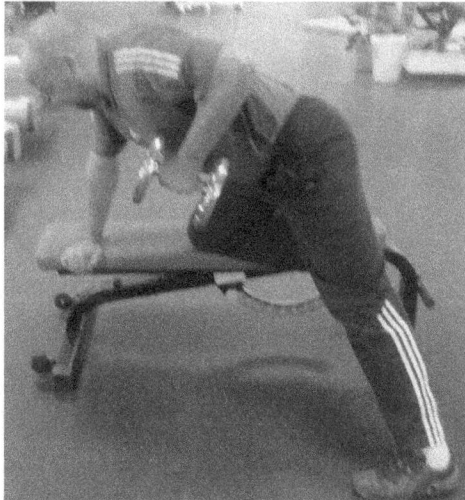

Select a weight that is low enough for you to master the technique first then kneel on a bench ensuring one foot is flat on the floor. Your hips, shoulders, head and eyes should be inline with your back perpendicular to the bench. Start off with your arm straight whilst holding the weight and pull it towards your waist whilst breathing out ensuring your shoulders are relaxed at all times. Attempt to initiate the movement via your abdominals but use your back muscles to pull the weight up with as little assistance from the biceps as possible. Return to the start position whilst breathing in and repeat accordingly.

Bent over row 2

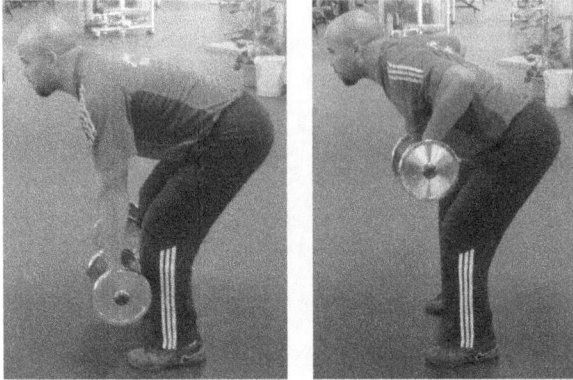

Select weights that are low enough for you to master the technique first then stand with your feet flat on the floor and around shoulder width apart. Your hips, shoulders, head and eyes should be inline with your back straight. Start off with your arms straight whilst holding the weights and then pull them towards your waist whilst breathing out ensuring your shoulders are relaxed at all times. Attempt to initiate the movement via your abdominals but use your back muscles to pull the weight up with as little assistance from the biceps as possible. Return to the start position whilst breathing in and repeat accordingly.

Dumbbell straight leg dead lift

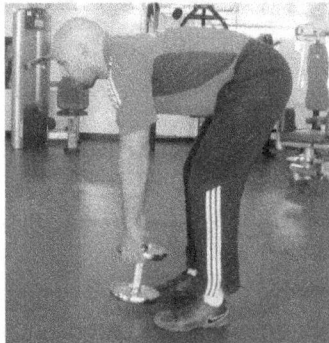

Select a weight that is low enough for you to master the technique first, and then stand with your feet flat on the floor for balance with a slight bend at the knee. Your hips, shoulders, head and eyes should be inline, with your back as straight as possible. Start off with your arms straight whilst holding the weight and then raise your upper body to the standing upright position whilst breathing out ensuring your shoulders are relaxed at all times. Attempt to initiate the movement via your abdominals but use your lower back muscles to raise your body upright. Return to the start position whilst breathing in and repeat accordingly.

Reverse flyes

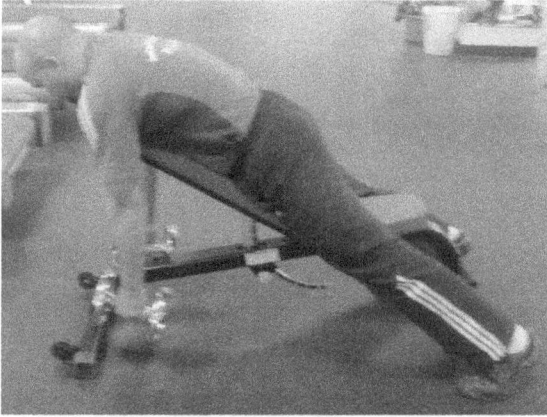

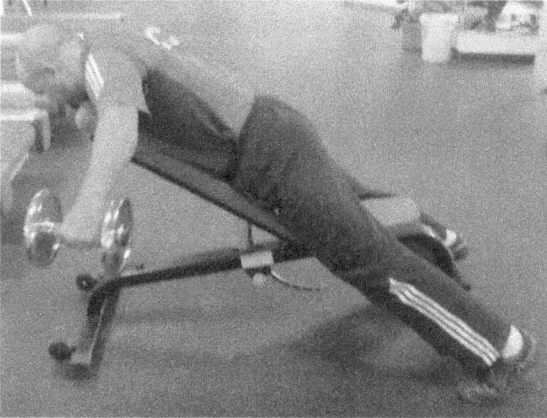

Select a weight that is low enough for you to master the technique first, and then lean onto an inclined bench and make sure your hips, shoulders, head and eyes are inline. Start off with your arms lowered towards the ground and pull the weights towards you with your arms outstretched to the side. Breathe out ensuring your elbows are slightly bent. Attempt to initiate the movement via your abdominals but use your upper back muscles to pull the dumbbells towards you as if you are bringing your shoulder blades together. There should be as little assistance from the shoulders as possible (no tension). Return to the start position whilst breathing in and repeat accordingly. This exercise is primarily for shoulders but also works the lats, rhomboids and mid traps, it can also be done on a flat bench.

Dumbbell pull

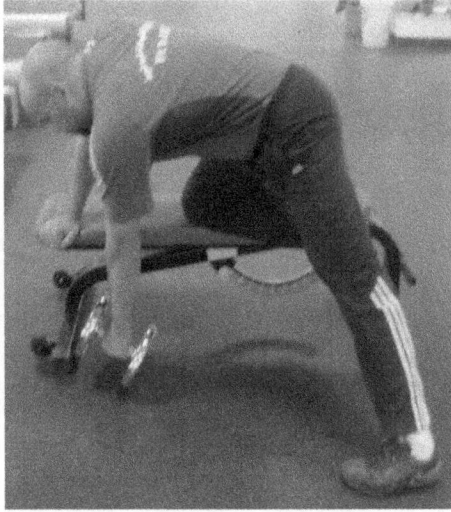

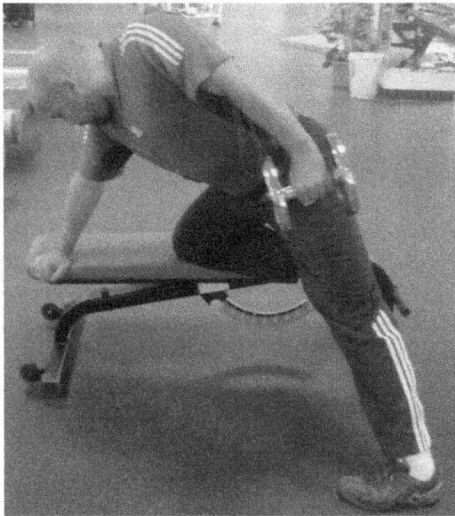

Select a weight that is low enough for you to master the technique first then kneel on a bench ensuring one foot is flat on the floor. Your hips, shoulders, head and eyes should be inline with your back perpendicular to the bench. Start off with your arm straight and in front of you whilst holding the weight and pull it towards your hips and beyond whilst breathing out ensuring your shoulders are relaxed at all times. Attempt to initiate the movement via your abdominals but use your back muscles only to pull the weight. Return to the start position whilst breathing in and repeat accordingly. This exercise will also work the rear deltoid.

MOST COMMON CHEST EXERCISES

USING YOUR OWN BODYWEIGHT

Pectoral Isometric hold

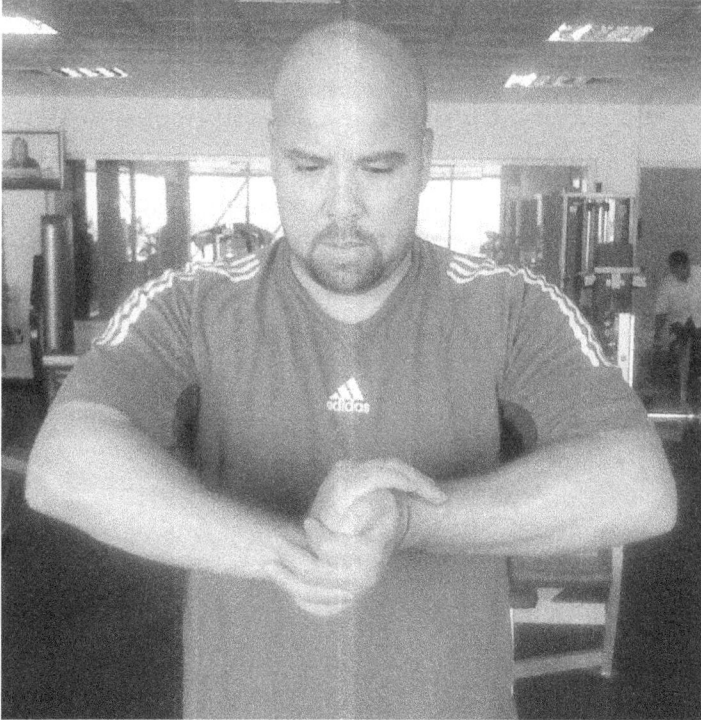

Place your hands together & level with your chest and ensure that your shoulders are relaxed whilst pushing your hands towards each other. Breathe consistently whilst pushing harder and contract your abdominals accordingly to ensure that you increase the power for better results. Your hands should only be slightly in front of your body.

Incline Push Ups

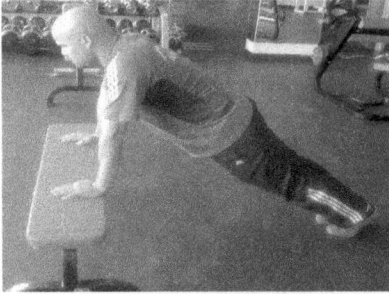

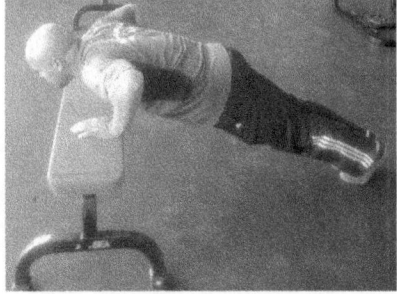

Lean onto a bench/stable object ensuring that your back is straight and your hands are level with your shoulders. Your shoulders should be relaxed and your hips and shoulders should remain facing towards the ground along with your head and eyes. Initiate the movement from the abdominals and lower your upper body until your chest is close to the bench/stable object whilst breathing in. Breathe out as you raise your upper body back to the start position. Maintaining control throughout the movement is important whilst breathing correctly.

Normal Push Ups

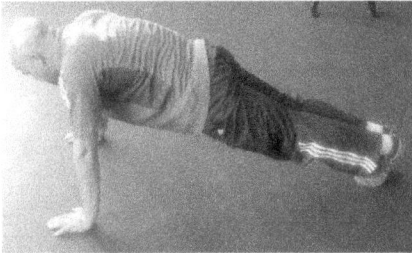

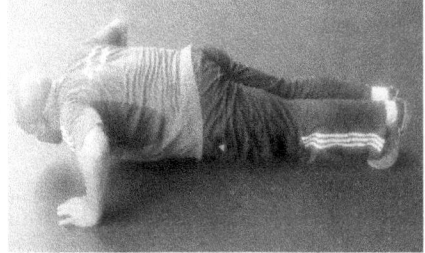

From the kneeling position ensure that your hands are level with your shoulders and your knees and hands are in line. Your shoulders should be relaxed and your hips and shoulders should remain facing towards the ground along with your head and eyes. Initiate the movement from the abdominals and lower your upper body until your chest is close to the floor whilst breathing in. Breathe out as you raise your upper body back to the start position. As you tire, concentrate on your breathing whilst compressing your abdominals and lower back; tense your whole body (not shoulders) to assist you in keeping good form. If this is too easy you can raise up from the floor whilst attempting to clap your hands together and return safely to the start position. Maintaining control throughout the movement is important whilst breathing correctly.

Decline Push Ups

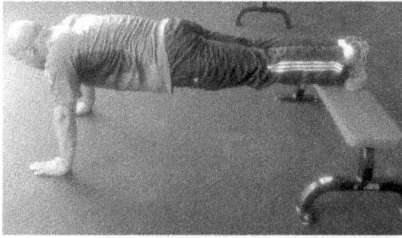

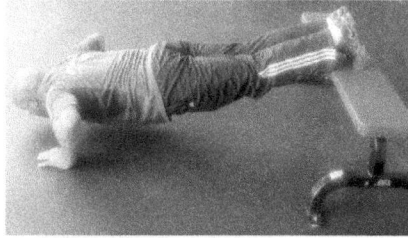

With your feet on a stable raised object ensure your hands are level with your shoulders and your knees and hands are in line. Your shoulders should be relaxed and your hips and shoulders should remain facing towards the ground along with your head and eyes. Initiate the movement from the abdominals and lower your upper body until your chest is close to the floor whilst breathing in. Breathe out as you raise your upper body back to the start position. Maintaining control throughout the movement is important whilst breathing correctly.

Bodyweight Dips

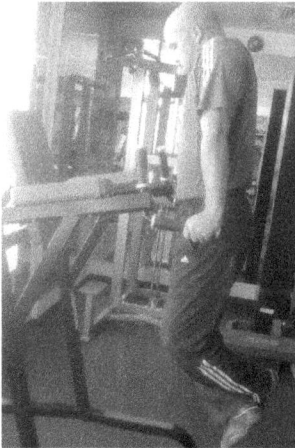

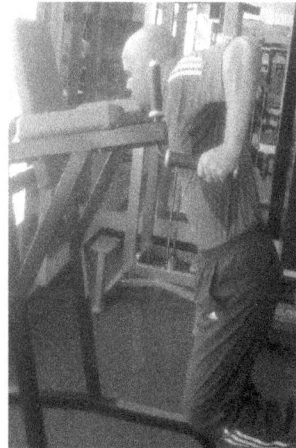

Find any object that is stable, safe and secure where you can bend your elbows fully behind your body. Your aim is to place the chest in a fully stretched position before raising your body upwards whilst breathing out and straightening your arms. You can use the apparatus above or place a chair/raised platform behind you and complete the same exercise, although the above apparatus is better to get primary results for the chest as opposed to chest and triceps.

CHEST EXERCISES USING RESISTANCE BANDS

Chest Press

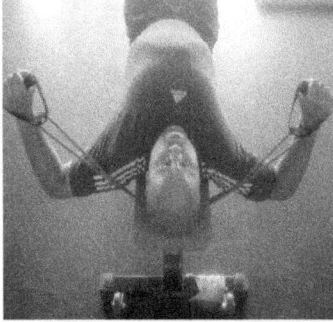

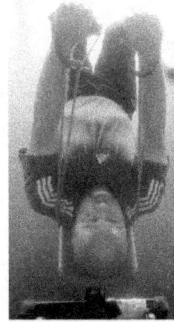

Safety should be your main priority especially when selecting the weight of the resistance band until you have mastered the technique and ensure that you secure the band safely around a solid object. Position yourself either on a flat surface or in the kneeling position and grip the bands firmly with one or both hands depending on the exercise. Once you have adjusted the resistance so that it is taught enough, position your hands level with the upper part of your chest with your elbows low where possible. As you breathe out, engage your abdominals and push the bands away from your body whilst straightening your arm(s). Breathe in as you return to the start position and repeat.

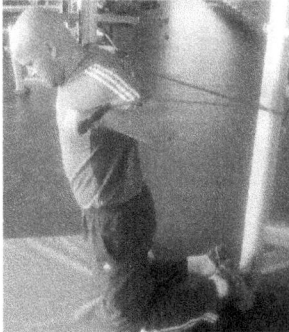

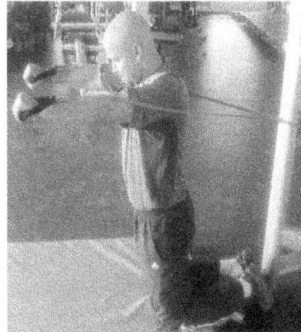

Flyes 1

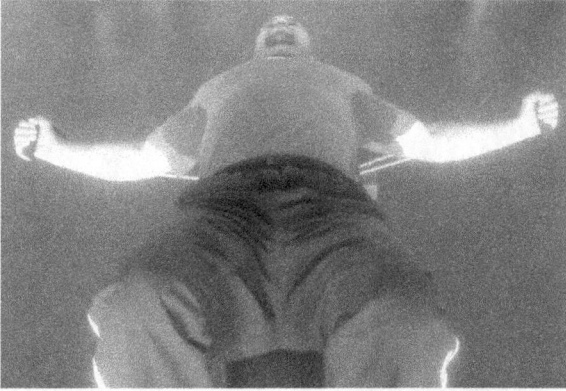

Safety should be your main priority especially when selecting the weight of the resistance band until you have mastered the technique and ensure that you secure the band safely around a solid object. Position yourself on a flat surface and grip the bands firmly with one or both hands depending on the exercise. Once you have adjusted the resistance so that it is taught enough, position your hands level with the upper part of your chest with your elbows low where possible and positioned out to the side of your body with outstretched arm(s) slightly below the level of your shoulder. As you breathe out, engage your abdominals and pull the bands up towards the midline of your body. Breathe in as you return to the start position and repeat. Attempt to keep your arm(s) straight albeit with a very slight bend at the elbow.

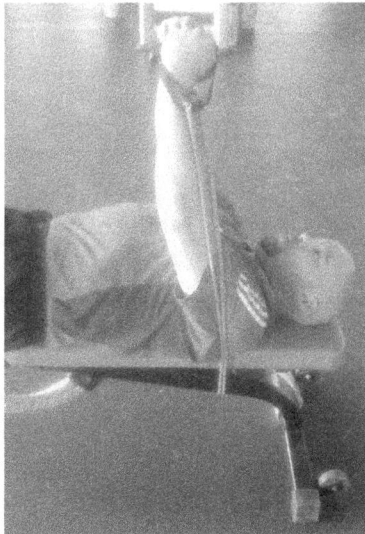

Flyes 2 & 3

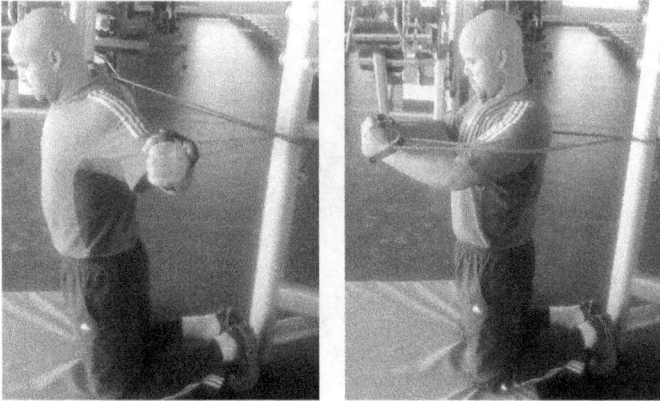

Safety should be your main priority especially when selecting the weight of the resistance band until you have mastered the technique and ensure that you secure the band safely around a solid object. Position yourself on your knees and grip the bands firmly with one or both hands depending on the exercise. Once you have adjusted the resistance so that it is taught enough, position your hands level with the upper part of your chest with your elbows low where possible and positioned out to the side of your body with outstretched arm(s) slightly below the level of your shoulder. As you breathe out, engage your abdominals and pull the bands forwards towards the midline of your body. Breathe in as you return to the start position and repeat. Attempt to keep a very slight bend at the elbow. Lean forward to work your chest at a different angle.

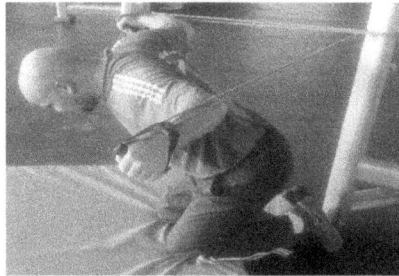

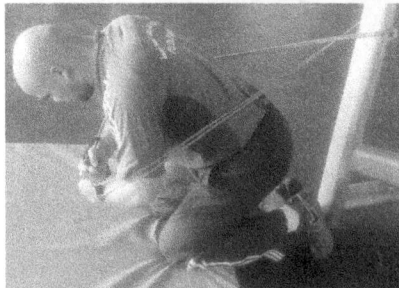

Pullovers

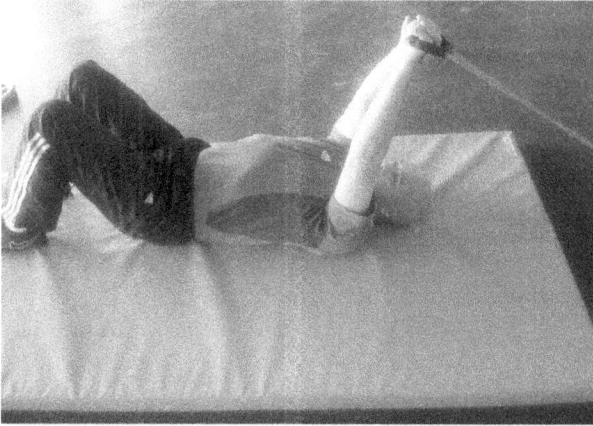

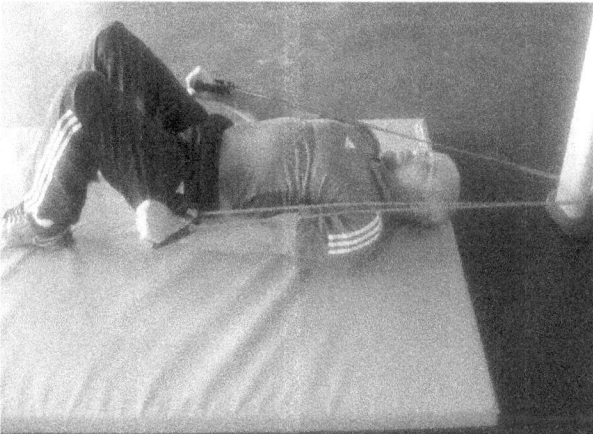

Select a safe weight to start with until you have mastered the technique and position yourself on a flat surface, preferably a mat or a bench and grip the band firmly with one or both hands depending on the exercise. Your arm(s) should be above your head and as you breathe out, engage your abdominals and pull the bands towards your hips. Your arm(s) should remain as straight as is comfortable, breathe in as you return to the start position and repeat.

CHEST EXERCISES USING A FIT-BALL

Chest Press

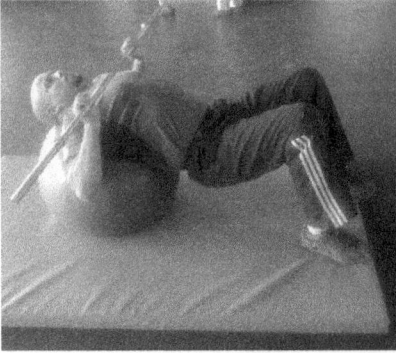

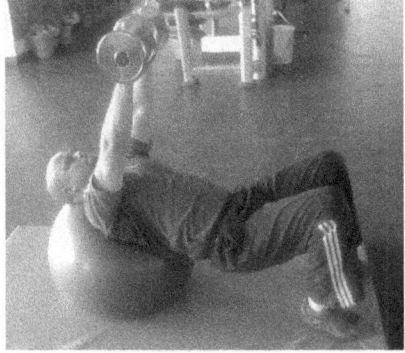

Safety should be your main priority especially when selecting the weight to start with until you have mastered the technique. Position yourself on the fit-ball so that the ball is in the centre of your back. Grip the weight firmly with one or both hands and once you have lifted the weight from the ground you should be positioned correctly on the ball with the weights level with the upper part of your chest and your elbows low where possible. As you breathe out, engage your abdominals and push the weights up whilst straightening your arm(s). Breathe in as you return to the start position and repeat.

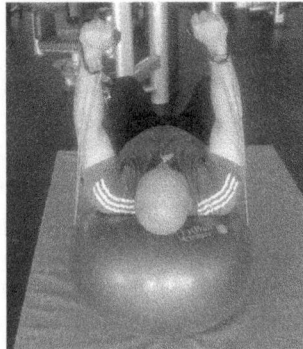

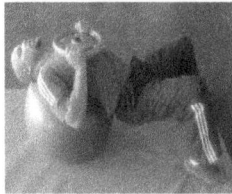

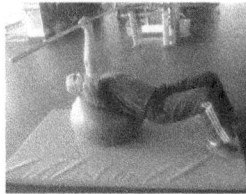

Flyes

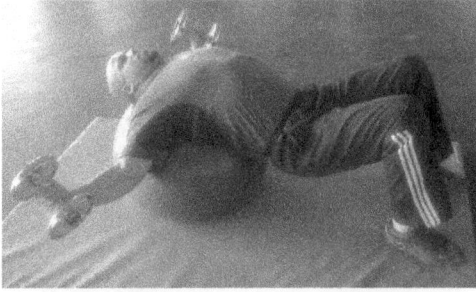

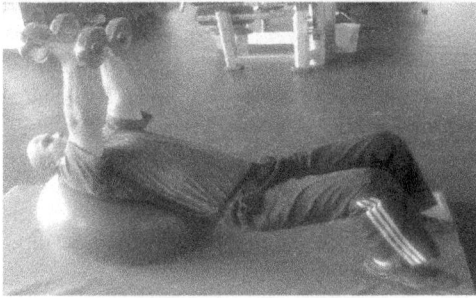

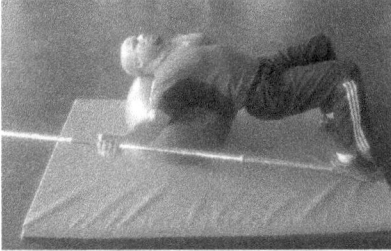

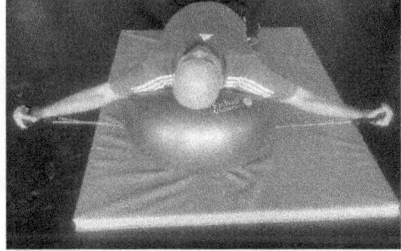

Safety should be your main priority especially when selecting the weight to start with until you have mastered the technique. Position yourself on the fit-ball so that the ball is in the centre of your back. Grip the weight firmly with one or both hands and once you have lifted the weight from the ground you should be positioned correctly on the ball with the weights level with the upper part of your chest and your elbows low where possible but more importantly with your arms outstretched to the side of your body with a slight bend at the elbows. As you breathe out, engage your abdominals and push the weight up with a straight arm(s). Breathe in as you return to the start position and repeat. Your hand position can vary from palms facing towards you or thumbs.

Pull Over

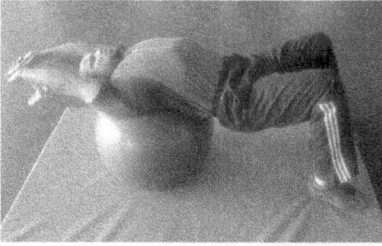
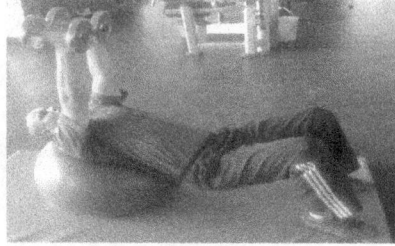

Safety should be your main priority especially when selecting a weight to start with until you have mastered the technique. Position yourself on the fit-ball so that the ball is in the centre of your back. Grip the weight firmly with one or both hands and once you have lifted the weight from the ground you should be positioned correctly on the ball with your arm(s) above your head and as you breathe out, engage your abdominals and pull the weight towards your lower chest. Your arm(s) should remain as straight as is comfortable, breathe in as you return to the start position and repeat.

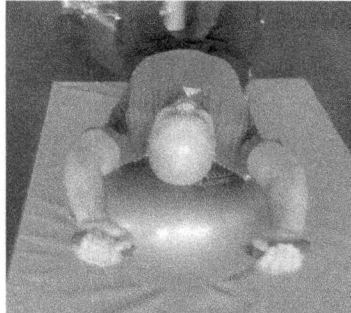

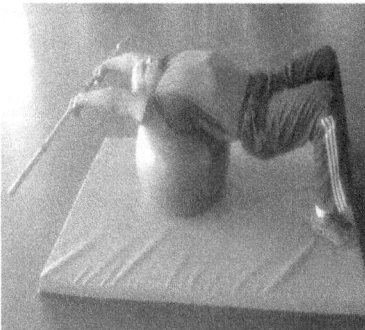
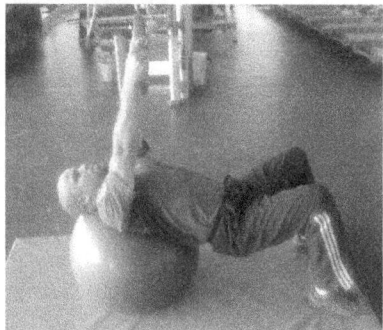

Push Up

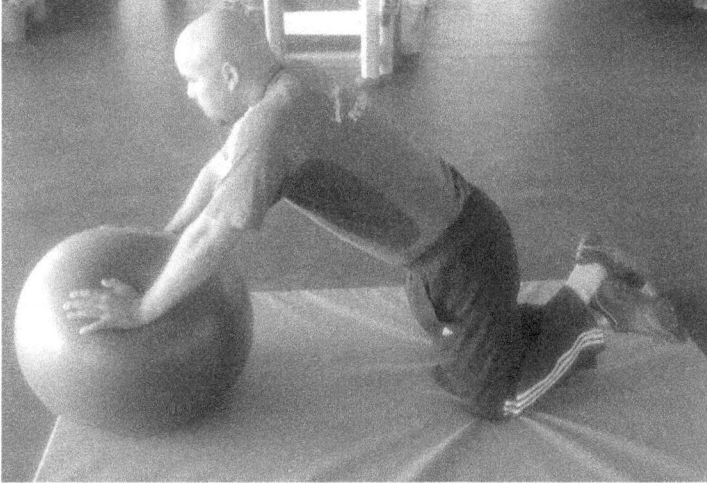

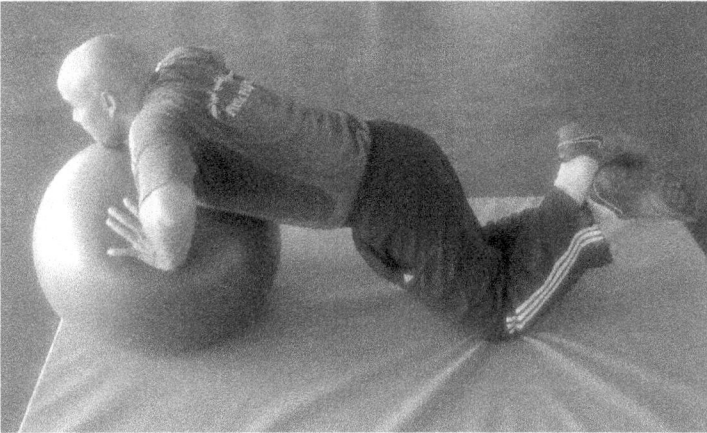

From the kneeling position ensure that your hands are level with your shoulders and that you lean onto the fit-ball. Your shoulders should be relaxed and your hips and shoulders should remain facing towards the ground along with your head and eyes. Initiate the movement from the abdominals and lower your upper body until your chest is close to the ball whilst breathing in. Breathe out as you raise your upper body back to the start position. As you tire, concentrate on your breathing whilst compressing your abdominals and lower back; tense your whole body (not shoulders) to assist you in keeping good form. If this is too easy you can begin by making it more difficult by re-placing your knees with your feet i.e. in the full push up position. Maintaining control throughout the movement is important whilst breathing correctly.

CHEST EXERCISES USING FITNESS MACHINES

Seated Press & Smiths Machine

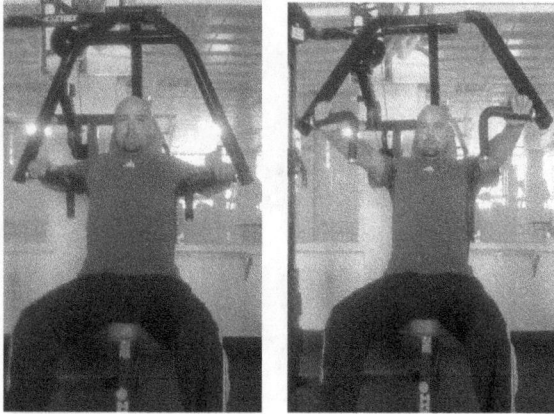

Select a weight that is safe so that you can master the technique and for the machine above adjust the position of the seat so that your hands are level with the upper part of your chest with your elbows as far back as possible. The same principles apply for the smith's machine below; just unhook the bar from the framework whilst on a bench. As you breathe out, engage your abdominals and push the weight forwards whilst straightening your arm(s). Breathe in as you return to the start position and repeat.

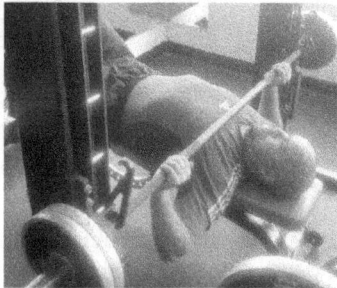

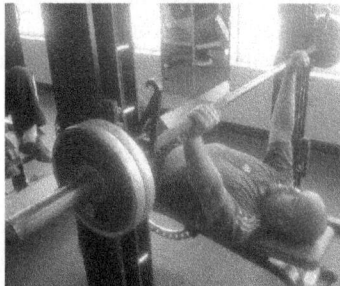

Seated Fly Machine

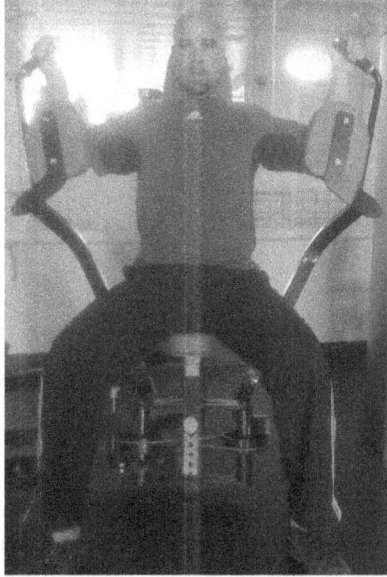

Select a weight that is safe so that you can master the technique; adjust the position of the seat so that your elbows are level with the upper part of your chest with your elbows as far back as possible slightly below the level of your shoulder. As you breathe out, engage your abdominals and pull the bars towards the midline of your body. Attempt to keep your lower back pressed up against the seat behind, breathe in as you return to the start position and repeat.

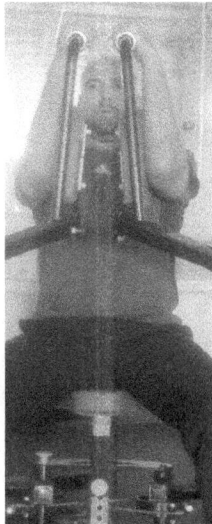

Cable Pullover

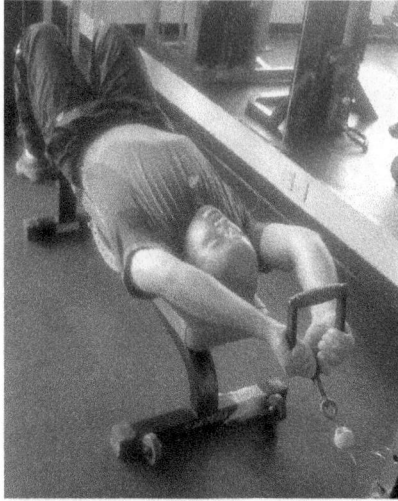

Safety should be your main priority especially when selecting a weight to start with until you have mastered the technique. Position yourself on a flat surface, preferably a bench and grip a weighted cable firmly with one or both hands depending on the exercise. Your arm(s) should be above your head and as you breathe out, engage your abdominals and pull the cable(s) towards your lower chest. Your arm(s) should remain as straight as is comfortable, breathe in as you return to the start position and repeat.

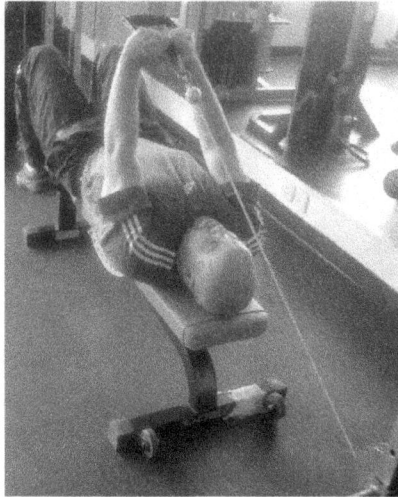

Cable Flyes 1 & 2

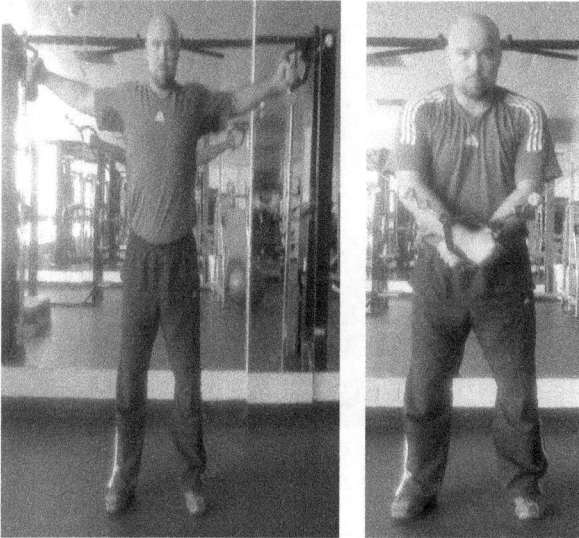

Safety should be your main priority especially when selecting a weight to start with until you have mastered the technique. Position yourself with your feet flat on the floor Grip the weighted cables firmly with one or both hands (outstretched) above your shoulders or level with your shoulders depending on the exercise. As you breathe out, engage your abdominals and pull the cables towards our hips. Your arm(s) should remain as straight as is comfortable, breathe in as you return to the start position and repeat. You can perform a double or single arm chest press using cables as well (refer to the technique of chest press).

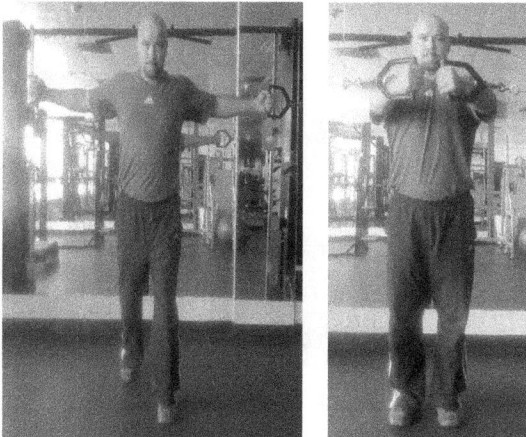

Cable Flyes 3, 4 & 5

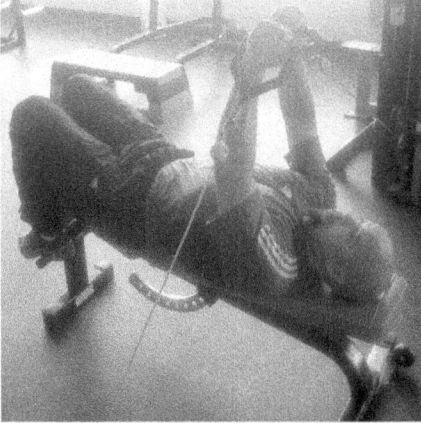

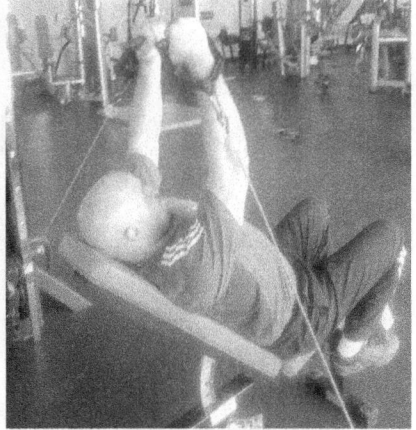

Select a safe weight to start with until you have mastered the technique and position yourself either on a flat surface or with your feet flat on the floor. Grip the weighted cables firmly with both hands. Your hands should be positioned out to the side of your body with an outstretched arm slightly below the level of your shoulder. As you breathe out, engage your abdominals and pull the cables up towards the midline of your body. Attempt to keep the cables levels, along with keeping your arms straight, albeit with a very slight bend at the elbow. Breathe in as you return to the start position and repeat.

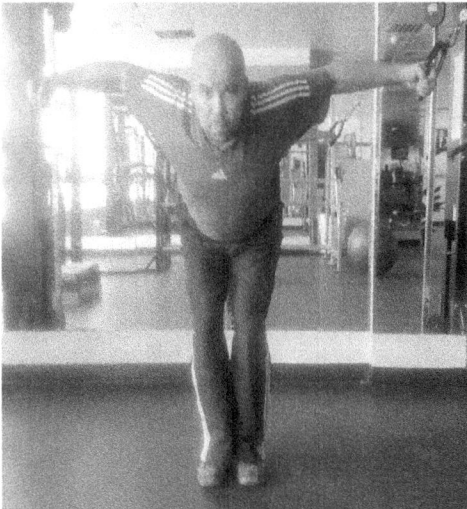

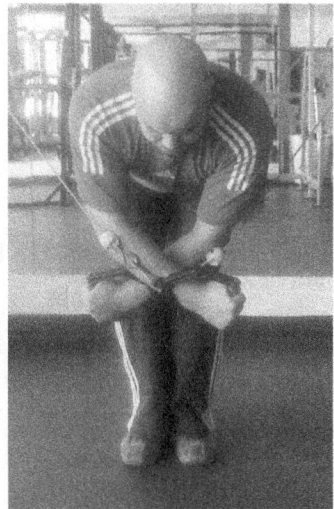

An alternative ex is the **cable push/pull exercise** – Stand upright facing the machine with the cables at waist h.t. Turn to your left so that your left arm is extended and your right is holding the handle at your chest. Your left foot should be forward & your right leg back. Pull with your left as you push with your right and rotate the shoulders as far as possible. Repeat on the other side by facing the other direction.

CHEST EXERCISES USING A BARBELL

Barbell Pull Over

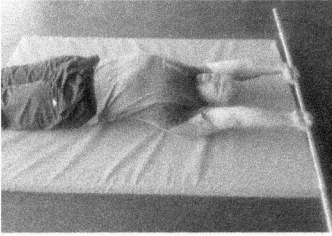

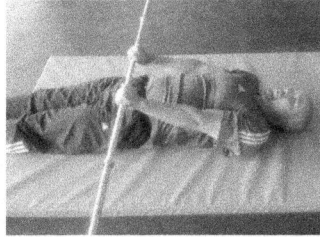

Safety should be your main priority especially when selecting a weight to start with until you have mastered the technique. Position yourself on a flat surface, preferably a bench and grip a weighted bar firmly with one or both hands depending on the exercise. Your arm(s) should be above your head and as you breathe out, engage your abdominals and pull the bar towards your hips. Your arm(s) should remain as straight as is comfortable, breathe in as you return to the start position and repeat.

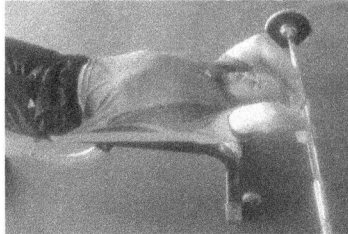

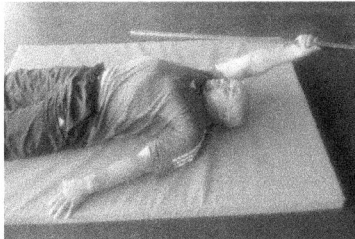

Bench Press

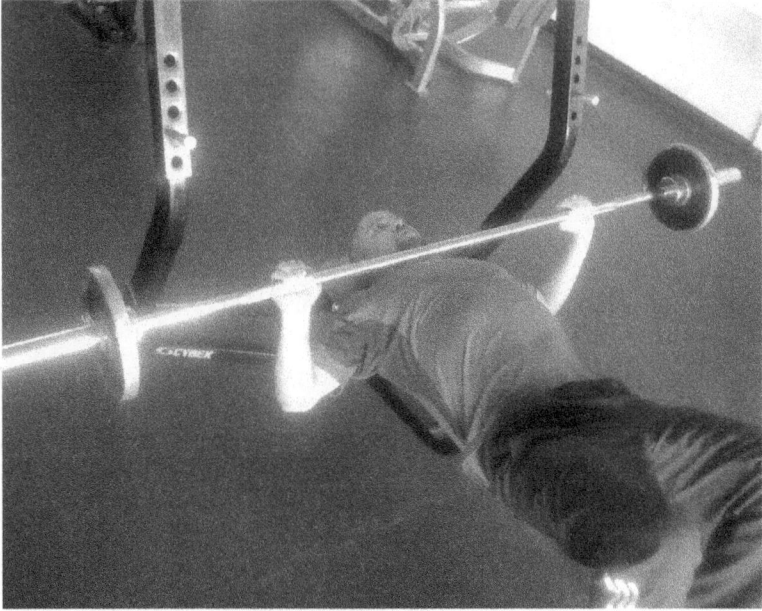

Safety should be your main priority especially when selecting a weight to start with until you have mastered the technique. Position yourself on a flat surface, preferably a bench and grip a weighted bar firmly with one or both hands depending on the exercise, your hands should be equal distance apart from each end unless you are doing a single arm press (diagram below right) then your hand should be in the centre. Once you have lifted the bar it should be positioned level with the upper part of your chest with your elbows low where possible. As you breathe out, engage your abdominals and push the bar up whilst straightening your arm(s). Breathe in as you return to the start position and repeat.

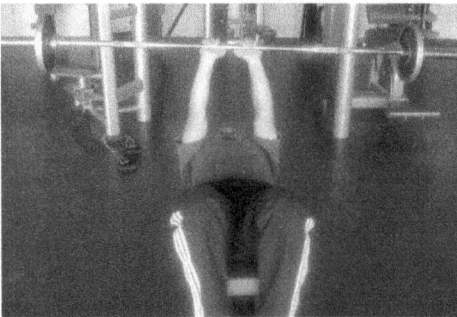
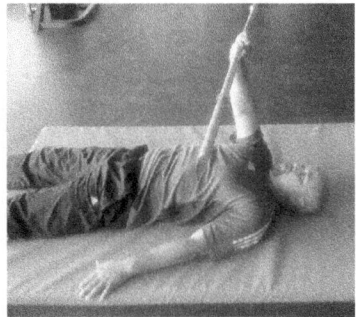

Incline Press

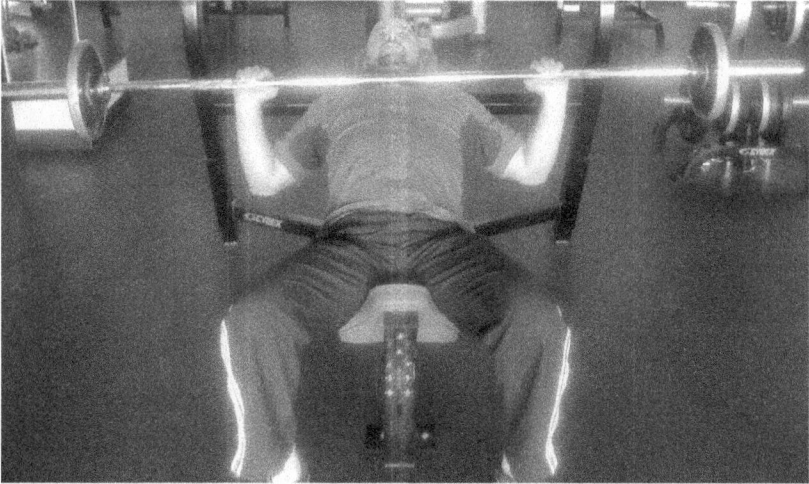

Explanation is the same as above, although on a bench where the height can be adjusted to approx. a 45 degree angle.

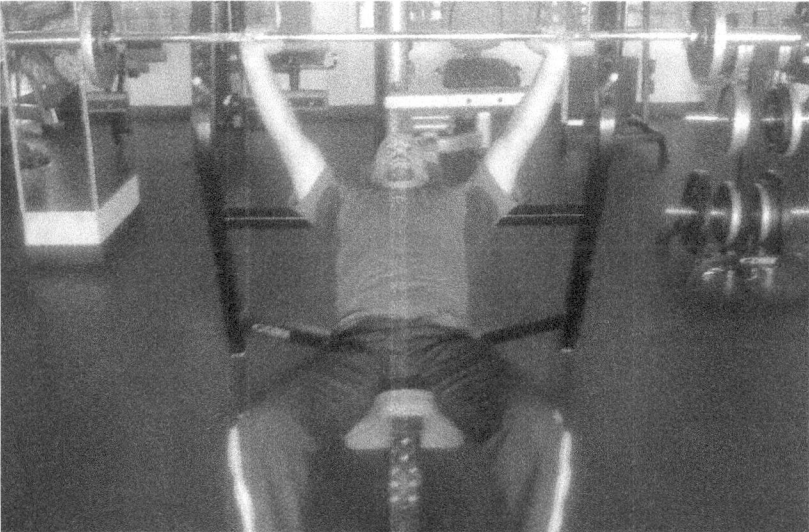

Decline Press

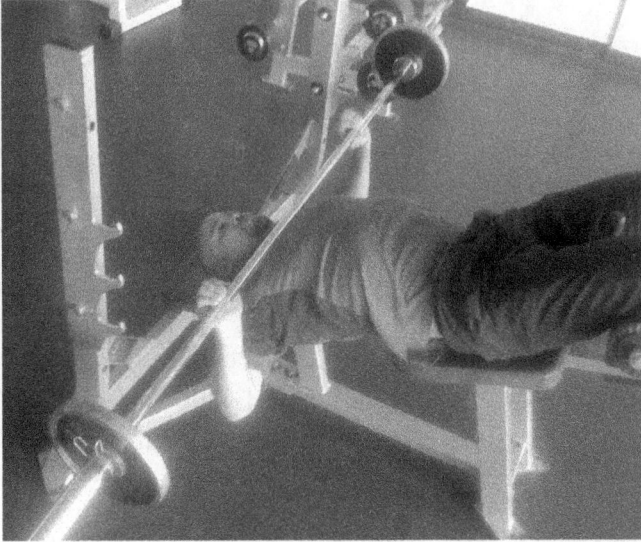

Explanation is the same as 2.2, although on a bench where the height can be adjusted to below the normal angle; ensure that your feet are fixed correctly

Barbell Fly

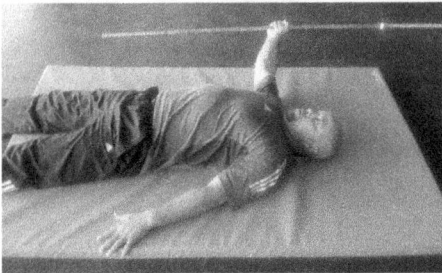

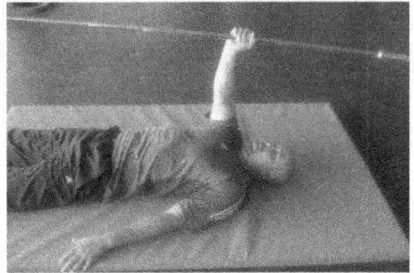

Select a safe weight to start with until you have mastered the technique and position yourself on a flat surface, preferably a floor or bench and grip a weighted bar firmly with one hand. Your hand should be in the centre of the bar and positioned out to the side of your body with an outstretched arm slightly below the level of your shoulder. As you breathe out, engage your abdominals and pull the bar up towards the midline of your body. Attempt to keep the bar level along with keeping your arm straight albeit with a very slight bend at the elbow. Breathe in as you return to the start position and repeat.

142

CHEST EXERCISES USING DUMBBELLS

Dumbbell Press

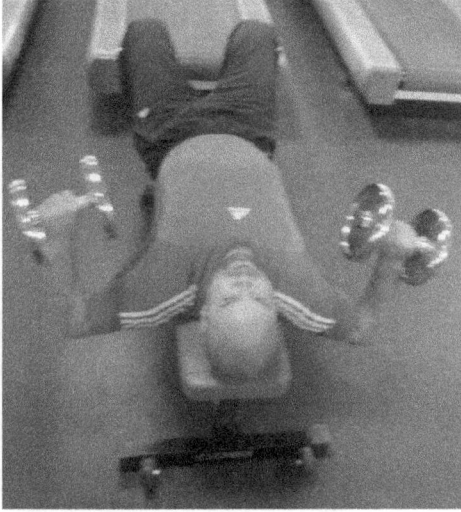

Safety should be your main priority especially when selecting weights to start with, until you have mastered the technique. Position yourself on a flat surface, preferably a bench and grip a set of weighted dumbbells firmly with both hands. Once you have lifted the dumbbells you should be positioned flat on the bench with the weights level with the upper part of your chest with your elbows low where possible. As you breathe out, engage your abdominals and push the weights up whilst straightening your arm(s). Breathe in as you return to the start position and repeat.

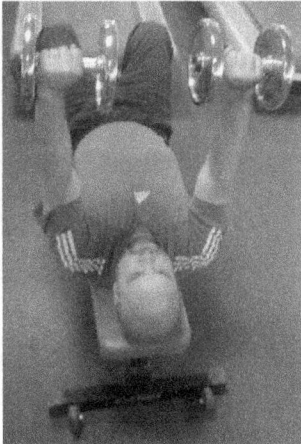

Incline Press

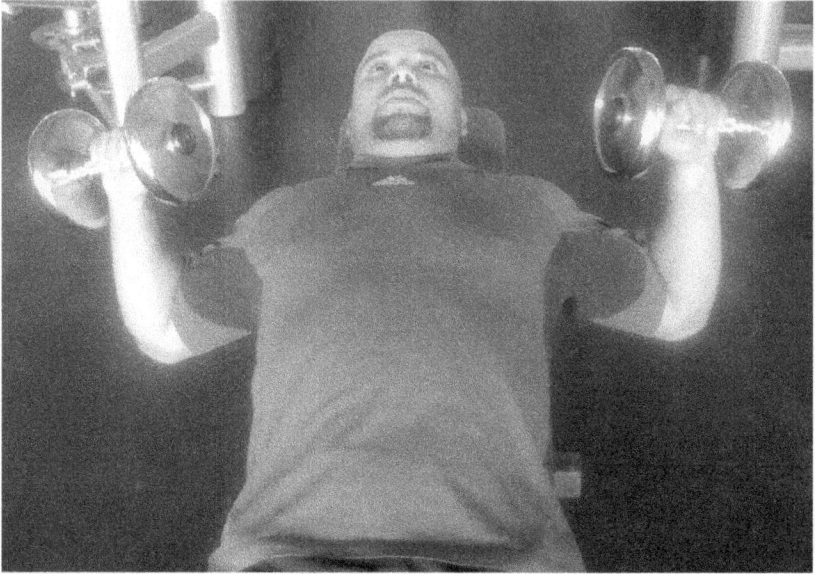

Explanation is the same as above, although on a bench where the height can be adjusted to approx. a 45 degree angle. For variety you can twist the weights so that your palms are facing inwards at the top of the movement.

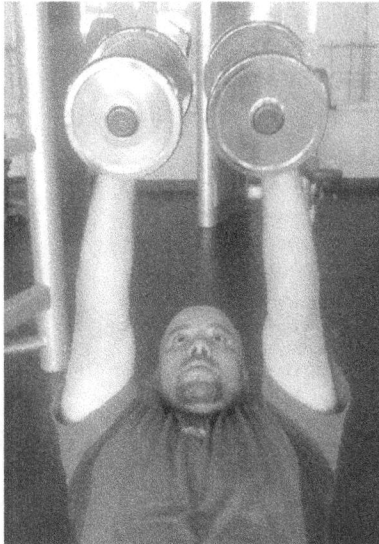

Decline Press

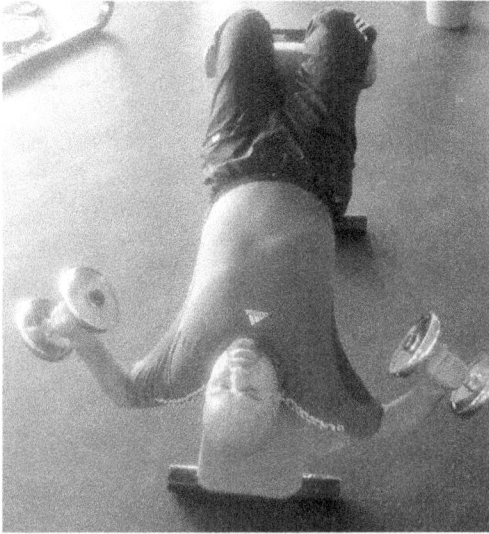

Safety should be your main priority especially when selecting weights to start with until you have mastered the technique. Position yourself on a bench where the height can be adjusted to below the normal angle; ensure that your feet are fixed correctly.

Grip a set of weighted dumbbells firmly with both hands and once you have lifted the dumbbells you should be positioned flat on the declined bench with the weights level with the upper part of your chest with your elbows low where possible.

As you breathe out, engage your abdominals and push the weights up whilst straightening your arm(s). Breathe in as you return to the start position and repeat.

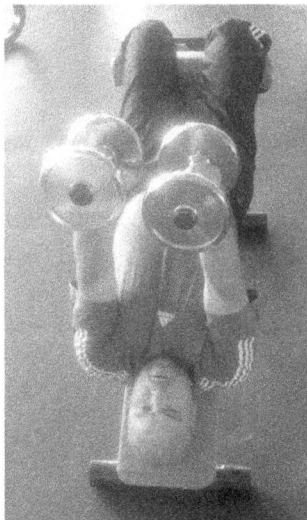

Pull Overs

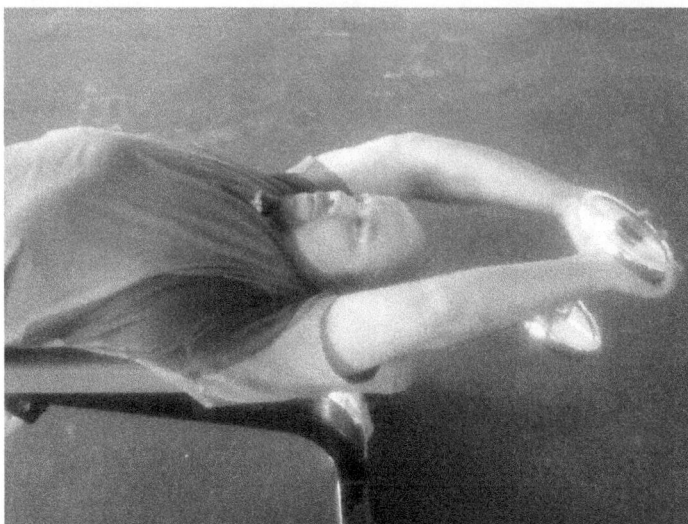

Safety should be your main priority especially when selecting a weight to start with until you have mastered the technique. Position yourself on either a flat, inclined or declined surface and grip a dumbbell firmly with both hands. Your arm(s) should be above your head and as you breathe out, engage your abdominals and pull the weight towards your lower chest. Your arm(s) should remain as straight as is comfortable, breathe in as you return to the start position and repeat.

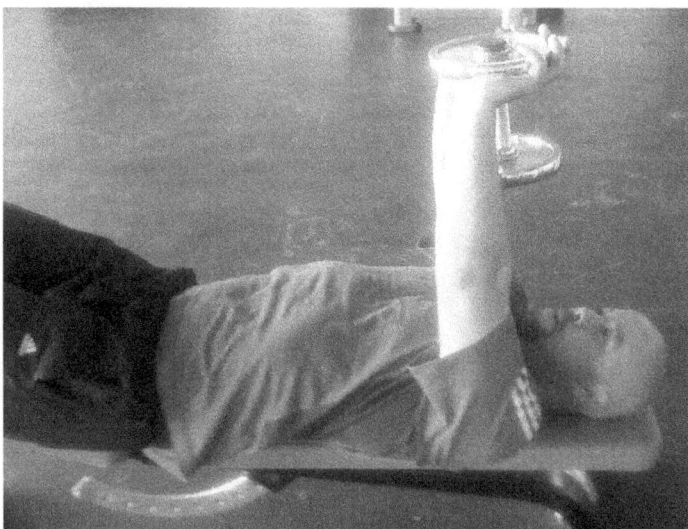

Flyes

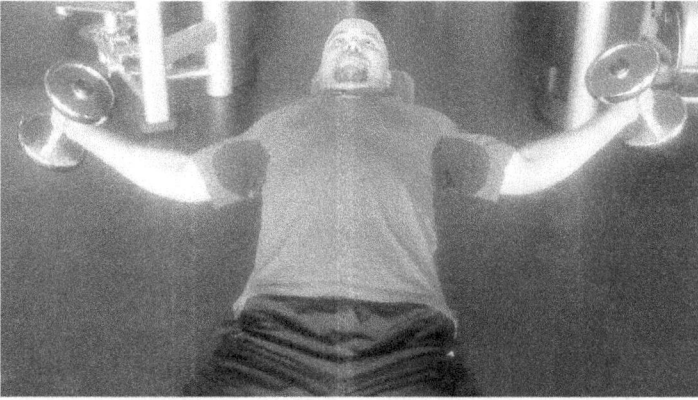

Safety should be your main priority especially when selecting weights to start with until you have mastered the technique. Position yourself on either a flat, inclined or declined surface and grip a dumbbell firmly with both hands. Once you have lifted the dumb-bells you should be positioned flat on the bench with the weights level with the upper part of your chest with your elbows low where possible but more importantly with your arms outstretched to the side of your body with a slight bend at the elbows. As you breathe out, engage your abdominals and push the weights up whilst straightening your arm(s). Breathe in as you return to the start position and repeat. Your hand position can vary from palms facing towards you or thumbs.

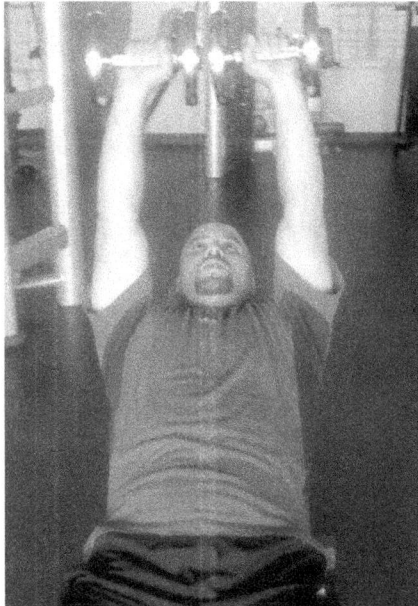

MOST COMMON SHOULDER EXERCISES

USING YOUR OWN BODYWEIGHT

Isometric Holds 1-4

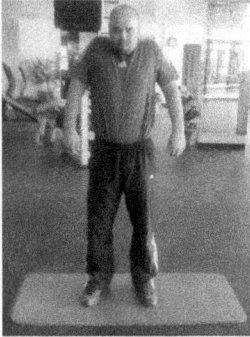

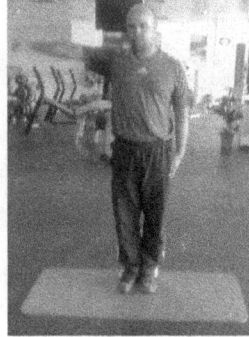

Whichever hold you are doing you must ensure that wherever possible your posture is good i.e. maintaining body alignment with your head, eyes, shoulders and hips inline and facing forwards as much as possible. Your abdominals should be initiated prior and during each hold with your shoulders relaxed as much as possible. All of the above movements are shoulder muscle actions; therefore all you are doing is moving the arm(s) in a particular direction and placing a hold within the range, your breathing should remain controlled and should not be forced.

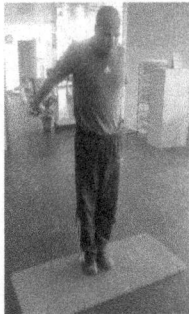

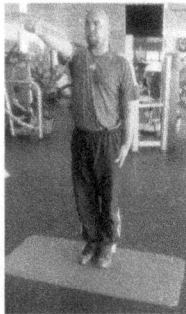

Advanced Hold

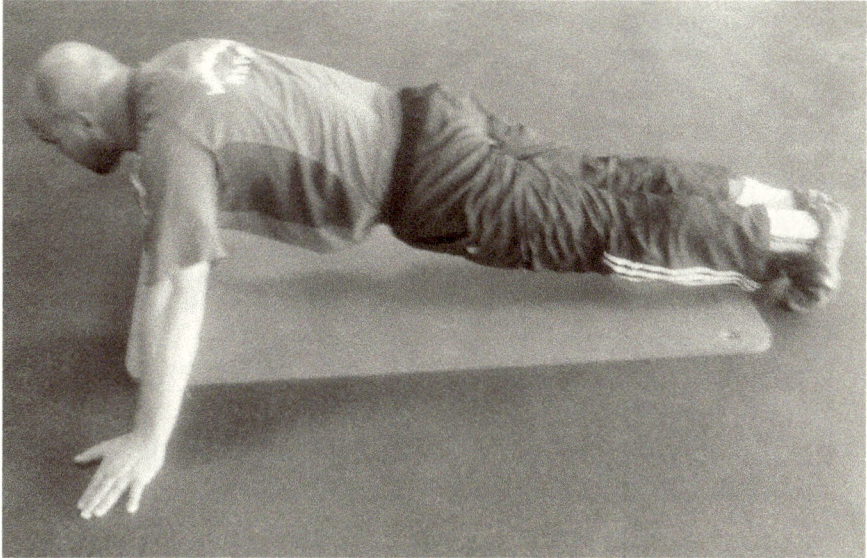

With this hold you must ensure that your posture is perfect i.e. maintaining body alignment with your head, eyes, shoulders and hips inline and facing forwards as much as possible. Your abdominals should be initiated prior and during the hold with your shoulders relaxed as much as possible. Your hands should be inline with the shoulders and your breathing should remain controlled and should not be forced. Hold the position for as long as possible without disrupting your body alignment and good form.

Partner Resisted Exercises

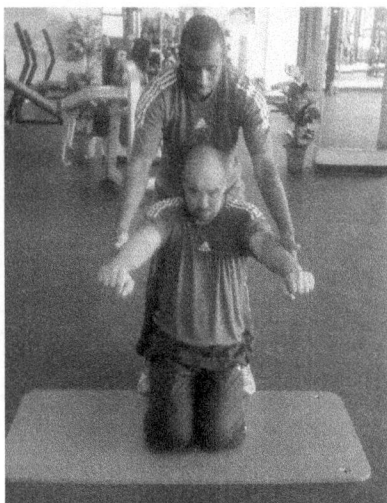

Pull arms down

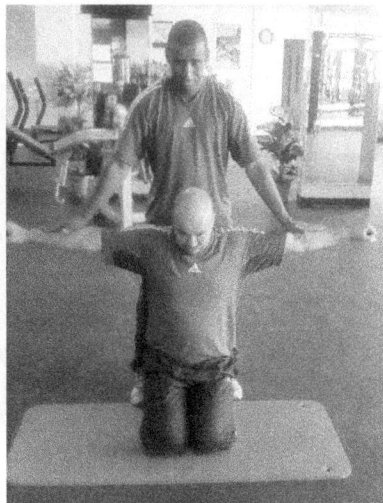

Push arms up

Most of the exercises shown are a variation of all the movements already covered (3.1), whether you are standing, or kneeling, your partner is just applying a resistance within a certain range whilst you attempt to raise, lower, push or pull against that resistance. You should always continue to breathe naturally and maintain good posture and form.

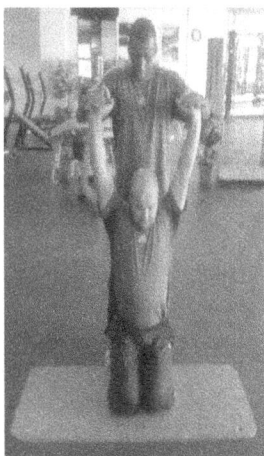

Push arms up

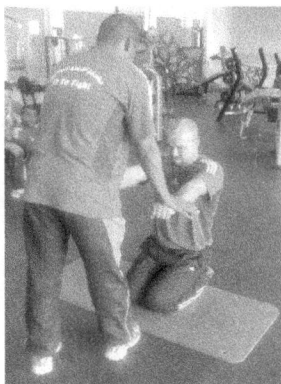

Push arms up

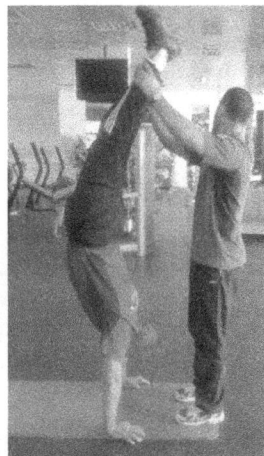

Hold or
Bend & Push

Caterpillar

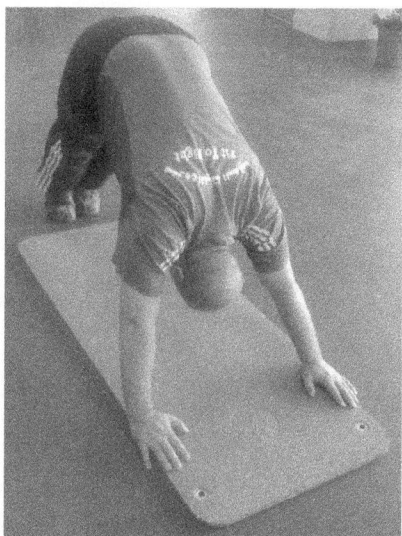

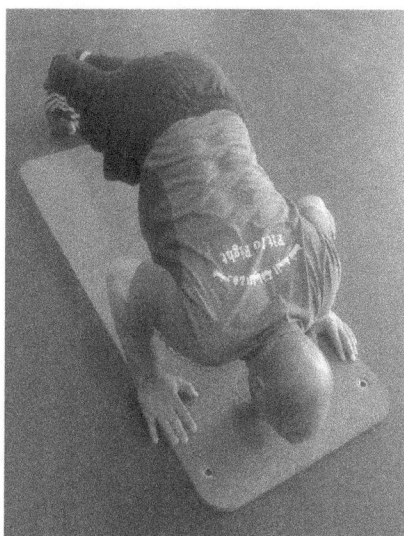

With your toes on the floor, your hands level on the floor and around shoulder width apart, hold your body in a V position as best you can with your backside raised up slightly. Throughout all 3 movements your abdominals should be initiated and as you breathe out you should roll your bodyweight forwards using only your shoulders, roll down and forwards bending your arms at the elbows until your chest almost brushes the ground and then roll upwards straightening your arms and hold. Breathe in until you reverse the movement by rolling your shoulders in the opposite direction until you are back in the start position. Repeat the movement but keep the shoulders pulled down and backwards as much as possible which will ensure that your upper spine and head are relaxed and not under too much tension.

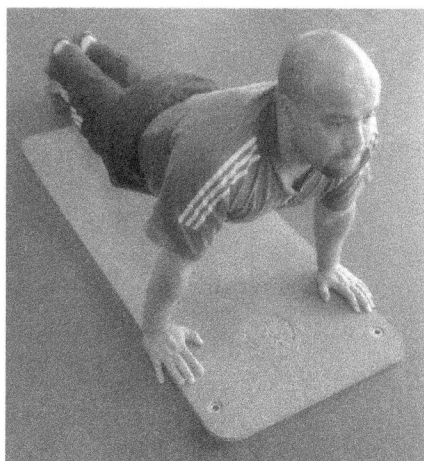

Additional Isometric Holds

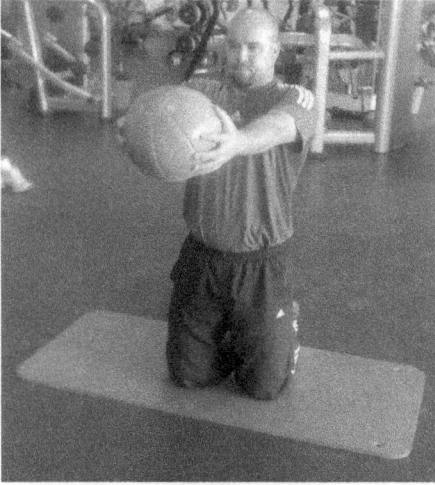

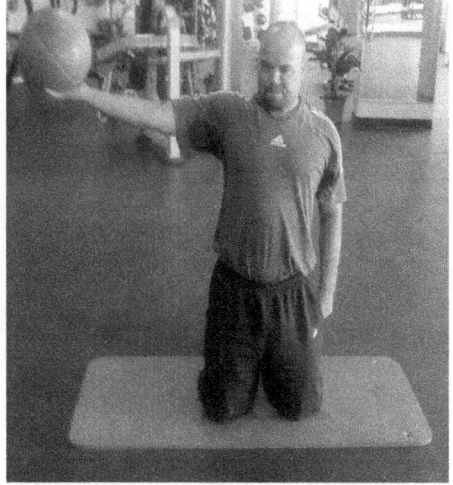

Select a low enough resistance to start with until you have mastered the technique and position yourself in the kneeling or standing position. Whichever hold you are attempting your shoulders should be relaxed with your breathing as per normal. Initially you should breathe out, engage your abdominals and raise the weight up, out to the side or in front of you and hold for as long as you can throughout the different ranges of motion whilst maintaining good posture. When you feel your posture and good form faltering, control your breathing throughout but most importantly (in) as you return to the start position and repeat.

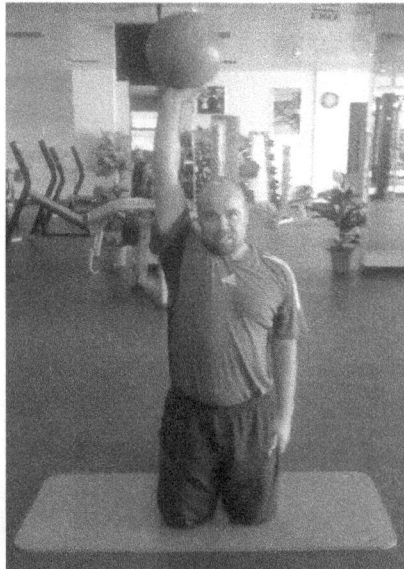

SHOULDER EXERCISES USING RESISTANCE BANDS

Isometric Holds

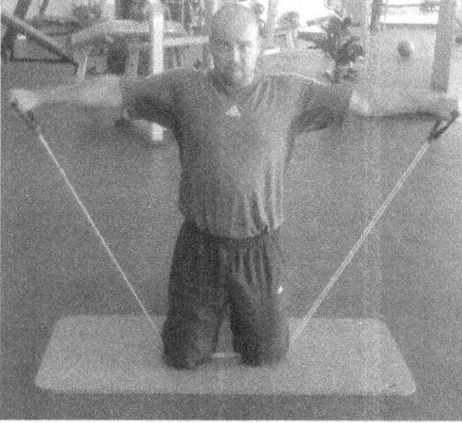

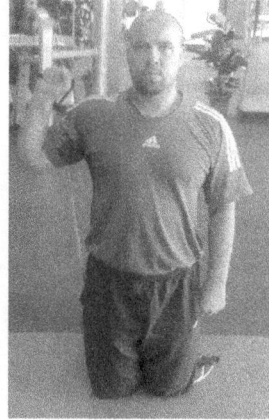

Select a low enough resistance to start with until you have mastered the technique and position yourself in the kneeling or standing position with the band secure & evenly fixed. Grip the band(s) firmly with one or both hands. Whichever hold you are attempting your shoulders should be relaxed with your breathing as per normal. Initially you should breathe out, engage your abdominals and raise the bands up, out to the side or behind you and hold for as long as you can throughout the different ranges of motion whilst maintaining good posture. When you feel your posture and good form faltering, control your breathing throughout but most importantly (in) as you return to the start position and repeat.

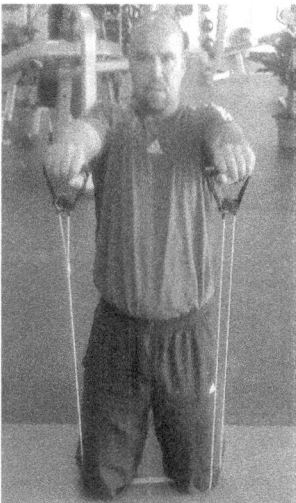

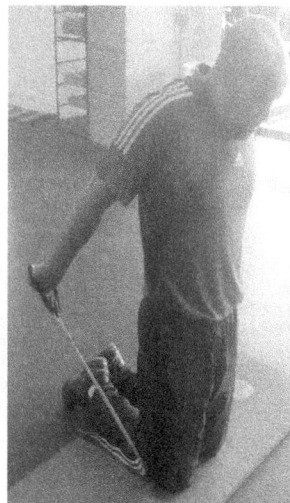

153

Shoulder Press

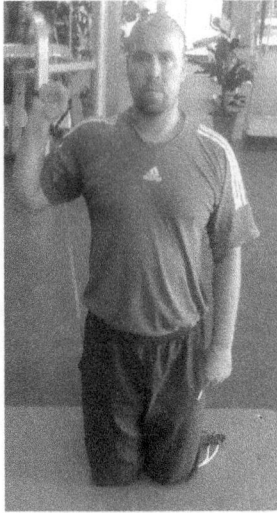

Select a low enough resistance to start with until you have mastered the technique and position yourself in the kneeling or standing position with the band secure & evenly fixed. Grip the band(s) firmly with one or both hands. Initially the bands should be positioned on either the front or rear of your shoulders with your elbows low and close to the side of your body. As you breathe out, engage your abdominals and raise the bands up and above your head with your arms outstretched and hold. Attempt to keep the bands level, along with keeping your arm(s) straight, breathe in as you return to the start position and repeat.

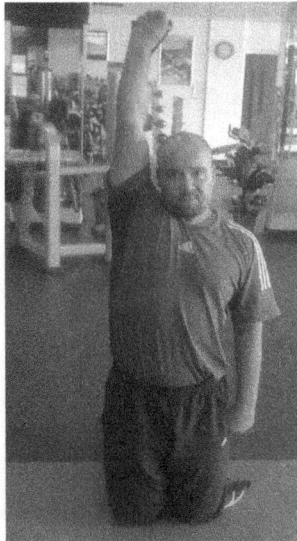

Frontal Raise

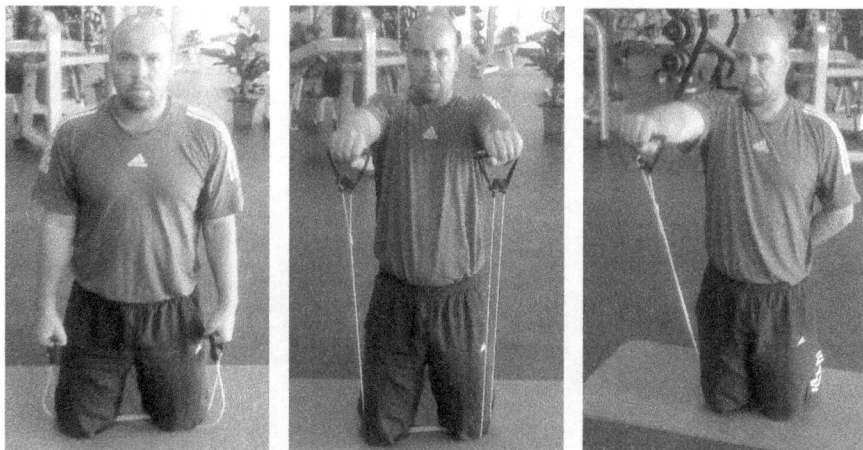

Select a low enough resistance to start with until you have mastered the technique and position yourself in the kneeling or standing position with the band secure & evenly fixed. Grip the band(s) firmly with one or both hands. Initially the bands should be positioned down and close to the front of the body with one or both arm(s) straight. As you breathe out, engage your abdominals and raise the bands up and level with your shoulders and hold. Attempt to keep the bands level along with keeping your arm(s) straight albeit with a very slight bend at the elbow to avoid injury. Breathe in as you return to the start position and repeat.

Rear Deltoid

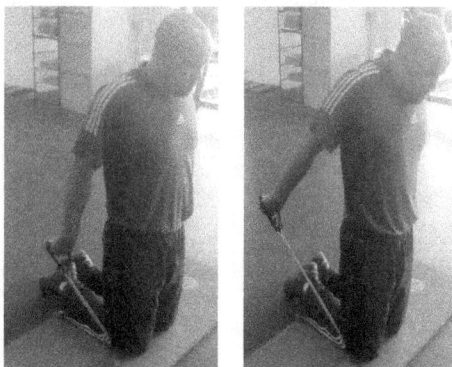

Select a low enough resistance to start with until you have mastered the technique and position yourself in the kneeling or standing position with the band secure & evenly fixed. Grip the band(s) firmly with one or both hands. As you breathe out, engage your abdominals and raise the bands away from the rear of your body and hold. Attempt to keep the band(s) level along with keeping your arms straight attempt to relax the shoulders and stick your chest out, breathe in as you return to the start position and repeat.

Lateral Raise

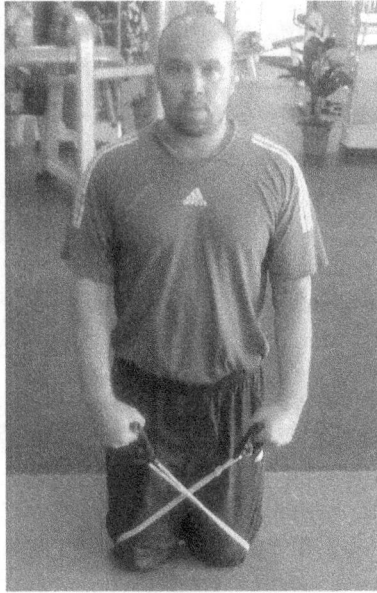

Select a low resistance to start with until you have mastered the technique and position yourself in the kneeling or standing position with the band secure, twisted but evenly fixed. Grip the bands firmly with both hands and the bands positioned down and close to the side of your body with straight arms. As you breathe out, engage your abdominals and raise the bands up, level with your shoulders with outstretched arms and hold. Attempt to keep the bands level and your arms straight albeit with a very slight bend at the elbow to avoid injury. Breathe in as you return to the start position and repeat.

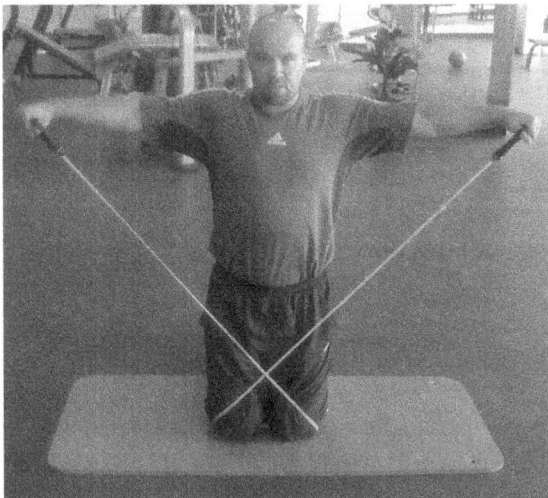

156

Upright row

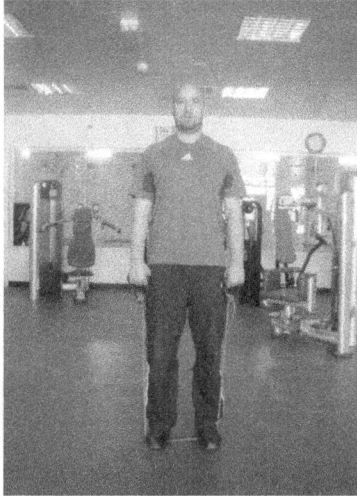

Select a low resistance to start with until you have mastered the technique and position yourself in the standing position with the band secure underneath your feet. Grip the bands firmly with both hands and the bands positioned down and close to the side of your body with straight arms. As you breathe out, engage your abdominals and raise the bands up, level with your shoulders with your elbows high and hold. Attempt to keep the bands level and your arms bent at the elbow. Breathe in as you return to the start position and repeat.

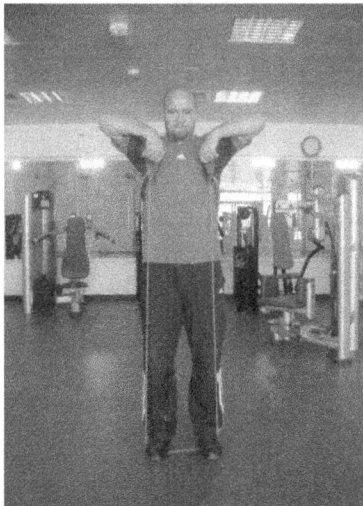

SHOULDER EXERCISES USING A FIT-BALL

Isometric Holds

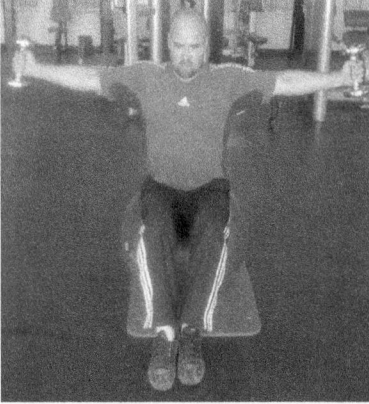
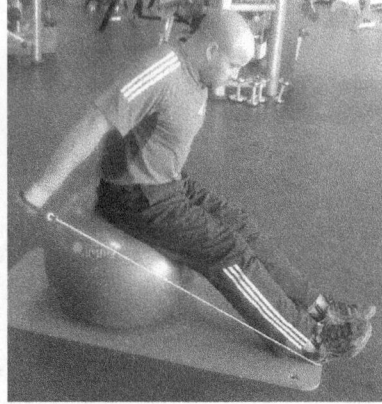

Whichever hold you are doing you must ensure that wherever possible your posture is good i.e. maintaining body alignment with your head, eyes, shoulders and hips inline and facing forwards as much as possible. Your abdominals should be initiated prior and during each hold with your shoulders relaxed as much as possible. All of the above movements are explained in the exercises to follow; therefore all you are doing is mimicking those muscle actions and placing a hold within the ranges, your breathing should remain controlled and should not be forced.

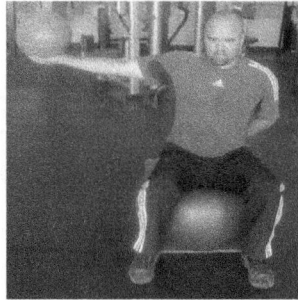
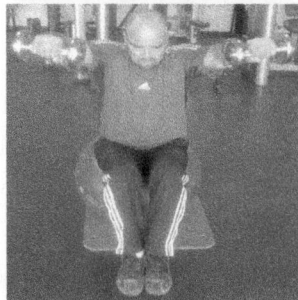

Shoulder Press

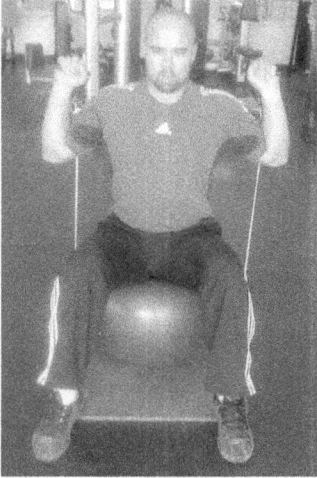

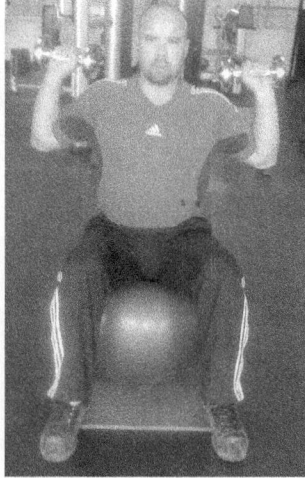

Select a safe weight to start with until you have mastered the technique and position yourself on the fit-ball with your feet flat on the floor and level. Grip the weights firmly with one or both hands and position your hand(s) just above the height of your shoulder(s) with your elbow(s) low and close to the side of your body. As you breathe out, engage your abdominals and raise the resistance up and above your head with your arms outstretched and hold, breathe in as you return to the start position and repeat

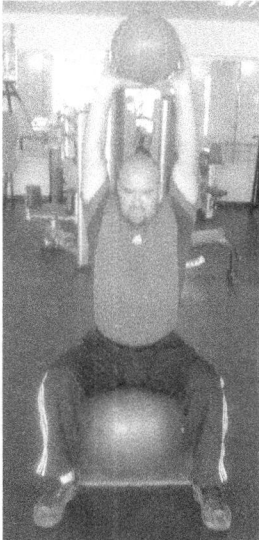

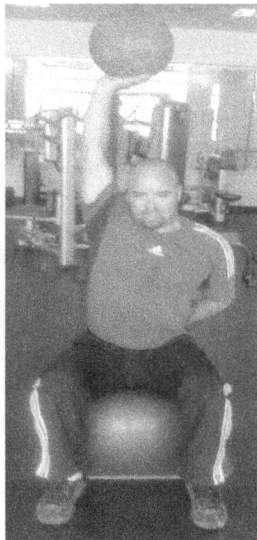

Frontal Raise

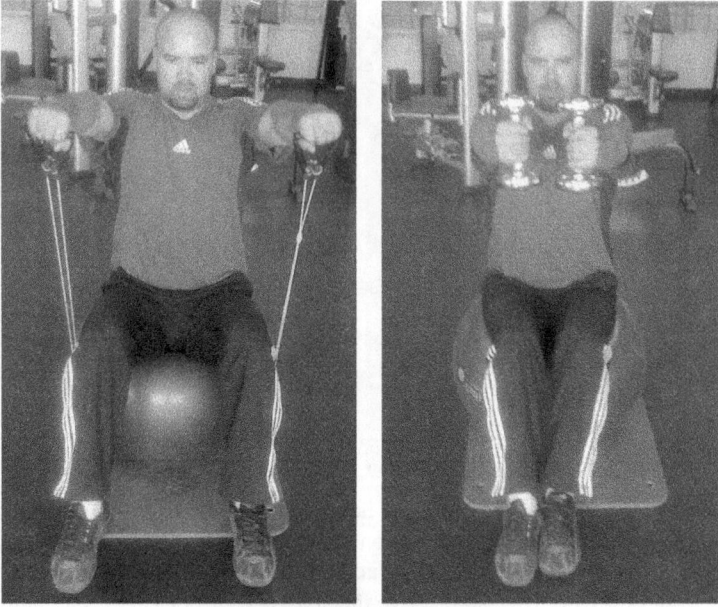

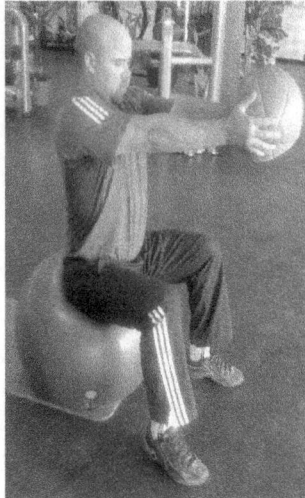

Select a safe weight to start with until you have mastered the technique and position yourself on the fit-ball with your feet flat on the floor and level. Grip the weights firmly with both hands and initially they should be positioned down and close to the front of the body with both arms straight. As you breathe out, engage your abdominals and raise the weights up and level with your shoulders and hold. Attempt to keep them level, along with keeping your arm straight, albeit with a very slight bend at the elbow to avoid injury. Keep your shoulders relaxed and breathe in as you return to the start position and repeat.

Lateral Raise

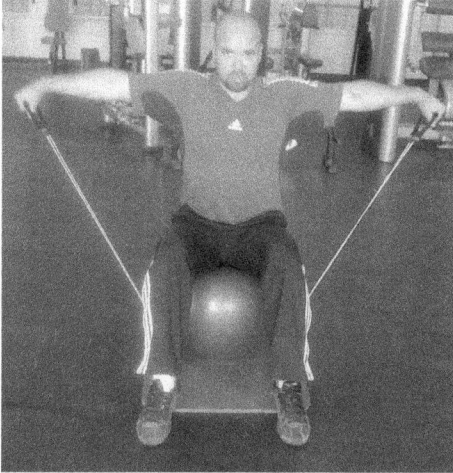

Select a safe weight to start with until you have mastered the technique and position yourself on the fit-ball with your feet flat on the floor and level. Grip the weights firmly with both hands and initially they should be positioned down and close to the side of the body with both arms straight. As you breathe out, engage your abdominals and raise the weights out to the side and level with your shoulders and hold. Attempt to keep them level, along with keeping your arm straight, albeit with a very slight bend at the elbow to avoid injury. Breathe in as you return to the start position and repeat.

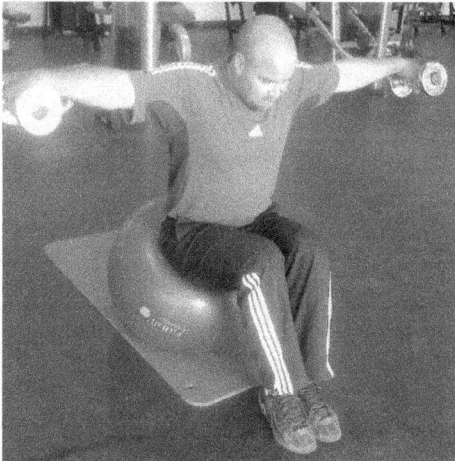

Prone lying raises

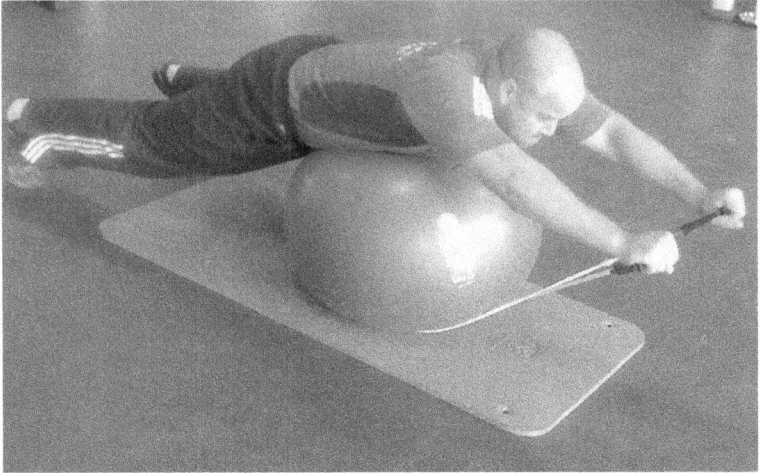

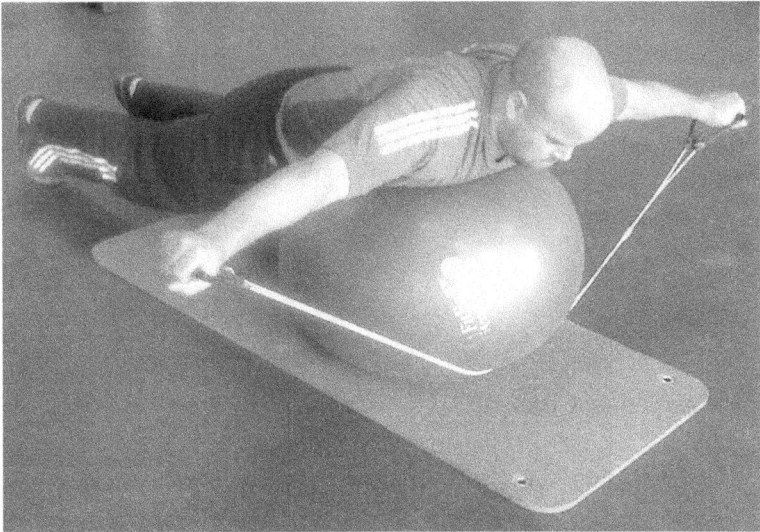

Select a safe resistance to start with until you have mastered the technique and position yourself lying on the ball with your legs in a stable position for balance but level. Grip the bands firmly with both hands and initially they should be positioned down and close to the ball with both arms relaxed. As you breathe out, engage your abdominals and raise the bands up level with your shoulders and beyond if possible and hold. Attempt to keep the bands level along with keeping your arms straight albeit with a very slight bend at the elbow to avoid injury. Breathe in as you return to the start position and repeat. Advance with your feet as you get more confident (read intro)

Fit-ball Caterpillar

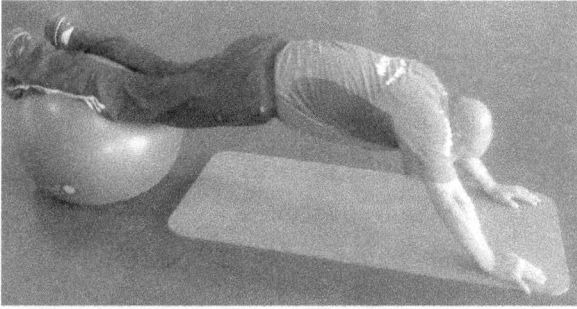

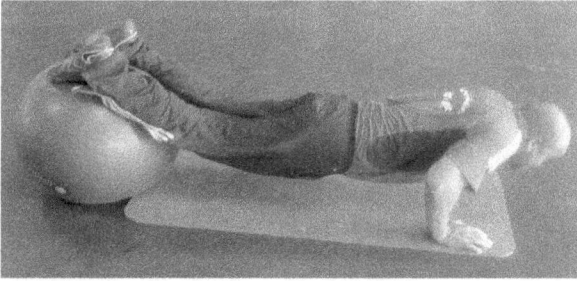

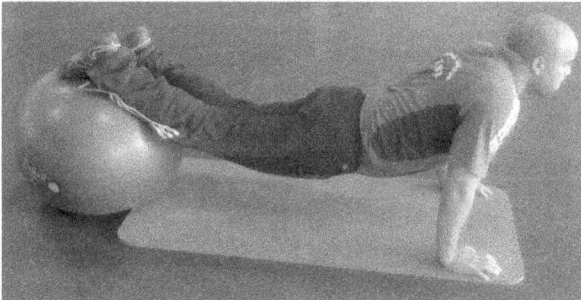

With your feet on the ball, your hands level on the floor and around shoulder width apart, hold your body in a V position as best you can with your backside raised up slightly. Throughout all 3 movements your abdominals should be initiated and as you breathe out you should roll your bodyweight forwards using only your shoulders, roll down and forwards bending your arms at the elbows until your chest almost brushes the ground and then roll upwards straightening your arms and hold. Breathe in until you reverse the movement by rolling your shoulders in the opposite direction until you are back in the start position. Repeat the movement but keep the shoulders pulled down and backwards as much as possible which will ensure that your upper spine and head are relaxed and not under too much tension.

SHOULDER EXERCISES USING MACHINES

Shoulder Press machines

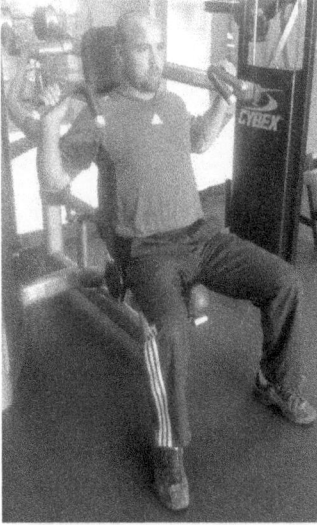

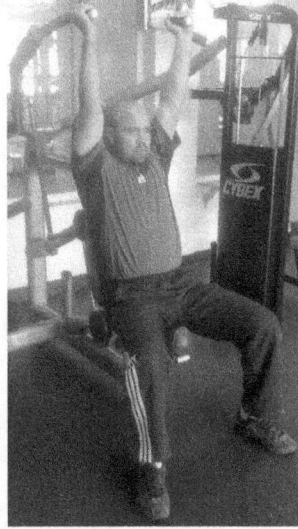

Select a safe weight to start with until you have mastered the technique and position yourself in the seated position with your hips/knees at 90 degrees and your back straight. Grip the bar firmly (choose grip-above) with the bar positioned on either the front or rear of your shoulders (dependant on machine) with your elbows low and close to the side of your body. As you breathe out, engage your abdominals and raise the bar up and above your head with your arms outstretched and hold. Be aware of keeping your arms straight, breathe in as you return to the start position and repeat.

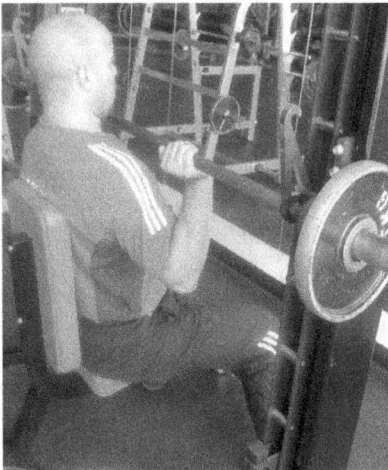

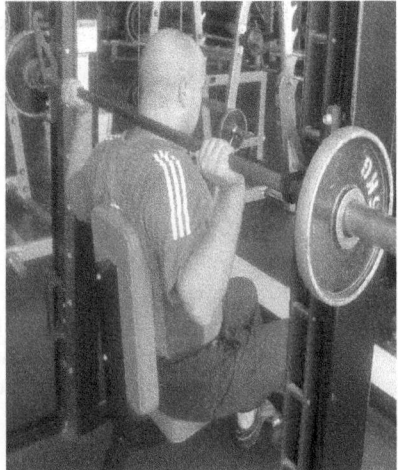

Forward raise (cable)

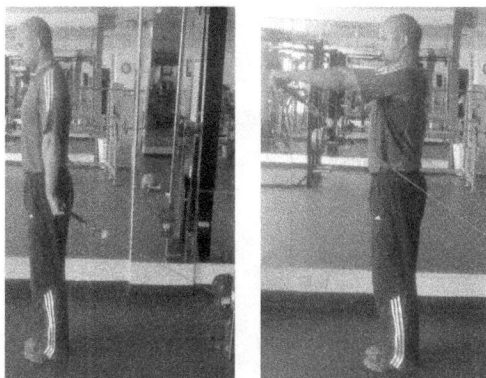

Select a safe weight to start with until you have mastered the technique and position yourself in the standing upright position with your knees slightly bent. Grip the cable firmly with it positioned behind you, close to the side of your body with your shoulders relaxed. As you breathe out, engage your abdominals and raise the cable up in front and level with your shoulder with an outstretched arm and hold. Attempt to keep the cable level, along with keeping your arm straight albeit with a very slight bend at the elbow to avoid injury. Breathe in as you return to the start position and repeat.

Rear Deltoid (cable)

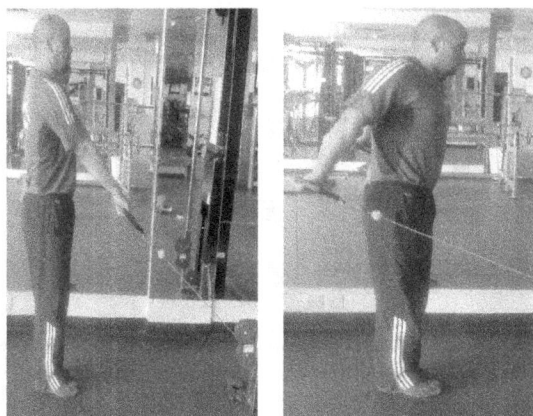

Select a safe weight to start with until you have mastered the technique and position yourself in the standing upright position with your legs around shoulder width apart and level. Grip the cable firmly with your arm outstretched in front of you, with your shoulders relaxed. As you breathe out, engage your abdominals and pull the cable to-wards you and then away from the rear of your body and hold. Keep your arm straight throughout the movement and the cable level, attempt to relax the shoulders and stick your chest out. Breathe in as you return to the start position and repeat.

Lateral Raise (cable)

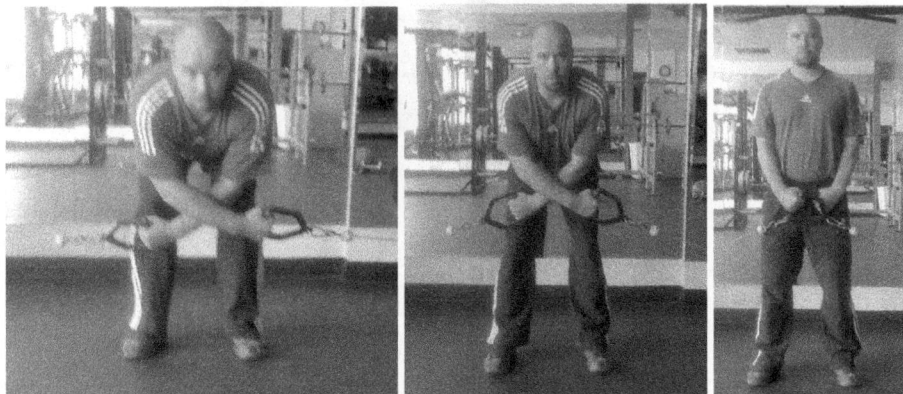

Select a safe weight to start with until you have mastered the technique and position yourself in either of the start positions above, with your legs around shoulder width apart and level. Grip the (crossed) cables firmly, positioned down and close to the centre of your body with semi straight arms. As you breathe out, engage your abdominals and raise the cables up and level with your shoulder (and slightly beyond if possible) with an outstretched arm and hold. Attempt to keep the cables level along with keeping your arms straight albeit with a very slight bend at the elbow to avoid injury. Breathe in as you return to the start position and repeat.

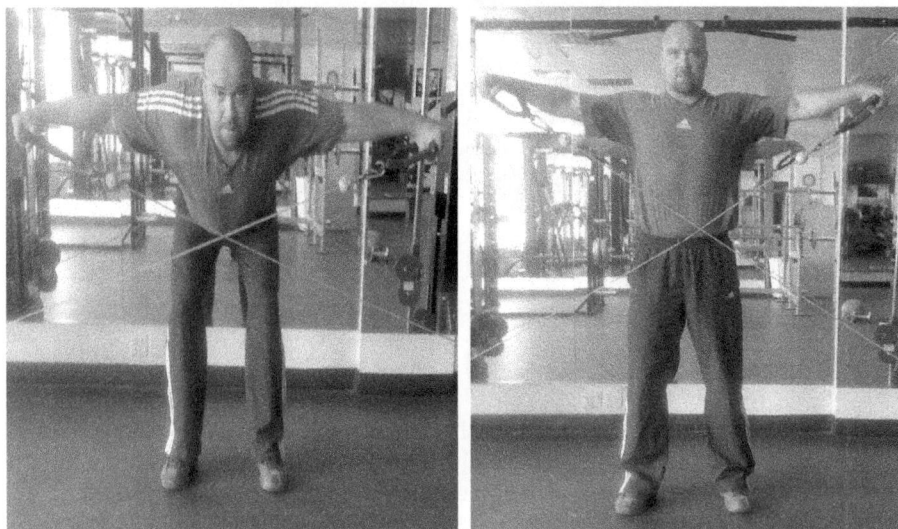

Medial Deltoid –Single Arm (cable)

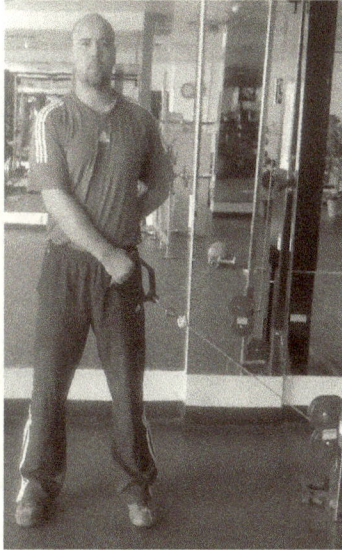

Select a safe weight to start with until you have mastered the technique and position yourself in the standing upright position with your legs around shoulder width apart and level. Grip the cable firmly with an outstretched arm, the cable should initially be positioned in front and down to the opposite side to the outstretched arm. Ensure that your body starts off with good form and posture and maintains it throughout. As you breathe out, engage your abdominals whilst raising the cable up, out to the side and level with your shoulder with an outstretched arm and hold. Attempt to keep the cable level, along with keeping your arm straight throughout the movement (albeit with a very slight bend at the elbow to avoid injury). Breathe in as you return to the start position and repeat.

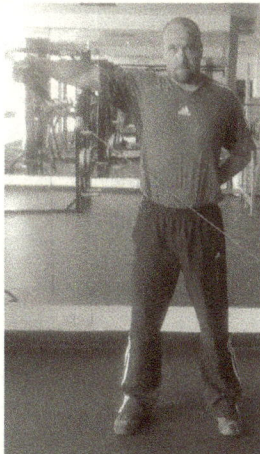

SHOULDER EXERCISES USING A BARBELL

Isometric holds

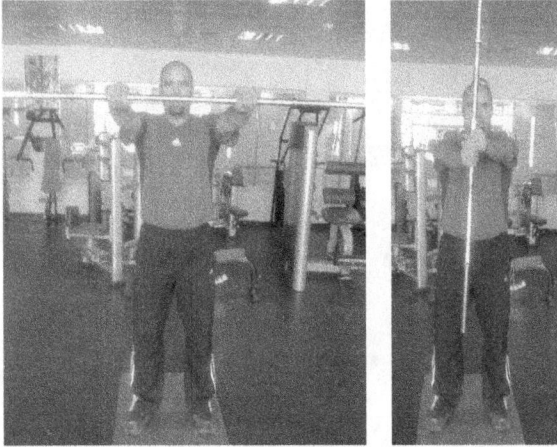

Select a safe weight to start with until you have mastered the technique and position yourself in the standing upright position with your legs around shoulder width apart and level. Grip a weighted bar firmly with one or both hands. Your hand should be either in the centre of the bar or equal distance apart from the centre. Initially the bar should be positioned close to the front of the body with straight arm(s). As you breathe out, engage your abdominals and raise the bar up and level with your shoulders and hold for as long as you can maintain good posture. Attempt to keep the bar level along with keeping your arm straight albeit with a very slight bend at the elbow to avoid injury. When you feel your posture and good form faltering, breathe in as you return to the start position and repeat.

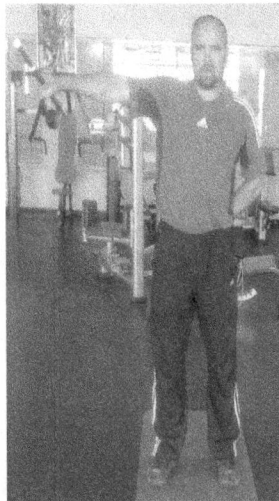

Frontal Raise

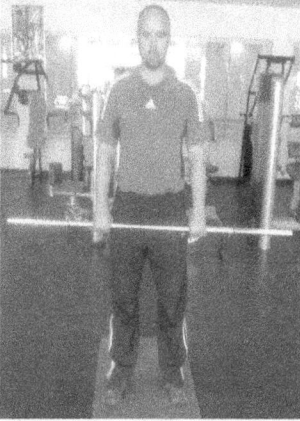

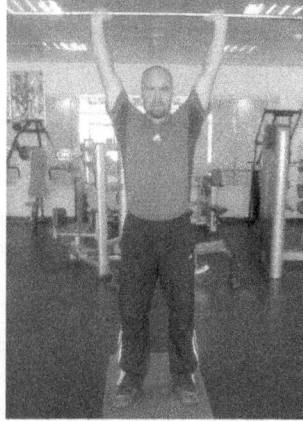

Select a safe weight to start with until you have mastered the technique and position yourself in the standing upright position with your legs around shoulder width apart and level. Grip a weighted bar firmly with one or both hands. Your hand(s) should be either in the centre of the bar or equal distance apart from the centre. Initially the bar should be positioned down and close to the front of the body with one or both straight arm(s). As you breathe out, engage your abdominals and raise the bar up and level with your shoulders and hold. Attempt to keep the bar level, along with keeping your arm straight, albeit with a very slight bend at the elbow to avoid injury. Breathe in as you return to the start position and repeat.

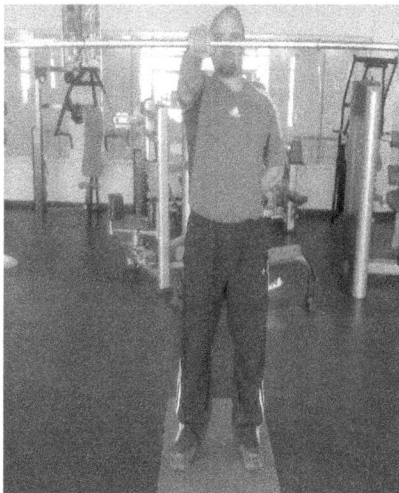

Rear Deltoid

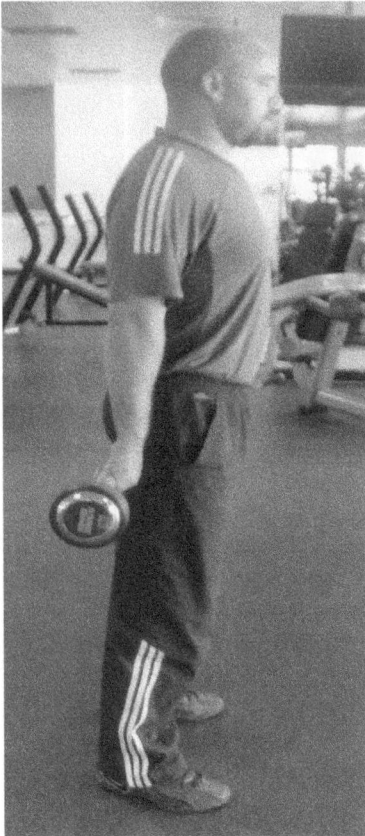

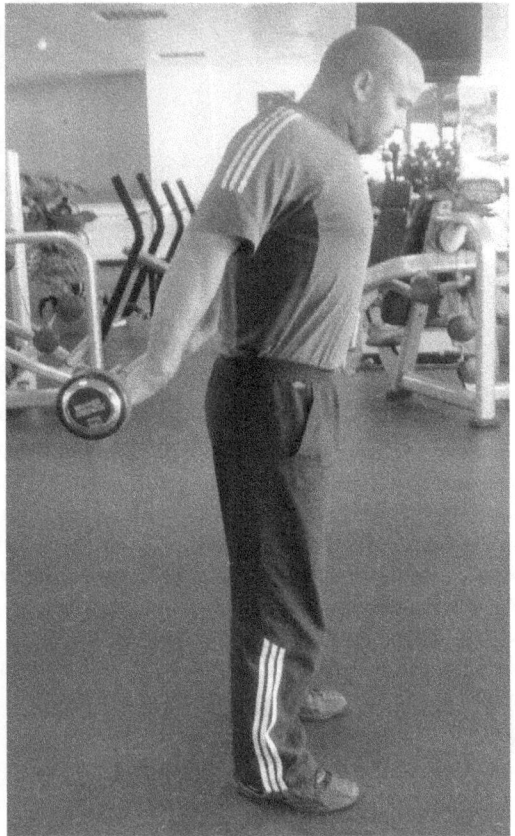

Select a safe weight to start with until you have mastered the technique and position yourself in the standing upright position with your legs around shoulder width apart and level. Grip a weighted bar firmly with both hands. Your hands should be equal distance apart from the centre of the bar and initially the bar should be positioned down and close to the rear of your body with straight arms. As you breathe out, engage your abdominals and raise the bar away from the rear of your body and hold. Attempt to keep the bar level, along with keeping your arms straight, attempt to relax the shoulders and stick your chest out. Breathe in as you return to the start position and repeat.

Shoulder Press

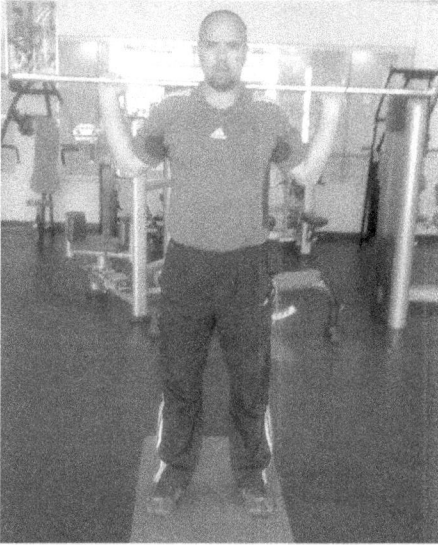

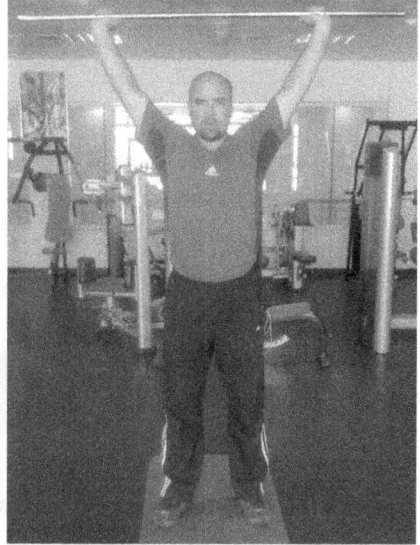

Select a safe weight to start with until you have mastered the technique and position yourself in the standing upright position with your legs around shoulder width apart and level. Grip a weighted bar firmly with both hands, your hands should be equal distance apart from the centre of the bar. Initially the bar should be positioned on either the front or rear of your shoulders with your elbows low and close to the side of your body. As you breathe out, engage your abdominals and raise the bar up and above your head with your arms outstretched and hold. Attempt to keep the bar level and breathe in as you return to the start position and repeat.

An alternative ex is the **push press exercise** – Start with the bar either in front of or behind the neck. Keep the body upright, dip downward until you are at about a quarter-squat position, and then forcefully drive upward with your legs, using this power and momentum to drive the weight over your head. Control the weight back as you lower it down to your shoulders. As you drive your legs on this movement shift onto your toes., and your legs should be straight when the weight is locked out over your head.

Lateral Raise

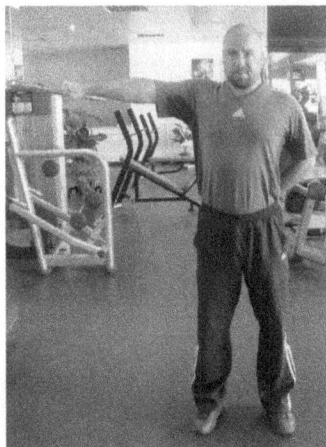

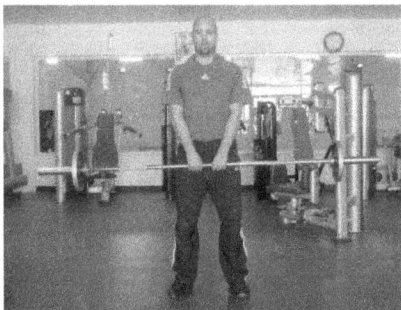

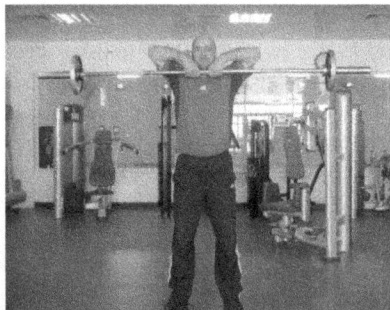

Select a safe weight to start with until you have mastered the technique and position yourself in the standing upright position with your legs around shoulder width apart and level. Grip a weighted bar firmly with one hand and ensure that your hand is in the centre of the bar. Initially the bar should be positioned down and close to the side of your body with a straight arm. As you breathe out, engage your abdominals and raise the bar up and level with your shoulder with an outstretched arm and hold. Attempt to keep the bar level, along with keeping your arm straight albeit with a very slight bend at the elbow to avoid injury. Breathe in as you return to the start position and repeat.

Upright row

Select a safe weight to start with until you have mastered the technique, and position yourself in the standing position with the bar in both hands positioned down and close to the front of your body with straight arms. As you breathe out, engage your abdominals and raise the bar up, level with your shoulders with your elbows high and hold. Attempt to keep the bar level and your arms bent at the elbow. Breathe in as you return to the start position and repeat.

SHOULDER EXERCISES USING DUMBBELLS

Shoulder Press

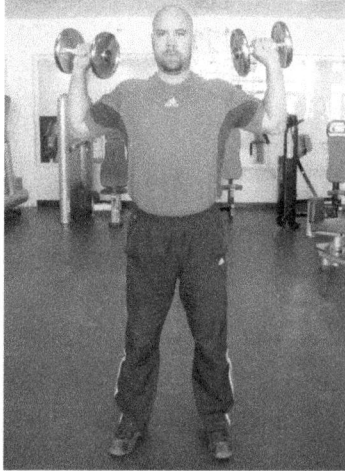

Select a safe weight to start with until you have mastered the technique and position yourself in the standing upright position with your legs around shoulder width apart and level, knees slightly bent. Grip the weights firmly with both hands and initially they should be positioned just above the height of your shoulders with your elbows low and close to the side of your body. As you breathe out, engage your abdominals and raise the weights up and above your head with your arms outstretched and hold. Attempt to keep the weights level along with keeping your arms straight, breathe in as you return to the start position and repeat.

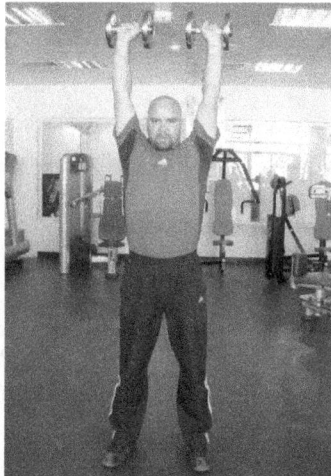

Forward Raise

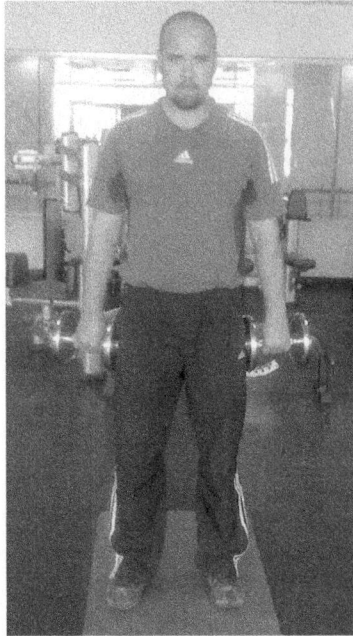

Select a safe weight to start with until you have mastered the technique and position yourself in the standing upright position with your legs around shoulder width apart and level, knees slightly bent. Grip the weights firmly with both hands and initially they should be positioned down and close to the front of the body with both arms straight. As you breathe out, engage your abdominals and raise the weights up and level with your shoulders and hold. Attempt to keep them level, along with keeping your arm straight, albeit with a very slight bend at the elbow to avoid injury. Breathe in as you return to the start position and repeat.

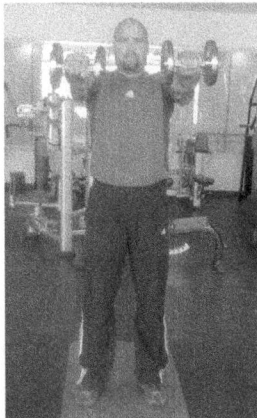

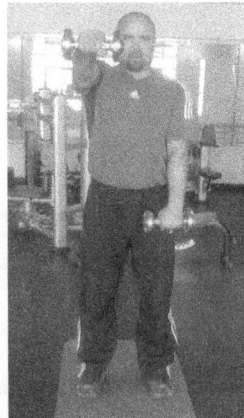

Rear Deltoid

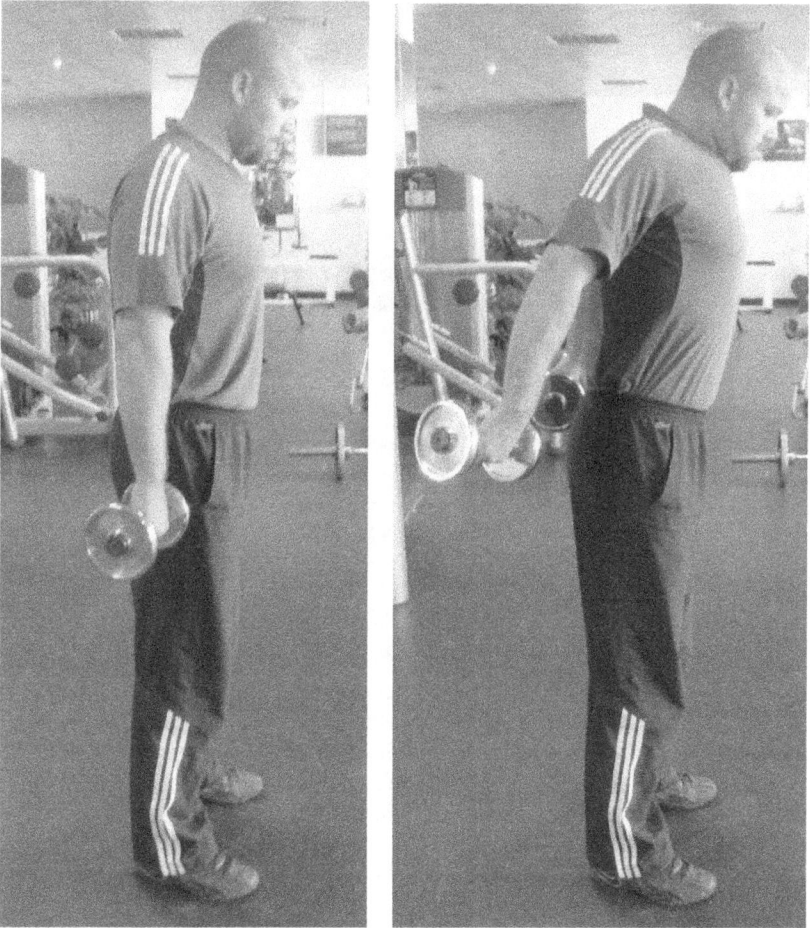

Select a safe weight to start with until you have mastered the technique and position yourself in the standing upright position with your legs around shoulder width apart and level, knees slightly bent. Grip the weights firmly with both hands and initially they should be positioned down and close to the rear of the body with both arms straight. As you breathe out, engage your abdominals and raise the weights away from your body and hold. Attempt to keep your arms straight, with your shoulders as relaxed as possible. Breathe in as you return to the start position and repeat.

Bent Over Flyes

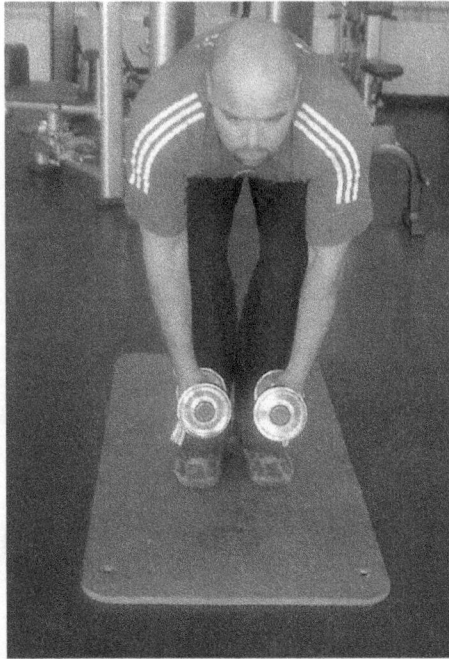

Select a safe weight to start with until you have mastered the technique and position yourself in the (forward) bent over position with your legs in a stable position for balance but level. Grip the weights firmly with both hands and initially they should be positioned down and close to the front of the body with both arms straight. As you breathe out, engage your abdominals and raise the weights up level with your shoulders and beyond if possible and hold. Attempt to keep the weights level along with keeping your arms straight albeit with a very slight bend at the elbow to avoid injury. Breathe in as you return to the start position and repeat.

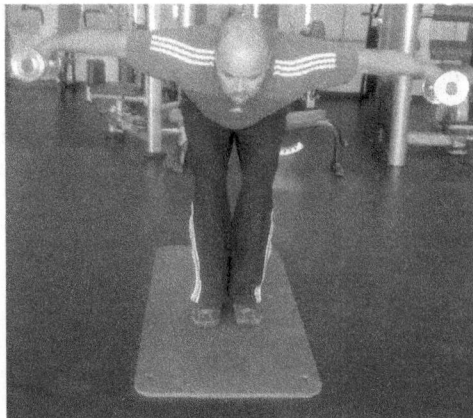

Lateral Raise

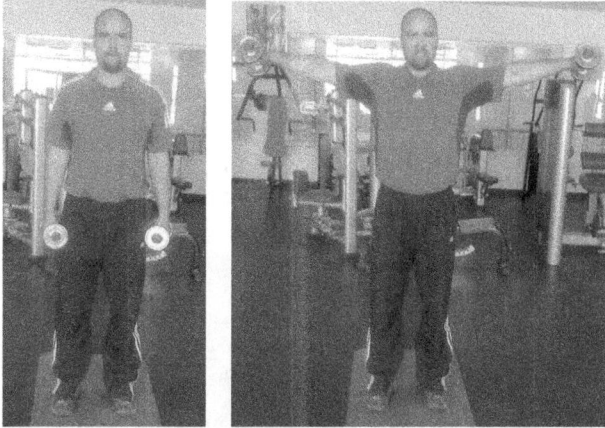

Select a safe weight to start with until you have mastered the technique and position yourself in the standing upright position with your legs around shoulder width apart and level, knees slightly bent. Grip the weights firmly with both hands and initially they should be positioned down and close to the side of the body with both arms straight. As you breathe out, engage your abdominals and raise the weights out to the side and level with your shoulders and hold. Attempt to keep them level, along with keeping your arm straight, albeit with a very slight bend at the elbow to avoid injury. Breathe in as you return to the start position and repeat.

Upright row

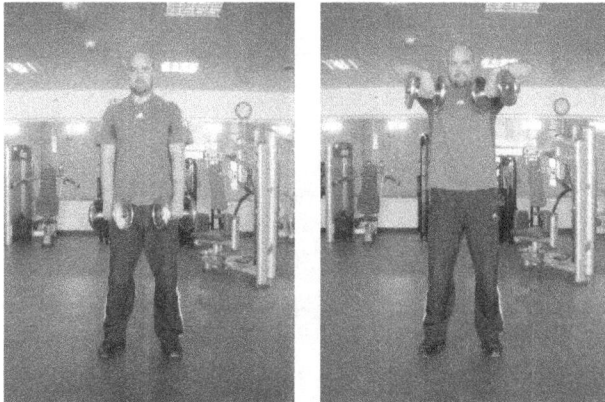

Select a safe weight to start with until you have mastered the technique, and position yourself in the standing position with the dumbbells in both hands positioned down and close to the front of your body with straight arms. As you breathe out, engage your abdominals and raise the dumbbells up, level with your shoulders with your elbows high and hold. Attempt to keep the dumbbells level and your arms bent at the elbow. Breathe in as you return to the start position and repeat.

MOST COMMON BICEP EXERCISES

USING YOUR OWN BODYWEIGHT

Isometric hold

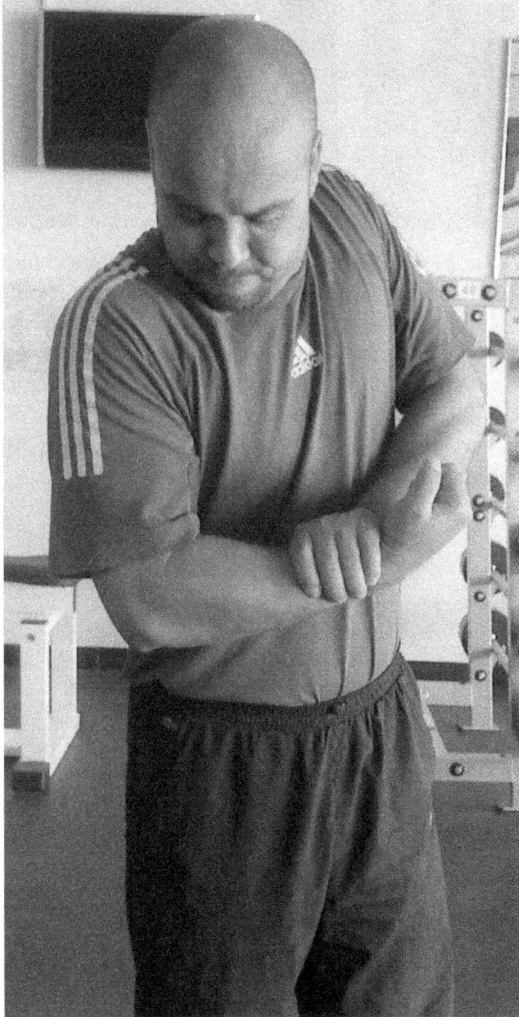

Bend one of your elbows at any range and hold the wrist with your other hand, apply a resistance and attempt to fully bend your arm whilst applying a greater force. Try resisting throughout all of the ranges, hold and repeat.

Partner Resisted Holds

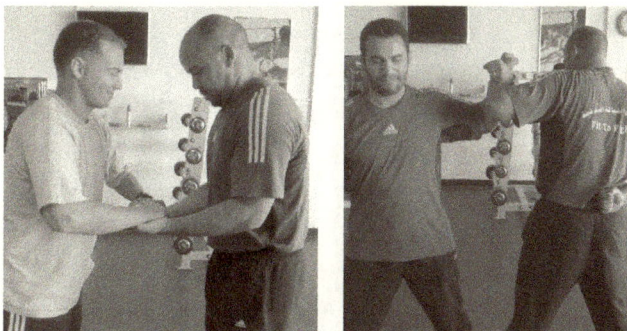

Bend one or both of your elbows at any range whilst your partner holds your arm(s) ensure he/she applies a resistance as you attempt to fully bend your arm(s) as your partner applies a greater force. Try resisting throughout all of the ranges; hold and repeat (attempt both methods, left & right pictures).

Under-grasp pull ups

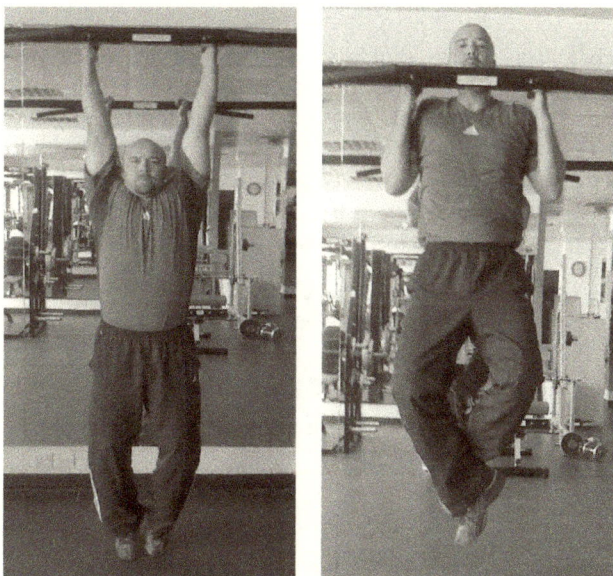

Allow your body to hang in a straight line (under grasp) as you ensure that you have a tight grip on the pull up bar. Initiate your abdominals as you breathe out, pull your bodyweight up and attempt to get your chin above your hands whilst bending your arms only. Hold the position for 2-3 seconds, breathe in, lower your body under control and repeat.

Behind the neck pull ups

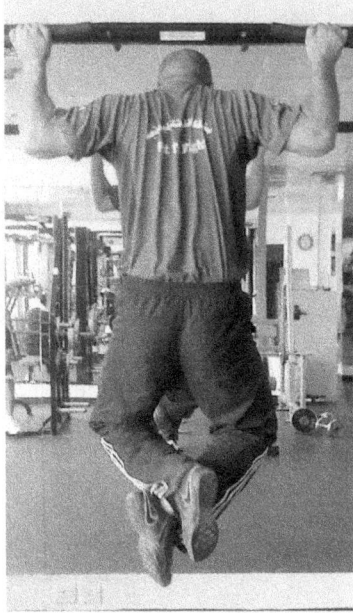

Allow your body to hang in a straight line (wide grip) as you ensure that you have a tight grip on the pull up bar. Initiate your abdominals as you breathe out, pull your bodyweight up and attempt to get the back of your neck level with your hands whilst bending your arms only. Hold the position for 2-3 seconds, breathe in, lower your body under control and repeat.

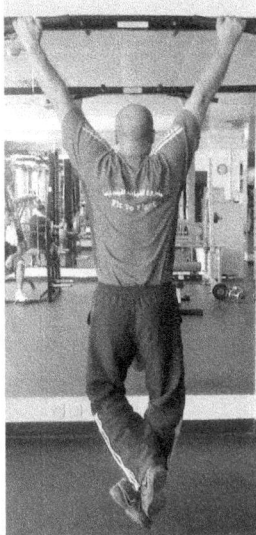

BICEP EXERCISES USING RESISTANCE BANDS

Isometric Hold

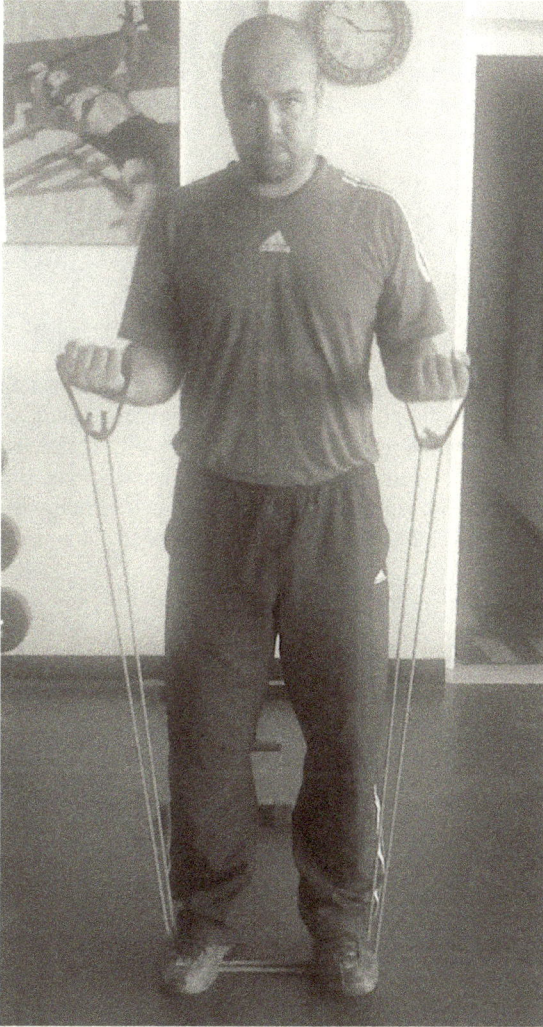

Select a safe resistance to start with until you have mastered the technique and position yourself in the standing upright position with your legs around shoulder width apart, slightly bent and level. Grip the resistance bands firmly with both hands and close to the side of your body with straight arms. As you breathe out, engage your abdominals and raise the bands up to the midway position by bending your elbows and hold. Attempt to hold for a long enough period and then breathe in as you slowly return to the start position and repeat.

Standing Curls

Both arms   Single arm

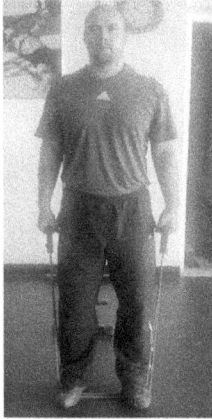 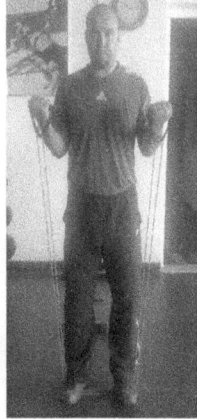 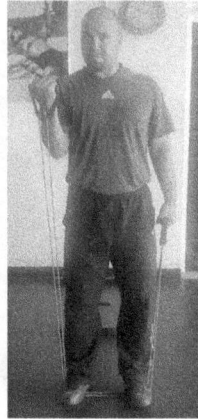

Select a safe resistance to start with until you have mastered the technique and position yourself in the standing upright position with your legs around shoulder width apart, slightly bent and level. Grip the resistance bands firmly with both hands and positioned down and close to the side of your body with straight arms. As you breathe out, engage your abdominals and raise the bands up fully by bending your elbows and hold. Attempt to keep the bands level and breathe in as you slowly return to the start position and repeat.

Overhead Pull

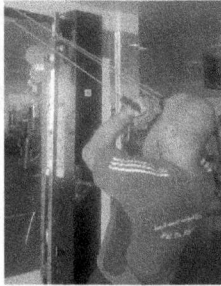 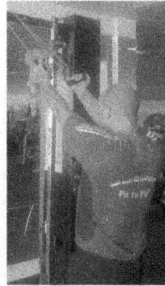

Select a safe resistance to start with until you have mastered the technique, position yourself in the standing position (leaning back slightly) with your legs around shoulder width apart, slightly bent and level. Hook the bands overhead to a sturdy object and grip the resistance bands firmly with both hands. Position the bands in front of you and above your head with straight arms (picture below). As you breathe out, engage your abdominals and pull the bands towards you fully by bending your elbows and hold. Attempt to keep the bands level and breathe in as you slowly return to the start position and repeat.

Bent over curl

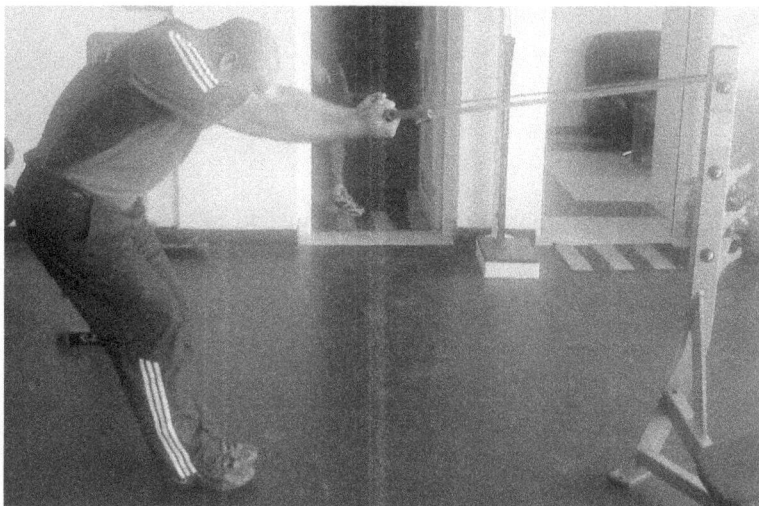

Select a safe resistance to start with until you have mastered the technique and position yourself in the standing position (bent over slightly) with your legs in a balanced stance, slightly bent and level. Hook the bands to a sturdy object around chest height and grip the resistance bands firmly with both hands. Position the bands in front of you and ensure your arms are straight (picture above). As you breathe out, engage your abdominals and pull the bands towards you fully by bending your elbows and hold. Attempt to keep the bands level and breathe in as you slowly return to the start position and repeat.

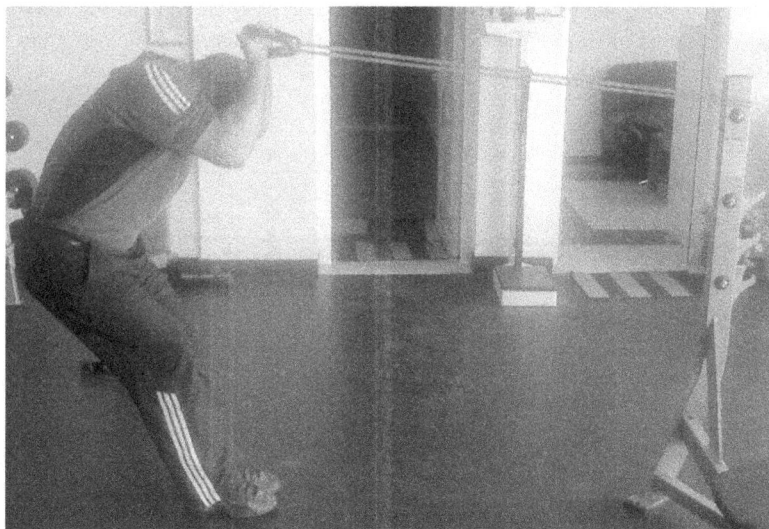

BICEP EXERCISES USING A FIT-BALL

Isometric Holds

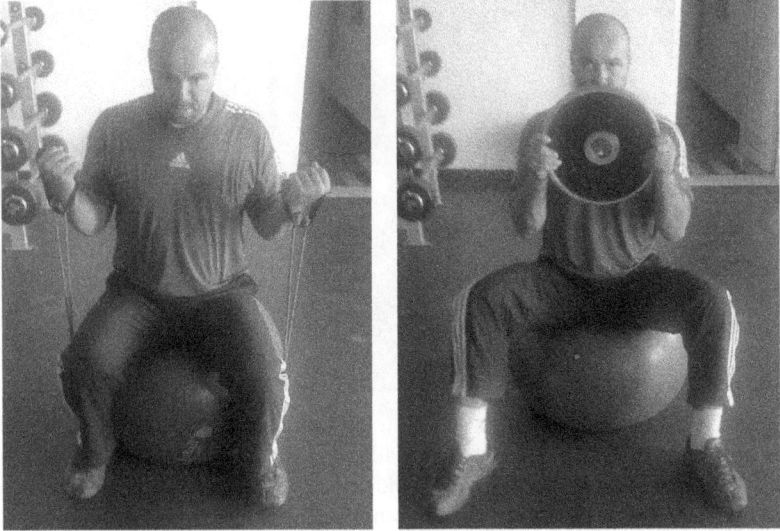

Select a safe resistance/weight to start with until you have mastered the technique and position yourself in the seated position on a fit-ball with your legs in a balanced position and level. Grip the bands/weight(s) firmly with one or both hand(s) and positioned down and close to the body with straight arms. As you breathe out, engage your abdominals and raise the resistance/weight(s) up by bending your elbows and hold. Attempt to hold for a challenging length of time and then breathe in as you slowly return to the start position and repeat. Attempt to vary the exercise by completing a single or double arm hold.

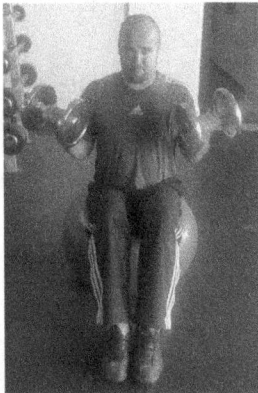

Resistance band curls

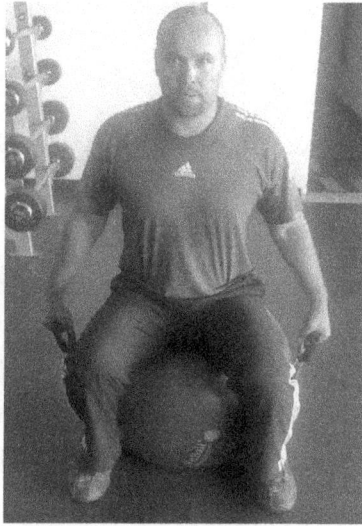

Select a safe resistance to start with until you have mastered the technique and position yourself in the seated position on a fit-ball with your legs in a balanced position and level. Grip the bands firmly with both hands and positioned down and close to the side of your body with straight arms. As you breathe out, engage your abdominals and raise the bands up by bending your elbows and hold. Attempt to keep the bands level and breathe in as you slowly return to the start position and repeat. Attempt to vary the exercise by completing a single or double arm curl.

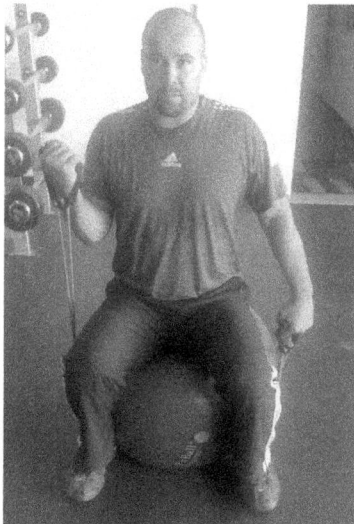

Hammer Curls

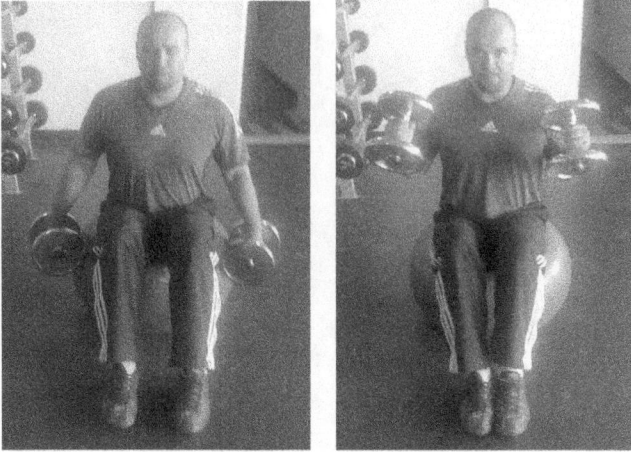

Select a safe weight to start with until you have mastered the technique and position yourself in the seated position on a fit-ball with your legs in a balanced position and level. Grip the weights firmly with both hands (knuckles facing outwards) and positioned down and close to the side of your body with straight arms. As you breathe out, engage your abdominals and raise the dumbbells up fully by bending your elbows and hold. Attempt to keep the weights level and breathe in as you slowly return to the start position and repeat. Attempt to vary the exercise by completing a single or double arm curl (picture below).

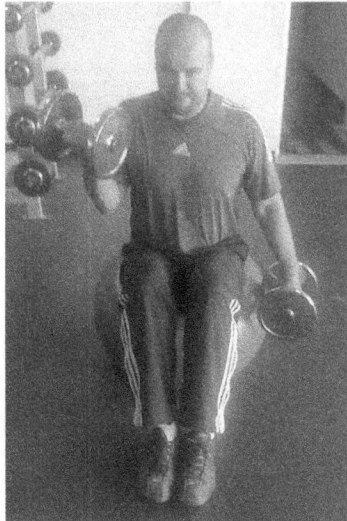

Variation of Curls

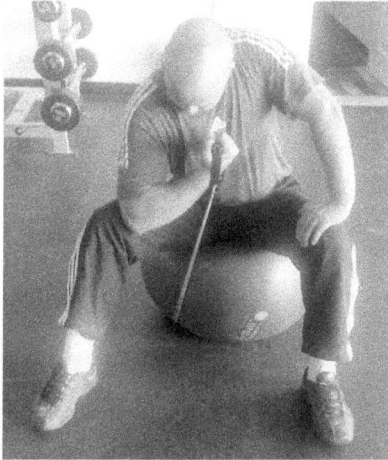

Whichever weight/resistance you use it should be safe enough to start with until you have mastered the technique and position yourself in the seated position on a fit-ball with your legs in a balanced position and level. Grip the resistance/ weight(s) firmly with one or both hands and positioned down with straight arms. As you breathe out, engage your abdominals and raise the resistance/weight(s) up fully by bending your elbows and hold. Attempt to keep the band(s)/weight(s) level and breathe in as you slowly return to the start position and repeat. Attempt to vary the exercise by completing a single or double arm curl (picture below).

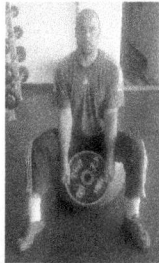

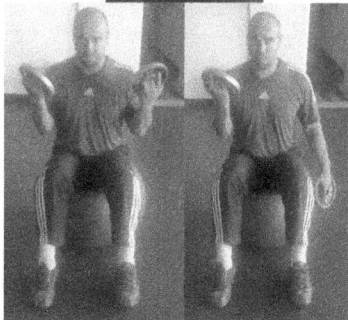

BICEP EXERCISES USING MACHINES

Seated Curls

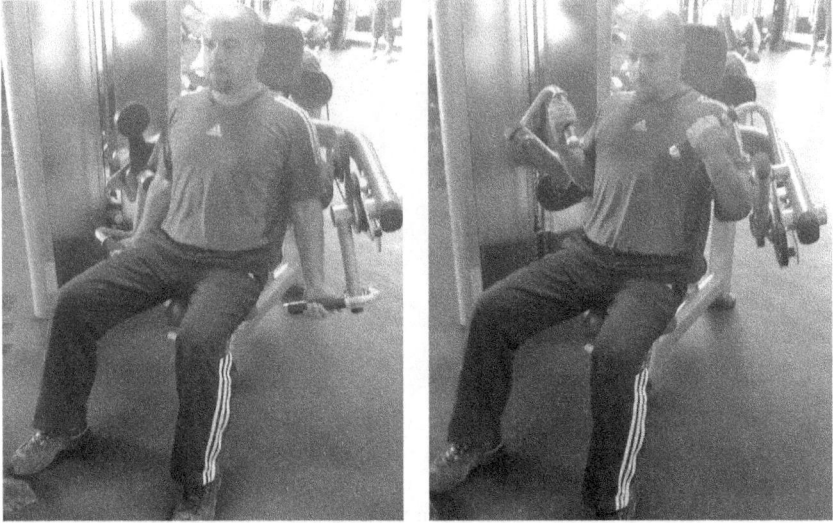

Select a safe weight to start with until you have mastered the technique and position yourself in the seated position with your legs and hips at a 90 degree angle. Grip the handles firmly with both hands with straight arms. As you breathe out, engage your abdominals and raise the resistance up by bending your elbows and hold. Attempt to keep the weights level and breathe in as you slowly return to the start position and repeat. Change to single arm curls (bottom picture).

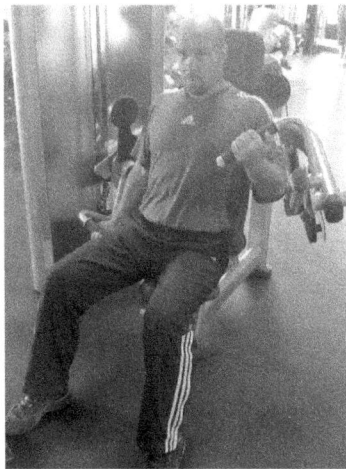

Standing Cable Curls

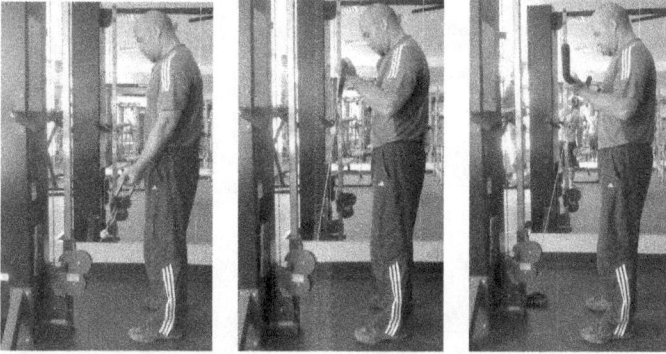

Select a safe weight to start with until you have mastered the technique and position yourself in the standing upright position with your legs around shoulder width apart, slightly bent and level. Grip the cable(s) or bar firmly with one or both hands and close to the side of your body with straight arm(s). As you breathe out, engage your abdominals and raise the resistance up by bending your elbows and hold. Attempt to keep the cable(s) or bar level and breathe in as you slowly return to the start position and repeat

Alternative overhead curls

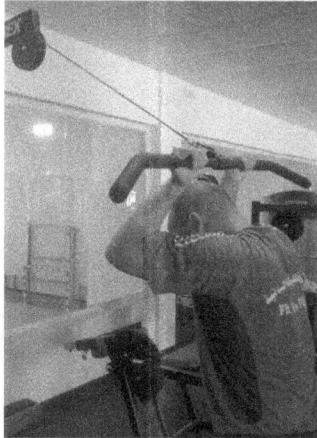

Select a safe weight to start with until you have mastered the technique and position yourself in the standing position behind the lat pull down machine. Grip the bar firmly in front of you but above your head with both hands with straight arms. As you breathe out, engage your abdominals and pull the bar towards you by bending your elbows and hold. Attempt to keep the bar level and breathe in as you slowly return to the start position and repeat.

189

Assisted under-grasp pull ups

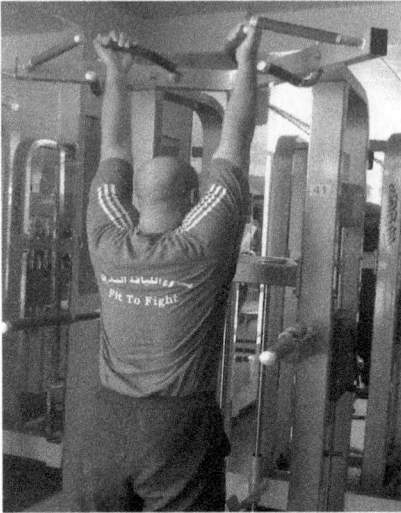

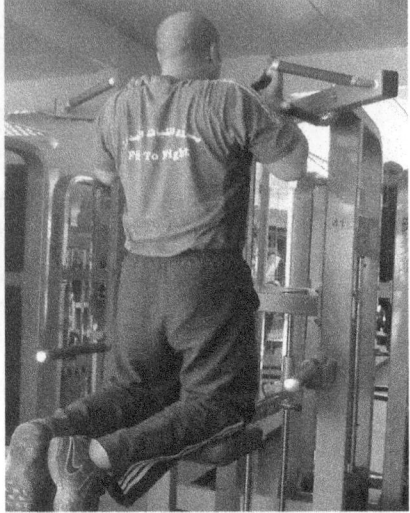

Select a weight that you would like to assist you, i.e. if you weigh 70 kg then you should not select anything higher than that as you will not be achieving anything. The aim is to master the technique first (with assistance) but to gain enough strength to be assisted as little as possible. Most people should be able (in time) to pull themselves up without assistance at all i.e. without this machine. You should start with your arms completely straight and as you breathe out raise up until your chin is level with your hands and breathe in as you lower down under control and repeat accordingly.

Different grips can be used (as shown below)

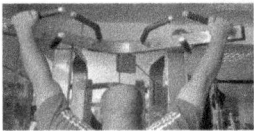

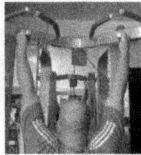

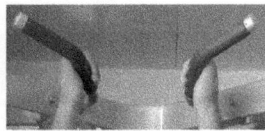

190

BICEP EXERCISES USING A BARBELL

Isometric Hold

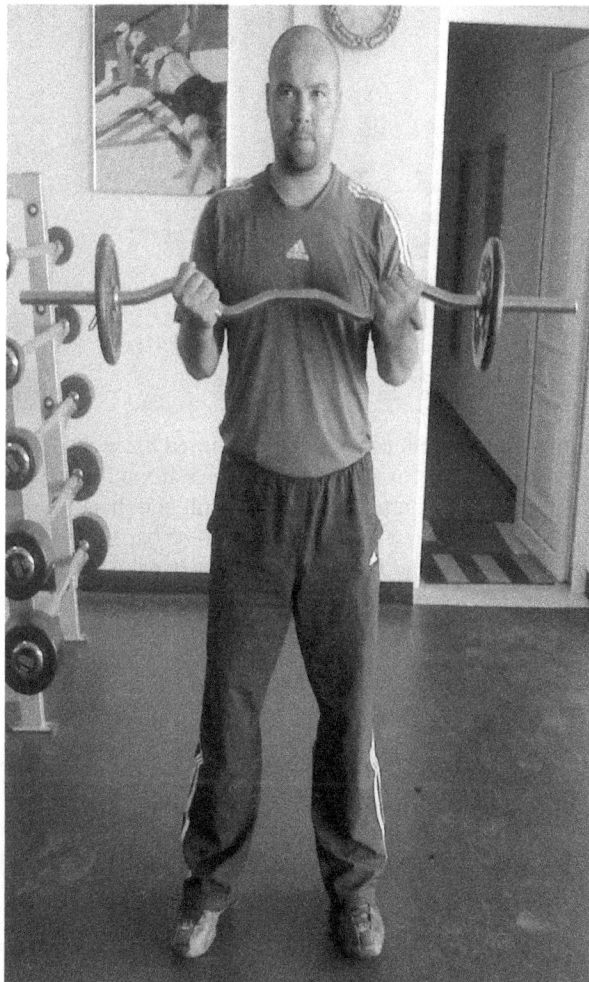

Select a safe weight to start with until you have mastered the technique and position yourself in the standing upright position with your legs around shoulder width apart, slightly bent and level. Grip any weighted bar firmly with both hands and ensure that they are equal distance from the centre of the bar. Initially the bar should be positioned down and close to the front of your body with straight arms. As you breathe out, engage your abdominals and raise the bar up to any range (normally midway) by bending your elbows and hold. Attempt to keep the bar level and hold for a comfortable amount of time, breathe in as you slowly return to the start position and repeat.

Standing Curls

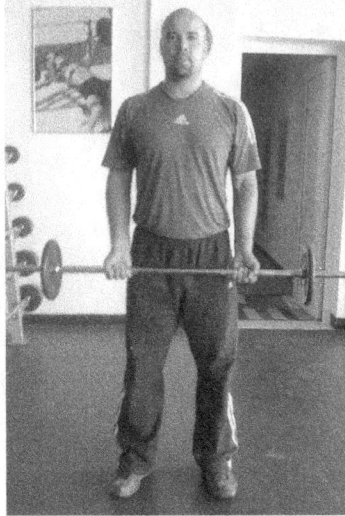

Select a safe weight to start with until you have mastered the technique and position yourself in the standing upright position with your legs around shoulder width apart, slightly bent and level. Grip a weighted bar firmly with both hands and ensure that they are equal distance from the centre of the bar. Initially the bar should be positioned down and close to the front of your body with straight arms. As you breathe out, engage your abdominals and raise the bar up by bending your elbows and hold. Attempt to keep the bar level and breathe in as you slowly return to the start position and repeat.

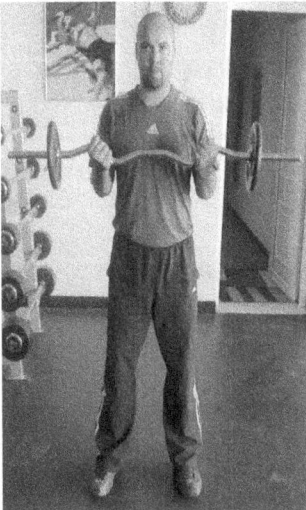

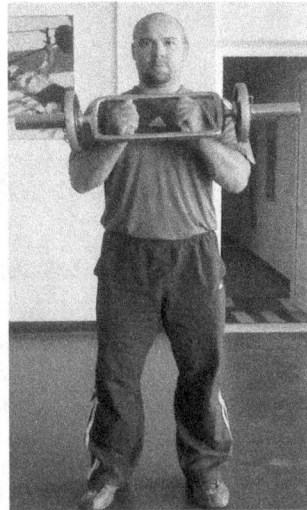

Preacher Curls

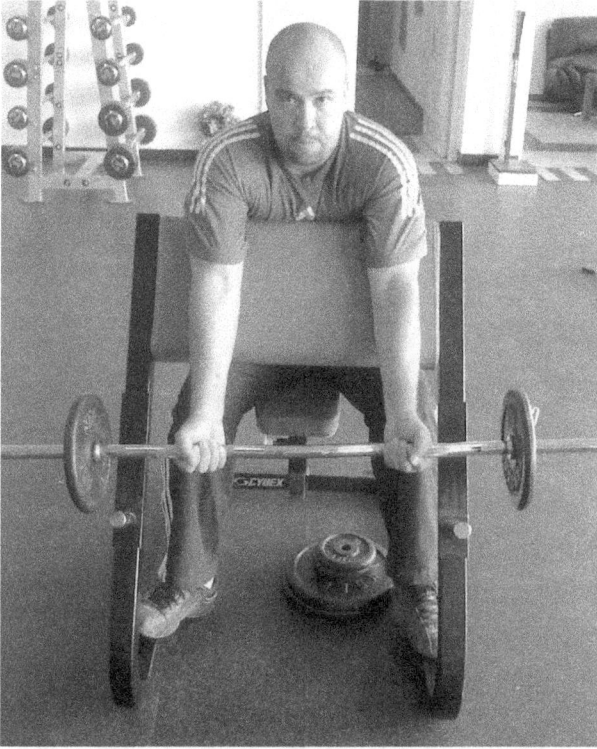

Select a safe weight to start with until you have mastered the technique and position yourself in the standing upright position with your legs around shoulder width apart, slightly bent and level. Grip a weighted bar firmly with both hands and ensure that they are equal distance from the centre of the bar. Initially the bar should be positioned down and close to the front of your body with straight arms. As you breathe out, engage your abdominals and raise the bar up by bending your elbows and hold. Attempt to keep the bar level and breathe in as you slowly return to the start position and repeat.

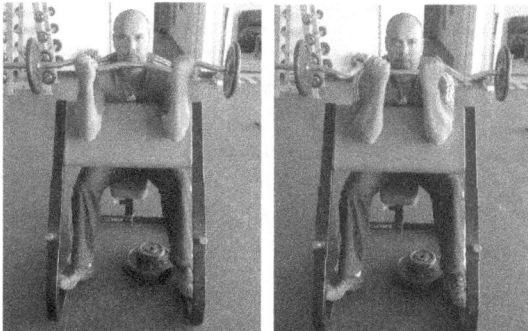

BICEP EXERCISES USING DUMBBELLS

Isometric Hold

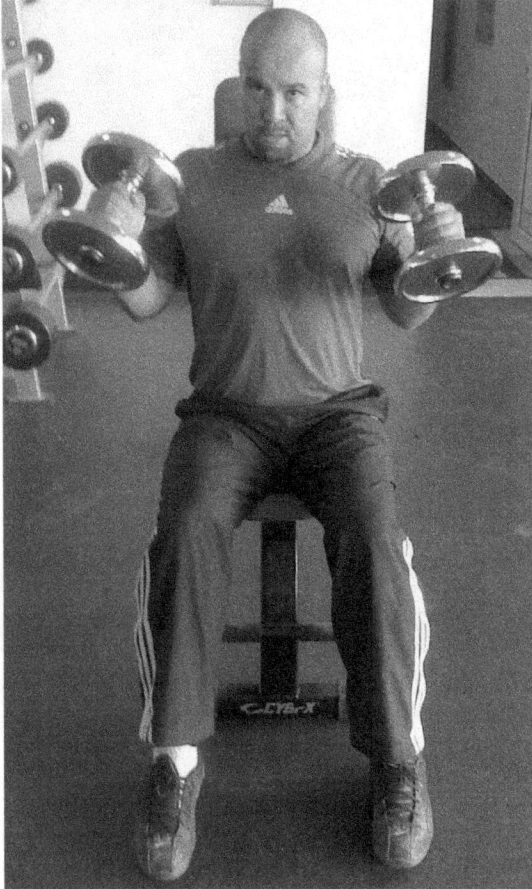

Select a safe weight to start with until you have mastered the technique and position yourself in any position and grip the dumbbell(s) firmly with one or both hands. Initially the weights should be positioned down and close to the side of your body with straight arms. As you breathe out, engage your abdominals and raise the weight(s) up to any range (normally midway) by bending your elbows and hold. Attempt to keep the weight(s) level and hold for a comfortable amount of time, breathe in as you slowly return to the start position and repeat.

Normal & Hammer Curls (standing)

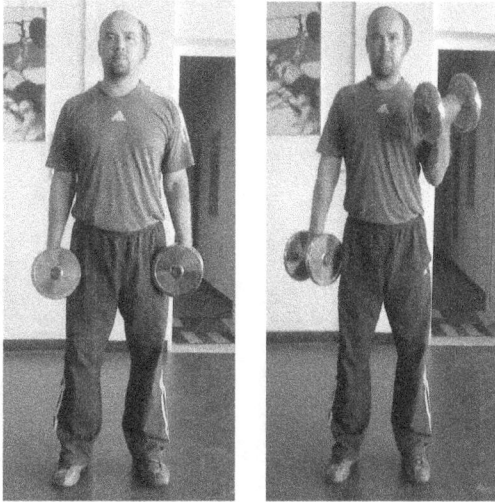

Select a safe weight to start with until you have mastered the technique and position yourself in the standing upright position with your legs around shoulder width apart, slightly bent and level. Grip the weights firmly with both hands and close to the side of your body with straight arms. As you breathe out, engage your abdominals and raise the weights up by bending your elbows and hold. Attempt to keep the weights level and breathe in as you slowly return to the start position and repeat. Change the hand position for hammer curls (right picture).

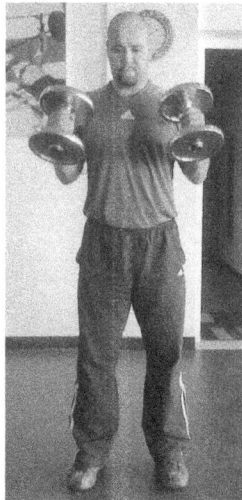

Preacher normal/hammer curls

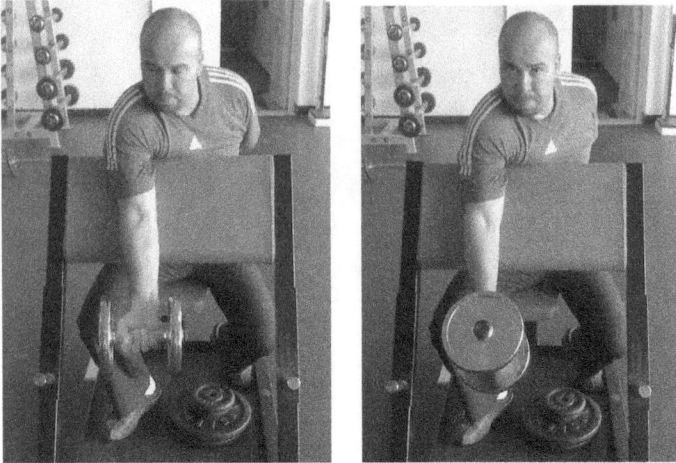

Select a safe weight to start with until you have mastered the technique and position yourself in the seated position within the preacher curl apparatus. Grip the weight(s) firmly with one or both hands on the platform with straight arm(s). As you breathe out, engage your abdominals and raise the weight(s) up by bending your elbows and hold. Attempt to keep the weight(s) level and breathe in as you slowly return to the start position and repeat. Change the hand position for hammer curls (right picture).

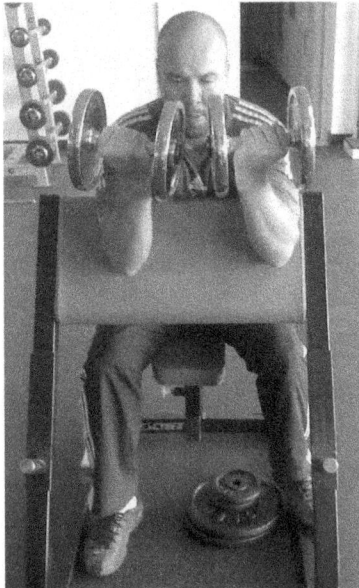

Normal & Hammer Curls (seated)

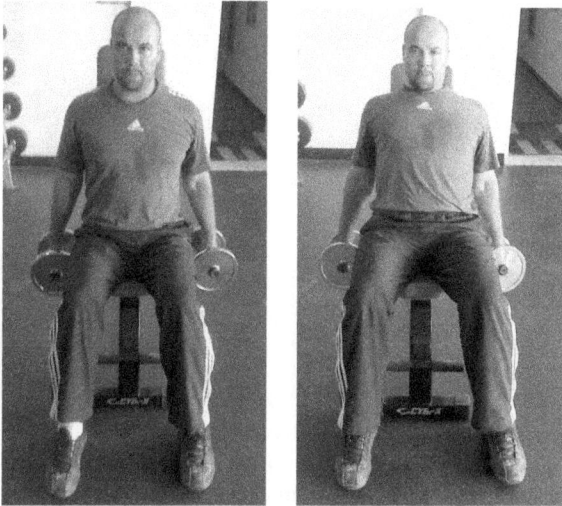

Select a safe weight to start with until you have mastered the technique and position yourself in the upright or inclined seated position. Grip the weight(s) firmly with one or both hands with straight arm(s). As you breathe out, engage your abdominals and raise the weight(s) up by bending your elbows and hold. Attempt to keep the weight(s) level and breathe in as you slowly return to the start position and repeat. Change the hand position for hammer curls (below right picture).

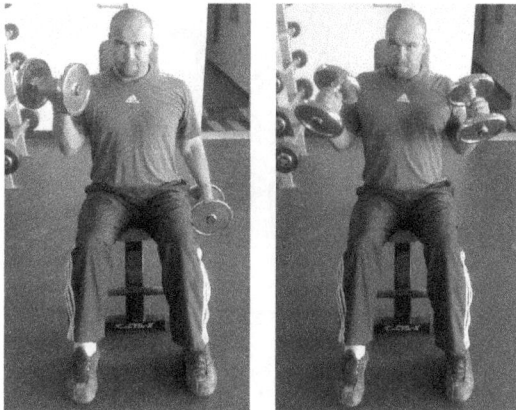

Seated or bent over curl

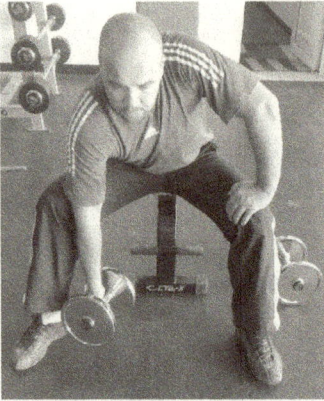

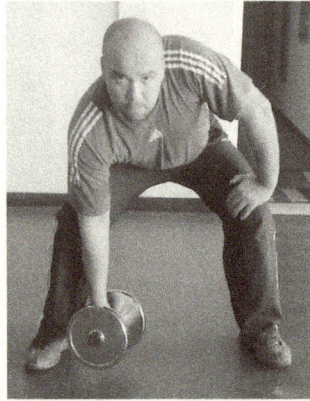

Select a safe weight to start with until you have mastered the technique and position yourself in the seated or bent over position. Grip the weight firmly with a straight arm and as you breathe out, engage your abdominals and raise the weight up by bending your elbow and hold. Attempt to keep the weight level and breathe in as you slowly return to the start position and repeat.

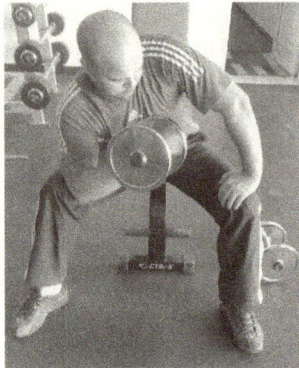

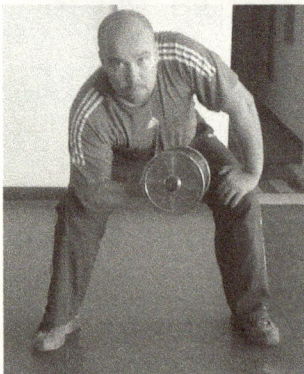

MOST COMMON TRICEP EXERCISES

USING YOUR OWN BODYWEIGHT

Bench Dips

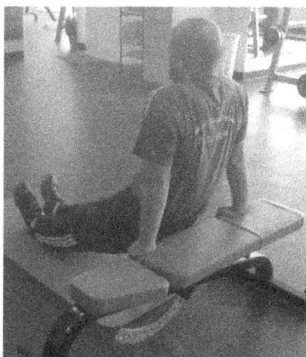

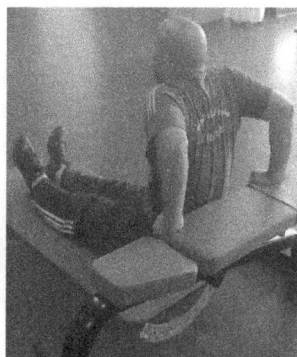

Find any object that is stable, safe and secure where you can bend your elbows fully behind your body. Your aim is to place your hands firmly behind you on the bench and fairly close together. Start off with your arms straight before bending at the elbow as you breathe in, then as you breathe out raise your body upwards whilst contracting your triceps by straightening your arms. You can use the bench as above or place a chair/raised platform behind you and complete the same exercise, repeat the movement. Elevate your feet to make it more difficult.

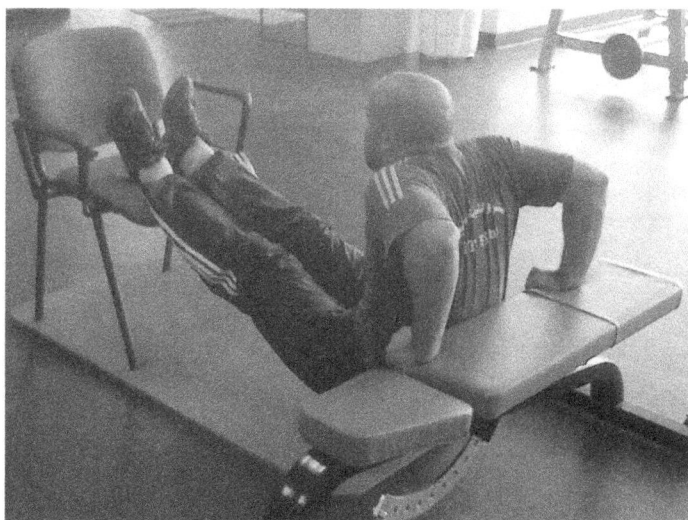

Incline press ups

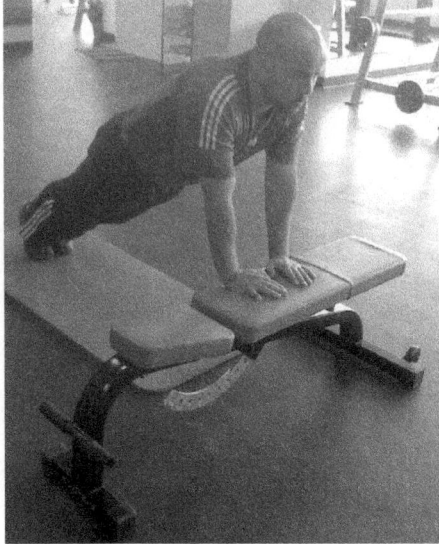

Lean onto a bench/stable object ensuring that your back is straight and your shoulders relaxed whilst your hips and shoulders remain facing towards the ground along with your head and eyes. Place your hands close together before you initiate the movement from the abdominals and lower your upper body until your chest is close to the bench/stable object whilst breathing in. Breathe out as you raise your upper body back to the start position. Maintaining control throughout the movement is important whilst breathing correctly. It is very important to keep your elbows as close to the body as possible.

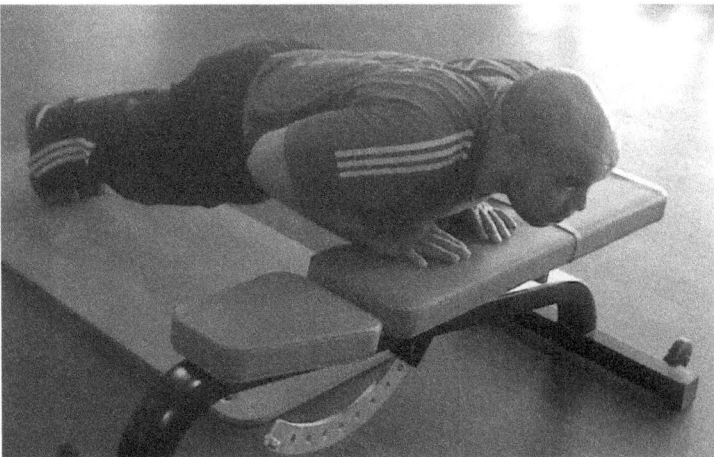

Advanced press ups

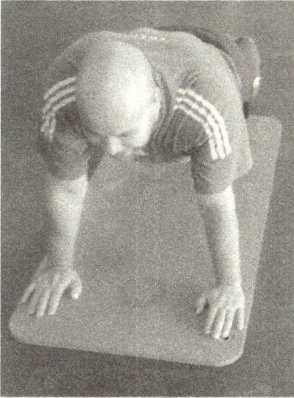

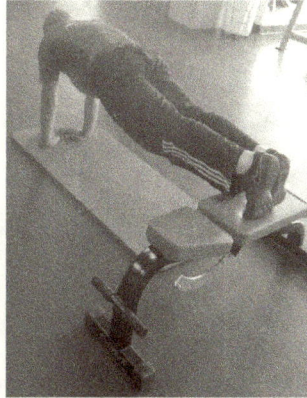

With your feet on a stable raised object ensure your hands are initially level with your shoulders and your knees and hands are in line. Your shoulders should be relaxed and your hips and shoulders should remain facing towards the ground along with your head and eyes. Progress until your hands are as close together as possible before you initiate the movement from the abdominals and lower your upper body until your chest is close to the floor whilst breathing in. Breathe out as you raise your upper body back to the start position. Maintaining control throughout the movement is important whilst breathing correctly. It is very important to keep your elbows as close to the body as possible. Progress further by elevating the legs on a stable platform or unstable platform such as the fit-ball.

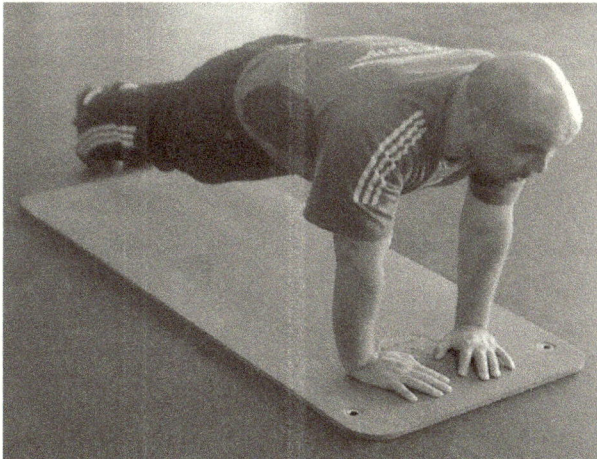

Partner walk

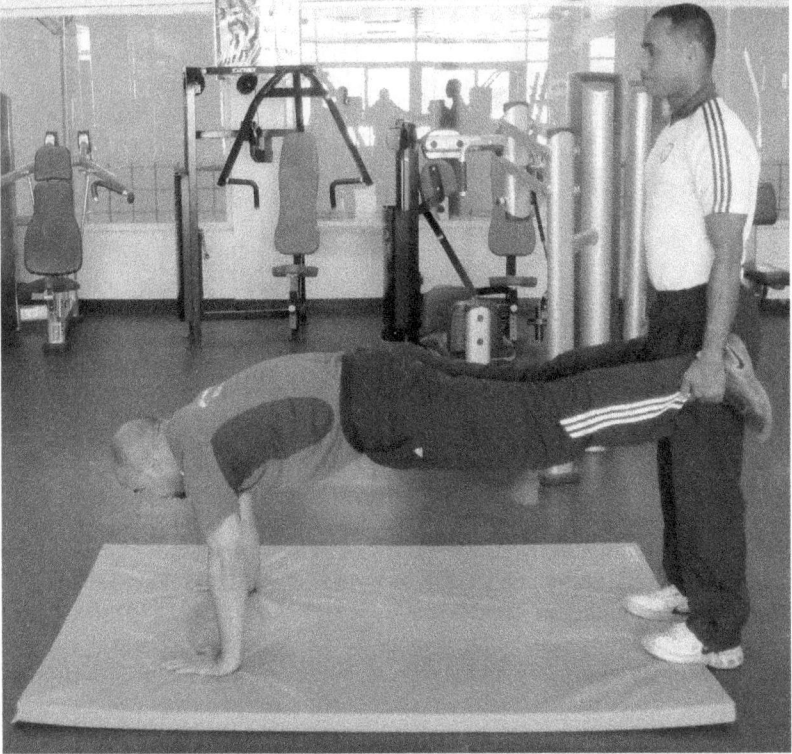

Get in the press up position as your partner takes a good grip of your legs, simply walk forwards in a straight line by using your hands only. Before walking, initiate the abdominals and endeavour to keep your back straight along with the head, eyes hips and shoulders. Relax your shoulders as much as possible.

Body raises

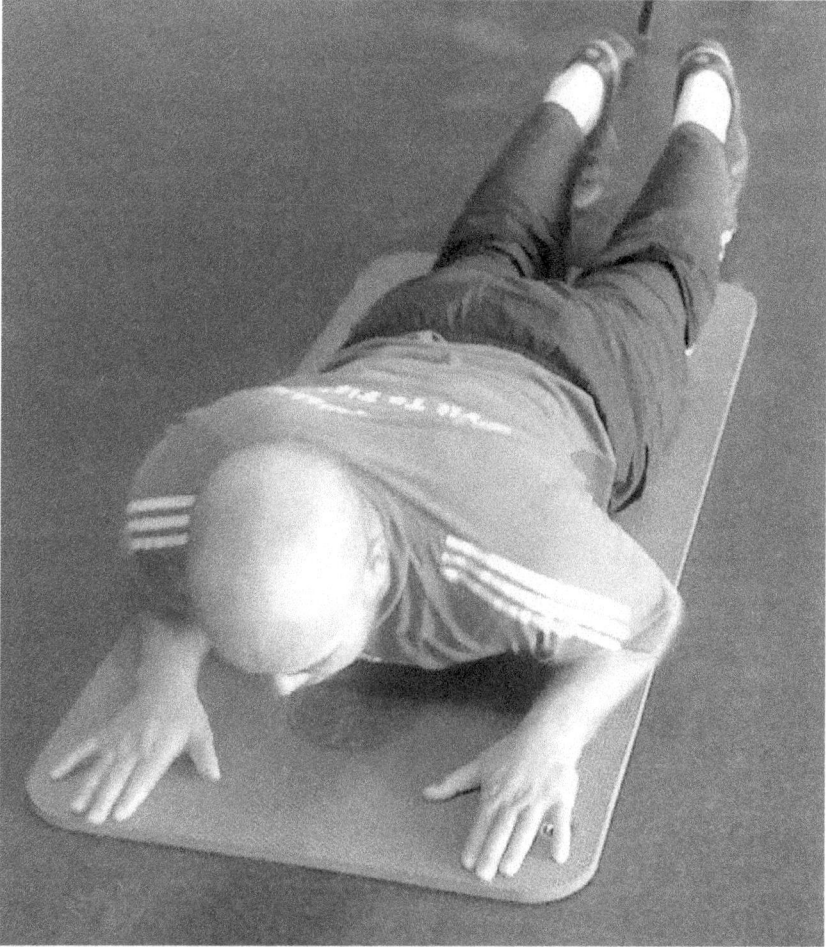

Start in the front lying position with your hands level with your head shoulder width apart and with your elbows close to the sides of your body. Whilst using the arms only, initiate the abdominals and breathe out as you straighten your arms. Endeavour to keep your shoulders down and relaxed as much as possible.

TRICEP EXERCISES USING RESISTANCE BANDS

Kneeling overhead press

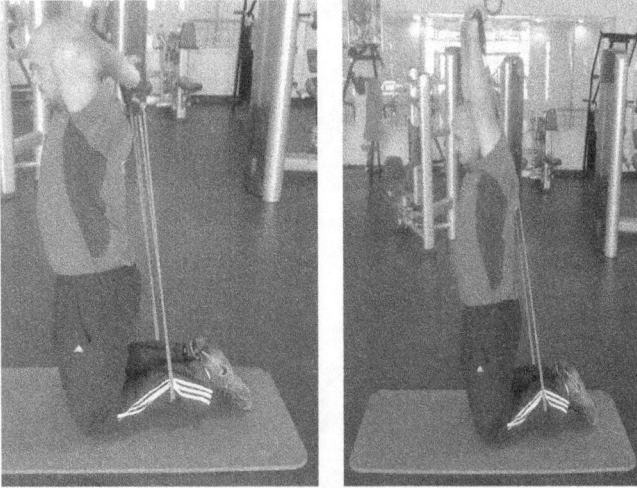

Select a safe resistance to start with until you have mastered the technique and position yourself in the kneeling or standing position. Ensure that the band is secure and has enough tension before you begin. Start with your arms fully bent at the elbows behind your head, initiate the abdominals as you breathe out and raise the bands above your head contracting your triceps as you straighten the arms. Breathe in & return back to the start position under control, repeat the movement.

Kickbacks

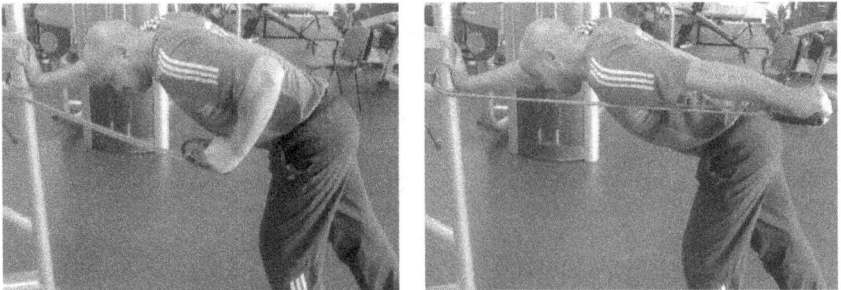

Select a safe resistance to start with until you have mastered the technique and position yourself in the standing position, leaning slightly forwards. Ensure that the band is secure and has enough tension before you begin. Start with one arm resting (for stability) and the other arm bent at the elbow with the band close to the body. Breathe out as you straighten the arm behind you whilst contracting your triceps, breathe in as you return the band back to the start position and change arms as you repeat the movement.

Over-head push

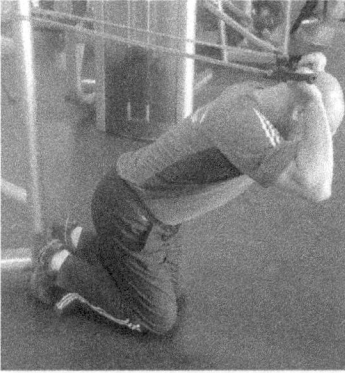

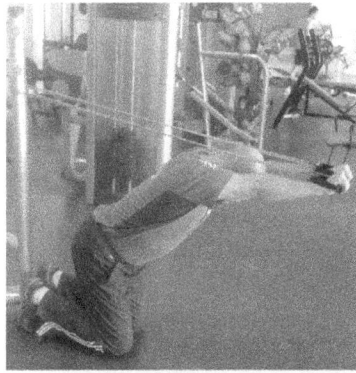

Select a safe resistance to start with until you have mastered the technique and position yourself in the kneeling position. Ensure that the band is secure and has enough tension before you begin. Start with your arms fully bent at the elbows behind your head, initiate the abdominals as you breathe out and push the bands in front of your head contracting your triceps as you straighten the arms. Breathe in & return back to the start position under control, repeat the movement. Move the arms only and relax the shoulders.

Forward press

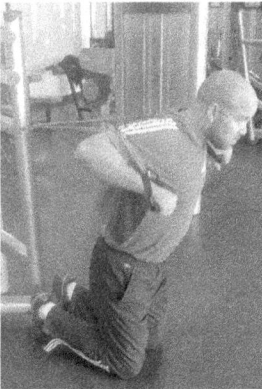

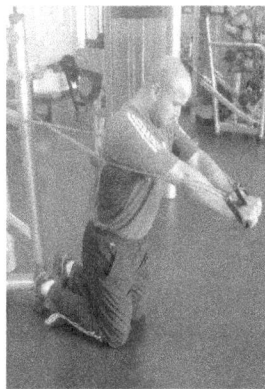

Select a safe resistance to start with until you have mastered the technique and position yourself in the kneeling position. Ensure that the band is secure and has enough tension before you begin. Start with your elbows behind you, shoulder blades close together with your hands holding the handles close to your chest. Initiate the abdominals as you breathe out and push the bands forwards as you straighten your arms to contract your triceps. Breathe in as you return back to the start position and repeat the movement.

TRICEP EXERCISES USING A FIT-BALL

Dumbbell overhead press (Back lying)

Both arms   **Single arm**

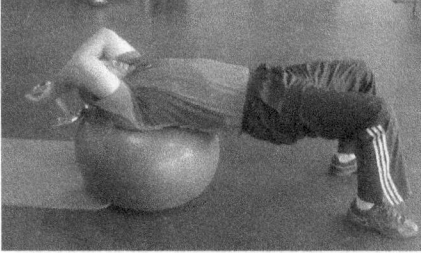 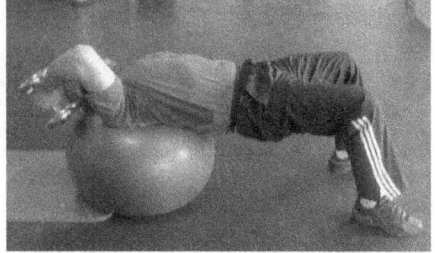

Select a safe weight to start with until you have mastered the technique and position yourself lying flat on the fit-ball with your arms straight and above your head. Breathe in and bend your arms at the elbow lowering the weight down whilst attempting to keep your elbows as close together as you can without moving the remainder of your arm. Initiate the abdominals as you breathe out and raise the weight back to the start position whilst contracting your triceps as you straighten the arms. As you get more confident move your feet closer together but keep your hips high at all times. Also, try single arm once you have perfected the technique with both.

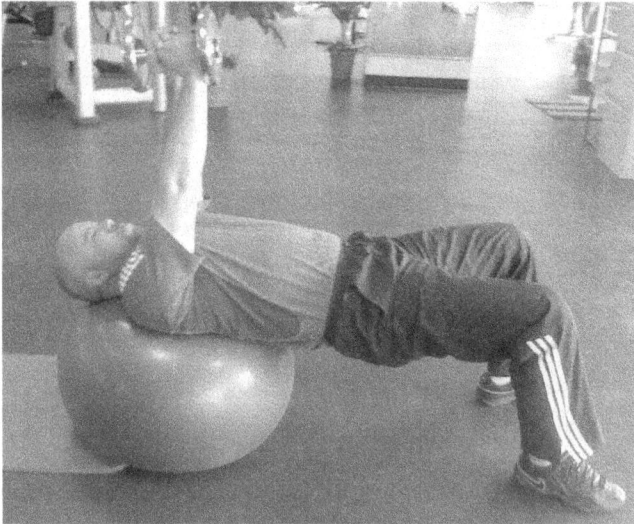

Barbell overhead press

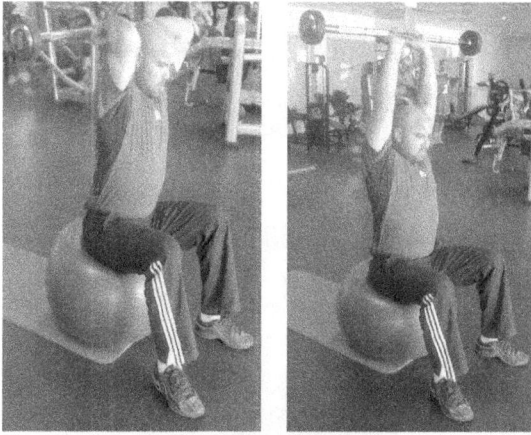

Select a safe weight to start with until you have mastered the technique and position yourself sat or lying on the fit-ball. Start with your arms straight above your head with your hands close together and equal distance from the centre of the bar. Breathe in and bend your arms at the elbow lowering the weight down behind you whilst attempting to keep your elbow as close together as you can without moving the remainder of your arms. Initiate the abdominals as you breathe out and raise the weight back to the start position whilst contracting your triceps as you straighten the arms, repeat the movement. As you get more confident move your feet closer together and if lying on the fit-ball keep your hips high at all times.

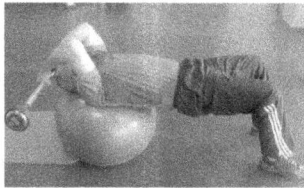

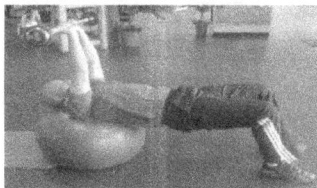

Kickbacks

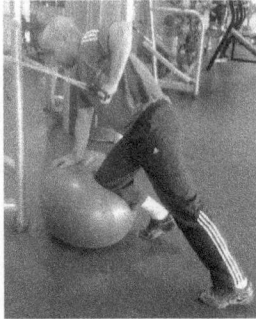

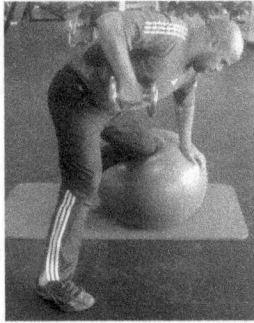

Select a safe weight to start with until you have mastered the technique and position yourself knelt on a fit-ball with your back straight and perpendicular to the bench. Start with one arm resting on the fit-ball (for stability) and the other arm bent at the elbow with the weight/band close to the body. Breathe out as you straighten the arm behind you whilst contracting your triceps, breathe in as you return the weight/band back to the start position and change arms as you repeat the movement. As you get more confident take your hand away from the fit-ball and/or move your leg closer to the ball.

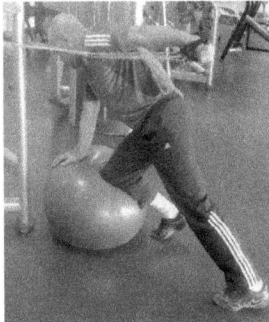

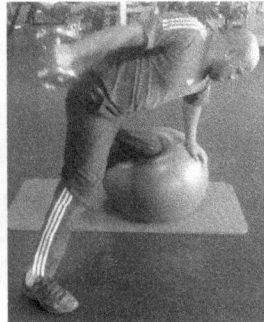

Close arm press

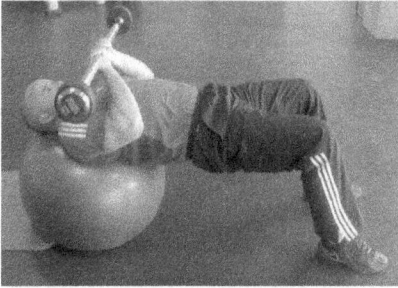
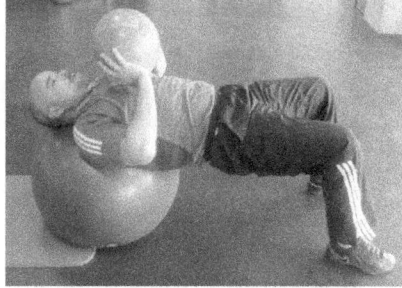

Select a safe weight to start with until you have mastered the technique and position yourself lying flat on a fit-ball with your hands positioned close together but equal distance from the centre of the weighted object. Start with the weight close to your chest; initiate the abdominals as you breathe out and raise the object up as you straighten your arms to contract your triceps. Breathe in as you lower the object back to the start position and repeat the movement. As you get more confident move your feet closer together and keep your hips high at all times.

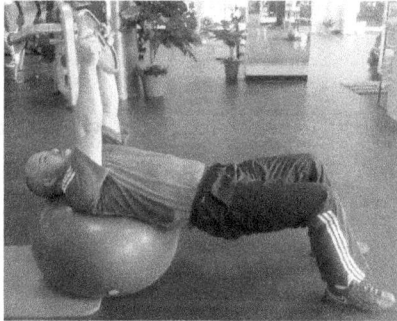

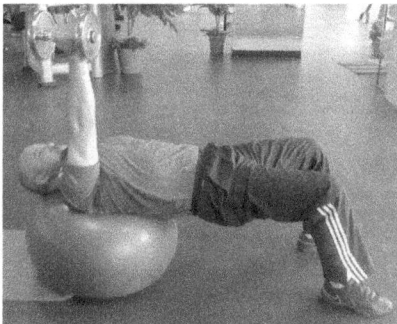

Other variations

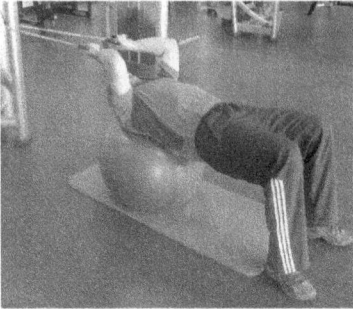

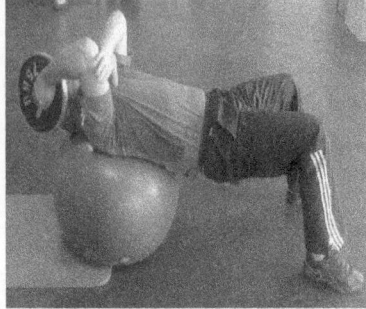

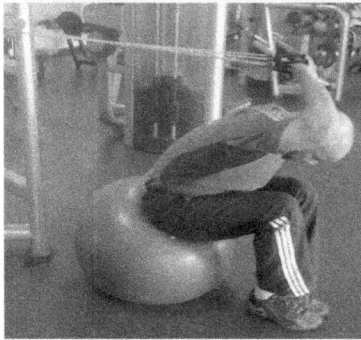

Select a safe weight to start with until you have mastered the technique and position yourself sat or lying on the fit-ball. Whichever exercise you are completing make sure that you start by breathing in whilst bending your arms at the elbow lowering the weight down behind you whilst attempting to keep your elbow as close together as you can without moving the remainder of your arms. Initiate the abdominals as you breathe out and raise the weight back to the start position whilst contracting your triceps as you straighten the arms, repeat the movement. As you get more confident move your feet closer together and if lying on the fit-ball keep your hips high at all times.

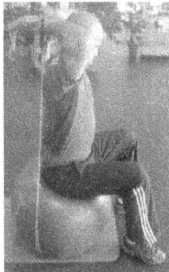

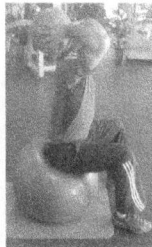

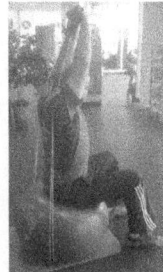

TRICEP EXERCISES USING MACHINES

Seated tricep push

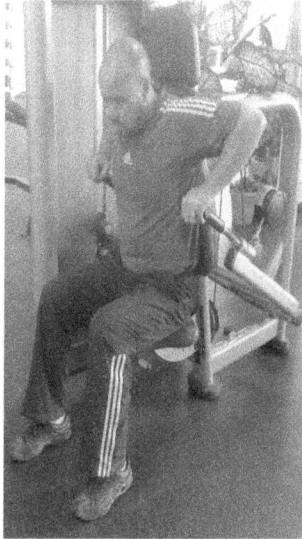

Select a safe weight to start with until you have mastered the technique and position yourself in the seated position with your hips/knees at 90 degrees and your back straight. Grip the bars firmly with the bars positioned so that your elbows are high but close to the midline of your body. As you breathe out, engage your abdominals and push the bars down by contracting your triceps until your arms are straight and hold. Breathe in as you return to the start position and repeat

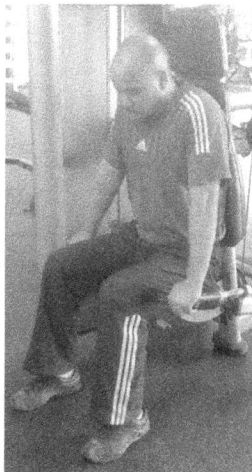

Overhead press

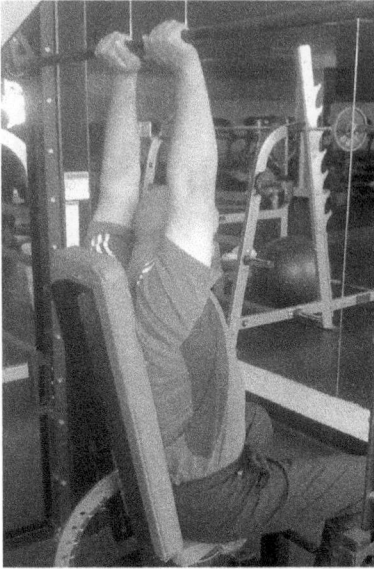

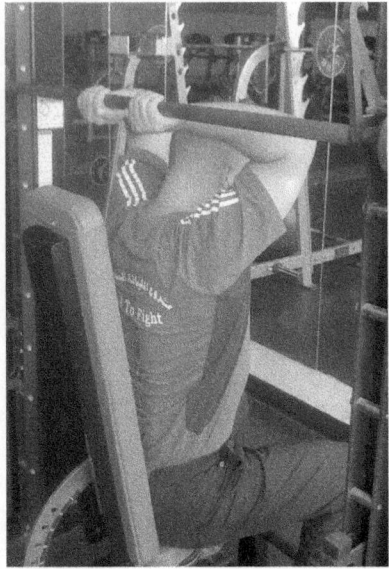

Select a safe weight to start with until you have mastered the technique and position yourself either sat on a bench, knelt down or stood with your back to a machine utilising cables or a bar. Start with your arms straight and above your head, unhook the bar or grip the cables and breathe in as you bend your arms at the elbow lowering the bar/cables down & behind you whilst attempting to keep your elbows as close together as you can without moving the remainder of your arm. Initiate the abdominals as you breathe out and raise the bar/cables back to the start position whilst contracting your triceps as you straighten the arms and repeat the movement. You can also use just one arm on the cable machine.

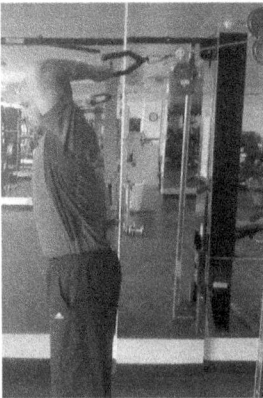

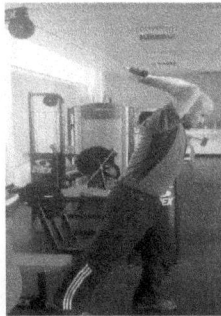

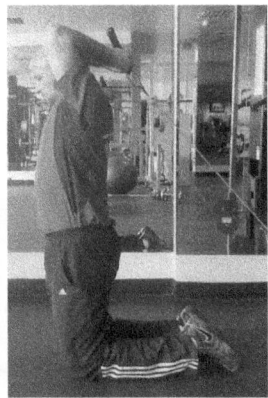

Pull downs

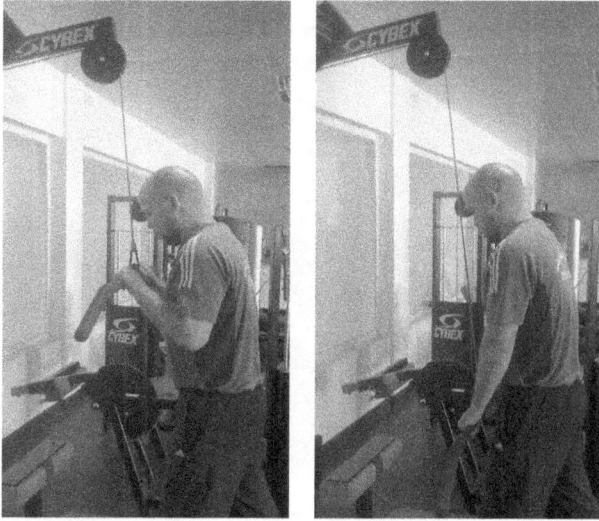

Select a safe weight to start with until you have mastered the technique and position yourself in front of or to the side of the cables or a bar. Start with your arms bent fully, grip the bar/cables and breathe out as you straighten your arms by pushing the bar/cables down whilst attempting to keep your elbows as close to your body as you can without moving the remainder of your arm, initiate the abdominals before and breathe in as you raise the bar/cables back to the start position, repeat the movement. You can also use just one arm on the cable machine and/or change the grip on either the bar or cable.

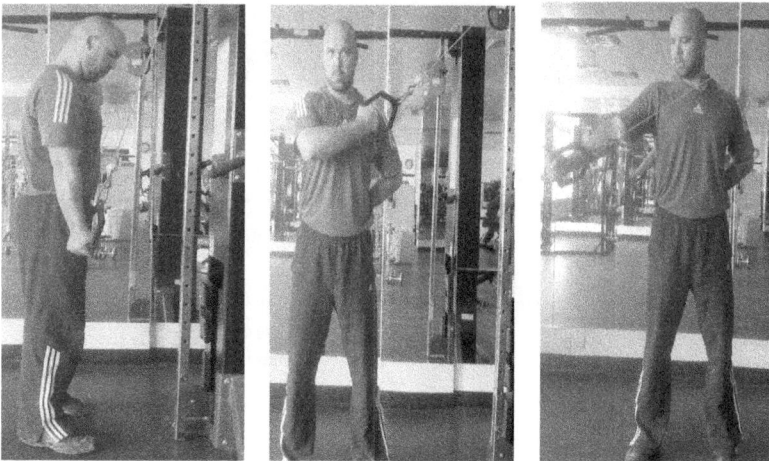

213

Close arm press

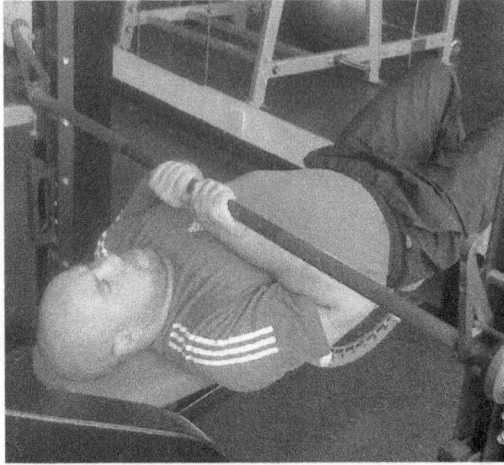

Select a safe weight to start with until you have mastered the technique and position yourself lying flat on a bench with your hands positioned close together but equal distance from the centre of the weighted bar. Start with the bar close to your chest; initiate the abdominals as you breathe out and raise the bar up as you straighten your arms to contract your triceps. Breathe in as you lower the bar back to the start position and repeat the movement.

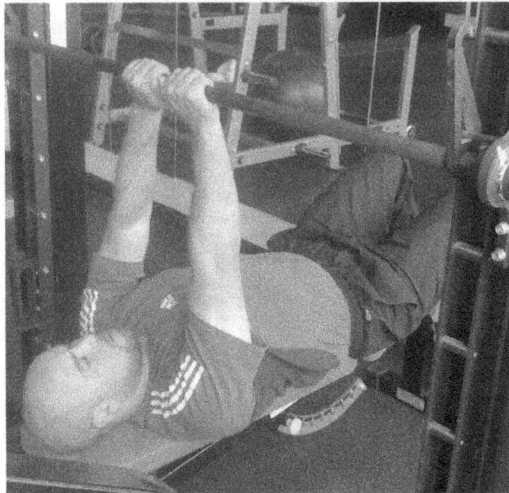

Dips

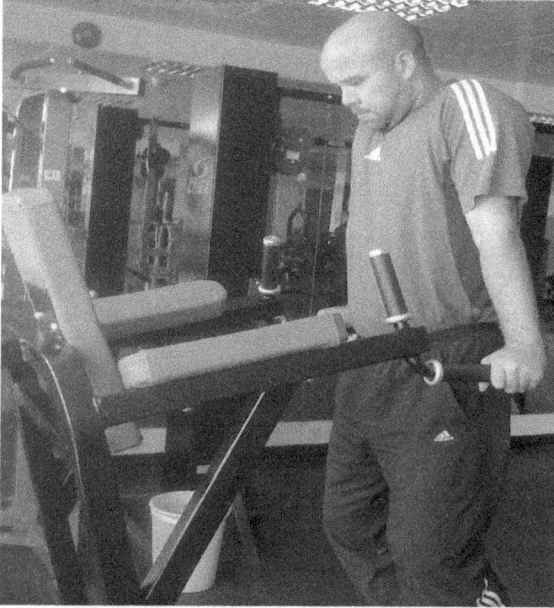

Position yourself on the apparatus so that you can bend your elbows fully behind your body. Your aim is to breathe in, bend the arms fully before breathing out and contracting your triceps until your arms are in the full outstretched position. Raise your body upwards by using your arms only. The above apparatus works the chest as well as your triceps.

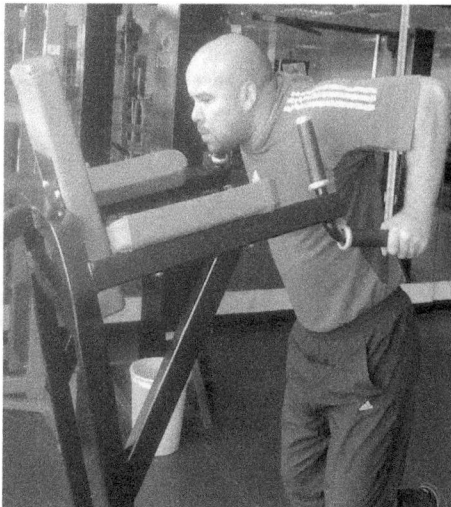

TRICEP EXERCISES USING A BARBELL

Lying overhead push

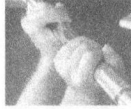

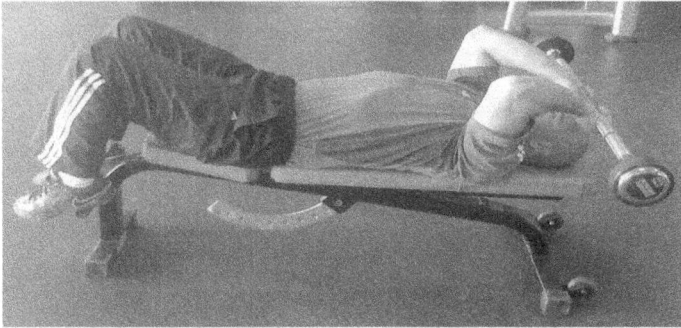

Select a safe weight to start with until you have mastered the technique and position yourself lying flat on a bench with your hands positioned close together but equal distance from the centre of the weighted bar. Start with your arms straight, breathe in and bend your arms at the elbow lowering the bar down whilst attempting to keep your elbows as close together as you can without moving the remainder of your arm. Initiate the abdominals as you breathe out as you raise the bar back to the start position whilst contracting your triceps as you straighten the arms. Repeat the movement....*you can also change the hand position.

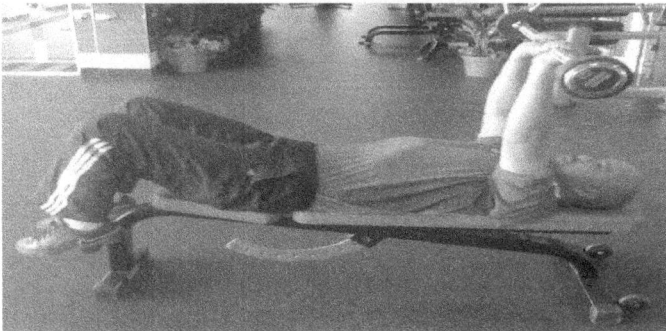

Seated press

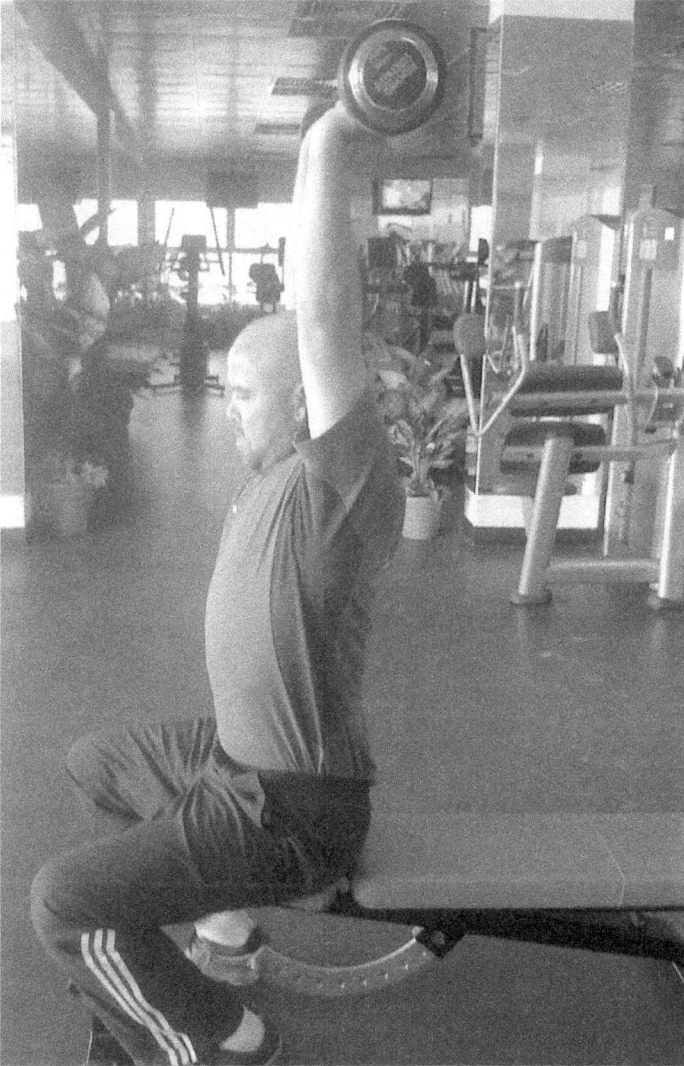

Select a safe weight to start with until you have mastered the technique and position yourself sat on a bench with your hands positioned close together but equal distance from the centre of the weighted bar. Start with your arms straight and above your head, breathe in and bend your arms at the elbow lowering the bar down behind you whilst attempting to keep your elbows as close together as you can without moving the remainder of your arm. Initiate the abdominals as you breathe out as you raise the bar back to the start position whilst contracting your triceps as you straighten the arms. Repeat the movement.

Close arm press

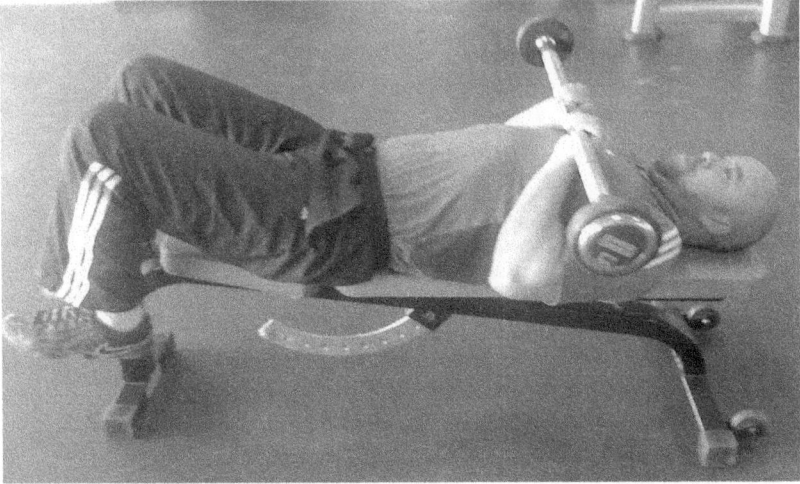

Select a safe weight to start with until you have mastered the technique and position yourself lying flat on a bench with your hands positioned close together but equal distance from the centre of the weighted bar. Start with the bar close to your chest; initiate the abdominals as you breathe out and raise the bar up as you straighten your arms to contract your triceps. Breathe in as you lower the bar back to the start position and repeat the movement.

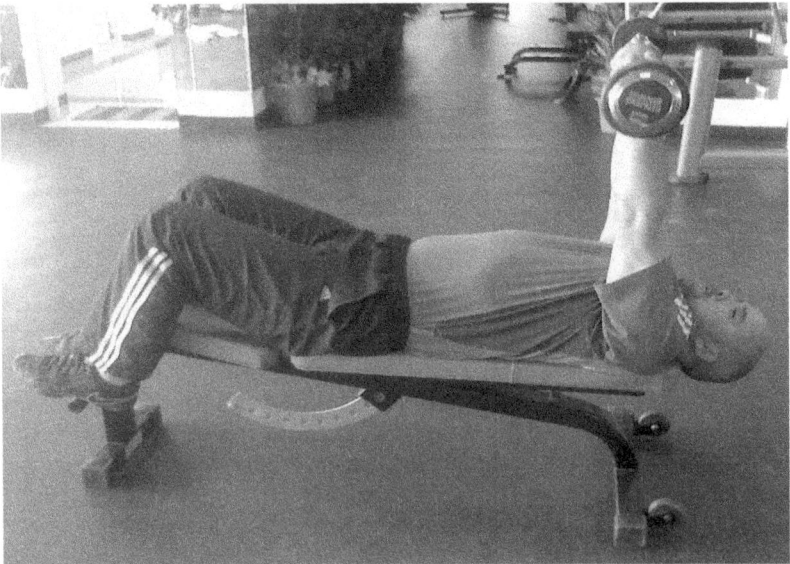

Tricep press (fixed bar)

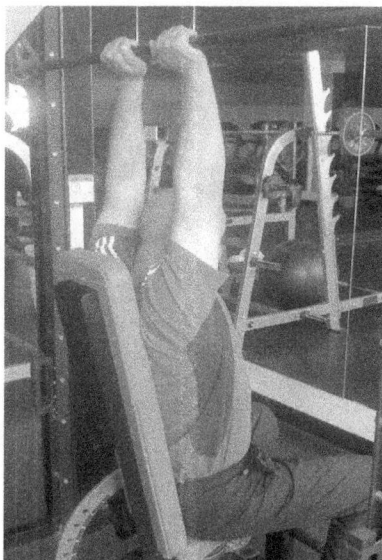

Select a safe weight to start with until you have mastered the technique and position yourself sat on a bench with your hands positioned close together but equal distance from the centre of the weighted bar.

Start with your arms straight and above your head, unhook the bar and breathe in as you bend your arms at the elbow lowering the bar down behind you whilst attempting to keep your elbows as close together as you can without moving the remainder of your arm. Initiate the abdominals as you breathe out and raise the bar back to the start position whilst contracting your triceps as you straighten the arms. Repeat the movement.

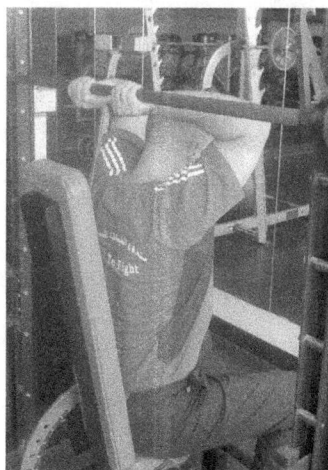

TRICEP EXERCISES USING DUMBBELLS

Seated overhead push

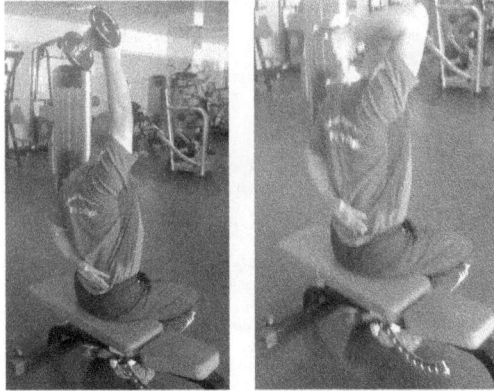

Select a safe weight to start with until you have mastered the technique and position yourself sat on a bench. Start with your arm straight and above your head, breathe in and bend your arm at the elbow lowering the weight down behind you whilst attempting to keep your elbow as close together as you can without moving the remainder of your arm. Initiate the abdominals as you breathe out as you raise the weight back to the start position whilst contracting your triceps as you straighten the arms. Change arms as you repeat the movement.

Kick backs

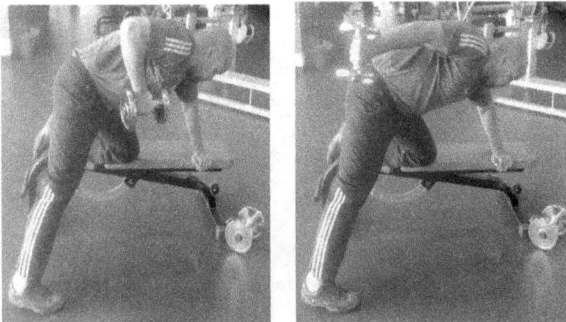

Select a safe weight to start with until you have mastered the technique and position yourself knelt on a bench with your back straight and perpendicular to the bench. Start with one arm resting on the bench (for stability) and the other arm bent at the elbow with the weight close to the body. Breathe out as you straighten the arm behind you whilst contracting your triceps, breathe in as you return the weight back to the start position and change arms as you repeat the movement.

Lying overhead press

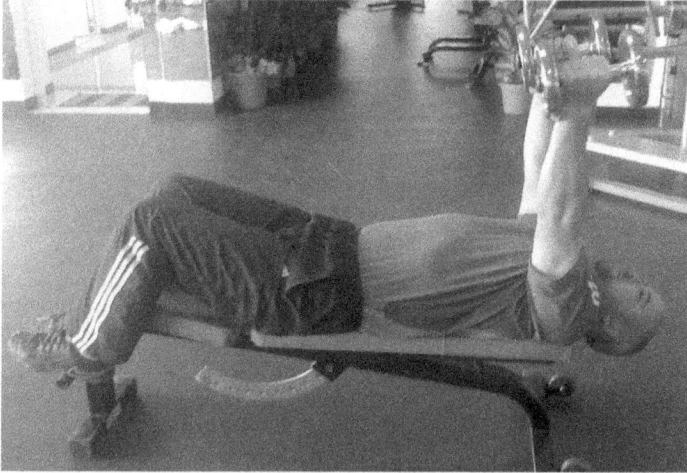

Select a safe weight to start with until you have mastered the technique and position yourself lying flat on a bench with your arms straight and above your head. Breathe in and bend your arms at the elbow lowering the weights down whilst attempting to keep your elbows as close together as you can without moving the remainder of your arm. Initiate the abdominals as you breathe out as you raise the weights back to the start position whilst contracting your triceps as you straighten the arms. Repeat the movement.

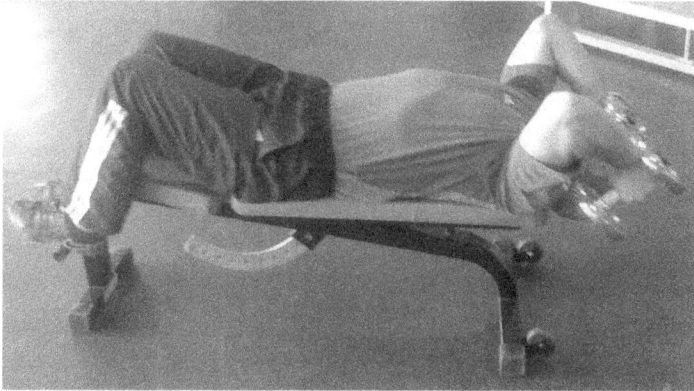

Double arm seated push

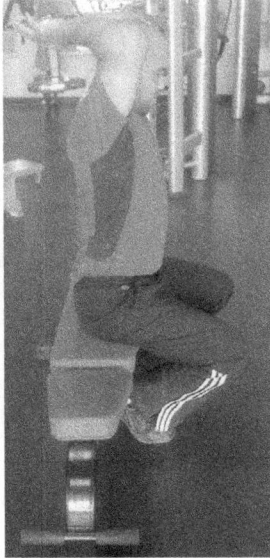

Select a safe weight to start with until you have mastered the technique and position yourself sat on a bench. Start with your arms straight and above your head, breathe in and bend your arms at the elbow lowering the weight down behind you whilst attempting to keep your elbow as close together as you can without moving the remainder of your arms. Initiate the abdominals as you breathe out and raise the weight back to the start position whilst contracting your triceps as you straighten the arms, repeat the movement.

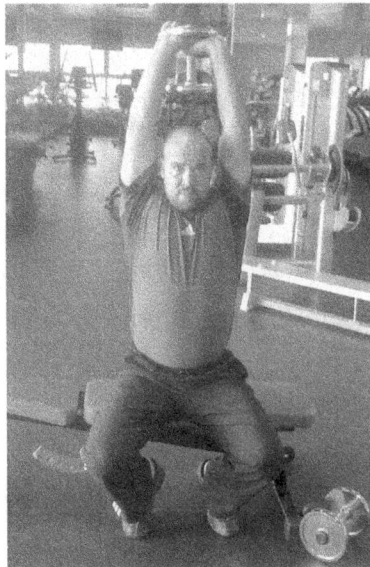

MOST COMMON LEG EXERCISES

USING YOUR OWN BODYWEIGHT

Static Hold

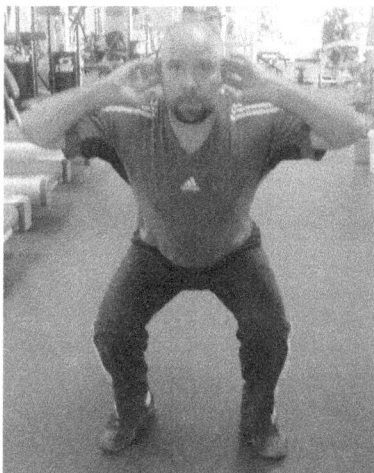

Ensure that you stand with your feet flat on the floor and wide enough to maintain good balance, (normally shoulder width apart) your thighs should be parallel to the ground. Ensure your hips, shoulders, head and eyes are inline. Squat down and backwards until your knees are level with your toes. Hold the position for as long as you can, whilst breathing in a controlled manner.

Bridge

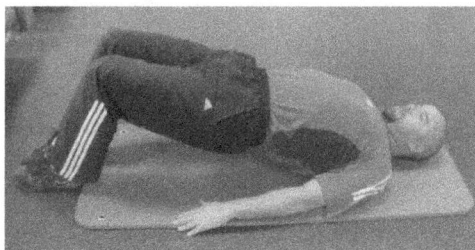

In the back lying position place your feet shoulder width apart and flat on the floor with your arms relaxed by your side. Your hips, shoulders, head and eyes should be inline prior to raising your hips off the ground whilst breathing out. Breathe in as you return to the start position. Concentrate on maintaining a good body position as you raise your hips high. Use the upper leg muscles to hold you in the position. Repeat the movement in a controlled manner.

Squat

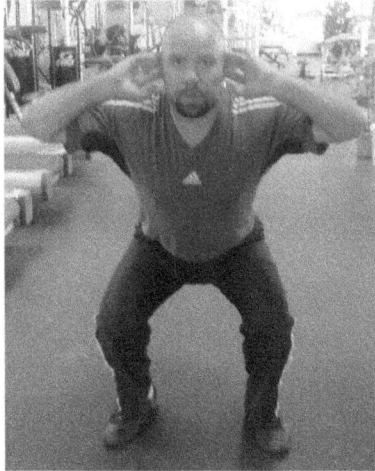

Stand with your feet flat on the floor and wide enough to maintain good balance. Your hips, shoulders, head and eyes should be inline as you squat down keeping your back straight, squat down and backwards until your thighs are parallel to the ground. Ensure your knees don't go too far beyond your toes as you hold the position for 2-3 seconds before returning to the start position. Breathe in a controlled manner.

Lunge

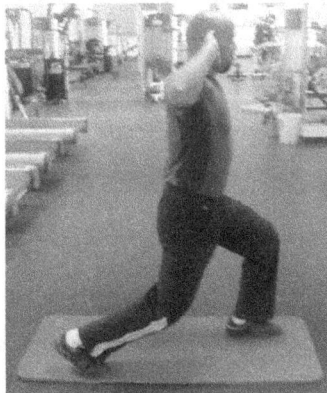

Stand with your feet flat on the floor and wide enough to maintain good balance. Step backwards with one leg until the thigh of the forward leg is parallel to the ground, your hips, shoulders, head and eyes should be inline and facing forwards. Initiate the movement via the abdominals whilst keeping the back straight and breathing out, breathe in as you return to the start position and repeat. All movements should be under control and safe!! This exercise can be changed so that you step forwards instead.

Step Up

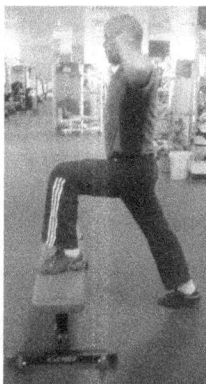

Stand with your feet flat on the floor and wide enough to maintain good balance. Choose a surface that is not too low or too high and your foot is flat on it before you step up. Your hips, shoulders, head and eyes should be inline and facing forwards. Initiate the movement via the abdominals and breathe out when you step up and attempt to stand upright. As always it is very important that your back remains straight at all times. Breathe in as you return to the start position and repeat. All movements should be under control and safe!!

Squat Jump

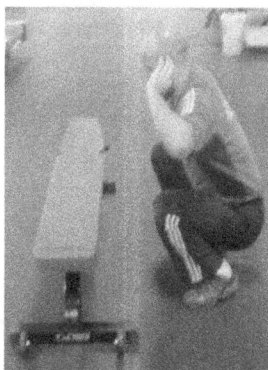

Choose a stable surface to use for this exercise and start off with it up against a wall. Stand with your feet flat on the floor and wide enough to maintain good balance. Your hips, shoulders, head and eyes should be inline as you squat down keeping your back straight, squat down and backwards until your thighs are close to the ground. Breathe out as you jump forward and upwards onto the stable surface. Progress in a safe manner onto a low surface first and gradually increase the height as you become more confident. Initiating the abdominals, keeping the back straight and your breathing are very important factors whilst attempting this exercise.

LEG EXERCISES USING RESISTANCE BANDS

Squats

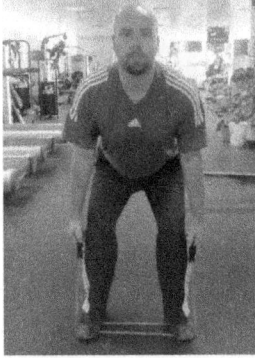

Firstly, choose a band that is the correct resistance for you and during the initial stages this will be a light weight until you master the technique. Stand with your feet flat on the floor and wide enough to maintain good balance with the band secure & under your feet. Your hips, shoulders, head and eyes should be inline as you squat down keeping your back straight, squat down and backwards until your thighs are parallel to the ground. Ensure your knees don't go too far beyond your toes as you hold the position for 2-3 seconds before returning to the start position. Breathe in a controlled manner.

Hip extension

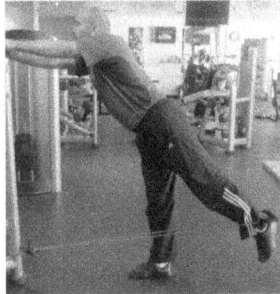

Firstly, choose a band that is the correct resistance for you and during the initial stages this will be a light weight until you master the technique. Attach the band to one of your legs whilst ensuring your other foot is firmly stable on the ground. Begin by holding onto something as you progress the exercise, although your aim should be to not do so and this will also work the stationary leg. Begin by standing as upright as possible, initiate your abdominals and pull the cable away from the midline of the body whilst breathing out. Breathe in as you return to the start position under control and repeat accordingly. Your leg should be as straight as possible. As you progress you can place your arms out to the side, by your side or across your chest.

226

Hip flexion

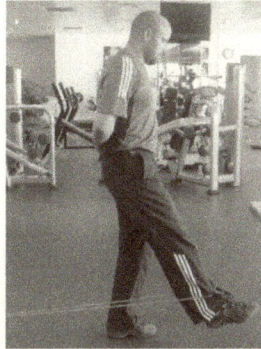

Firstly, choose a band that is the correct resistance for you and during the initial stages this will be a light weight until you master the technique. Attach the band to one of your legs whilst ensuring your other foot is firmly stable on the ground. Begin by holding onto something as you progress the exercise, although your aim should be to not do so and this will also work the stationary leg. Begin by standing as upright as possible, initiate your abdominals and pull the cable away from the midline of the body whilst breathing out. Breathe in as you return to the start position under control and repeat accordingly. Your leg should be as straight as possible. As you progress you can place your arms out to the side, by your side or across your chest.

Abduction / Adduction

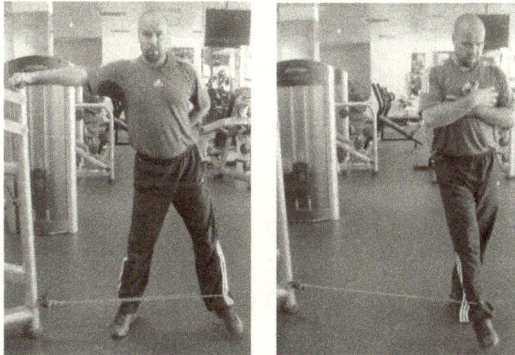

Firstly, choose a band that is the correct resistance for you and during the initial stages this will be a light weight until you master the technique. Attach the band to one of your legs whilst ensuring your other foot is firmly stable on the ground. Begin by holding onto something as you progress the exercise, although your aim should be to not do so and this will also work the stationary leg. Begin by standing as upright as possible, initiate your abdominals and pull the cable away from the midline of the body whilst breathing out. Breathe in as you return to the start position under control and repeat accordingly. Your leg should be as straight as possible. As you progress you can place your arms out to the side, by your side or across your chest.

227

LEG EXERCISES USING A FIT-BALL

Hip Flexors

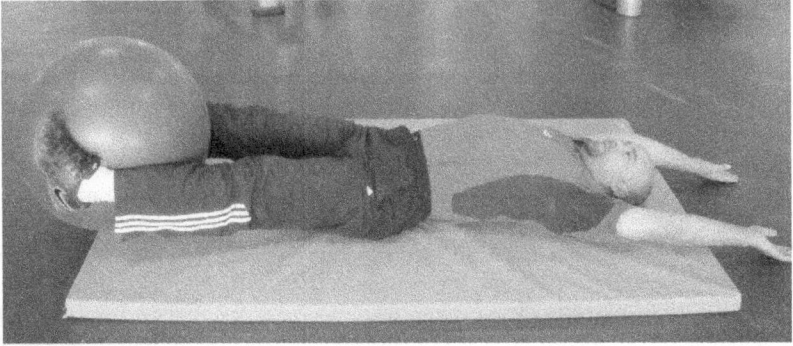

Lying on your back, place the ball in between your legs, squeeze the ball with your legs and raise your legs up and inline with your hips. Ensure at all times that you contract your abdominals and press the small of your back towards the ground whilst breathing out. Lower your legs under control whilst breathing in and repeat accordingly. Your aim should be to keep the legs from touching the floor and to apply a 3-5 second hold whilst keeping the legs as straight as possible.

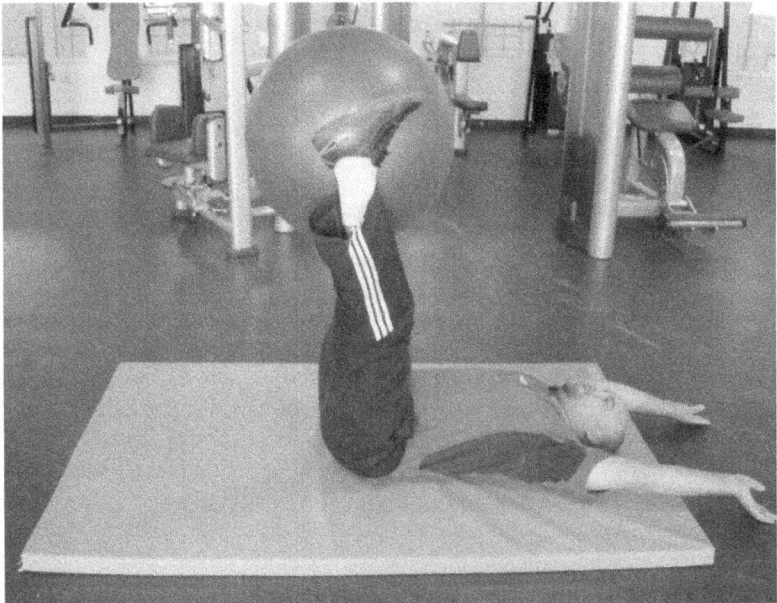

Leg Bridge

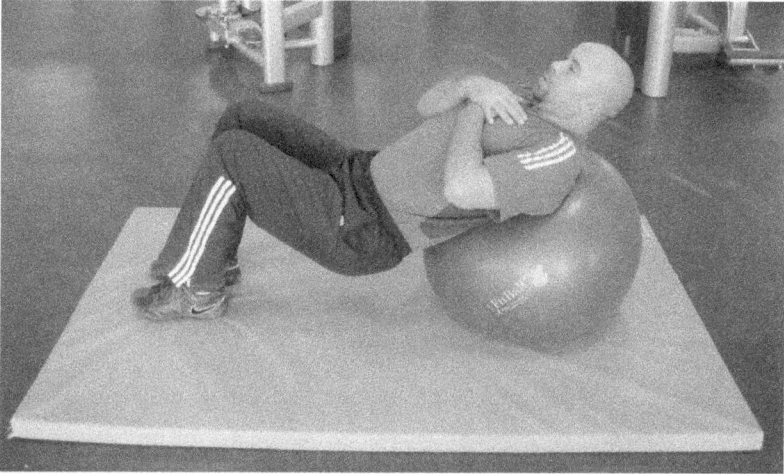

Lie on the ball with your arms outstretched (at first) and place your feet firmly on the floor (not too close together) initiate the movement from the abdominals and raise your hips until they are inline with the shoulders and tops of the knees, breathe out and hold for 3-5 seconds. Return to the start position whilst breathing in and repeat the exercise, progress accordingly with the arms.

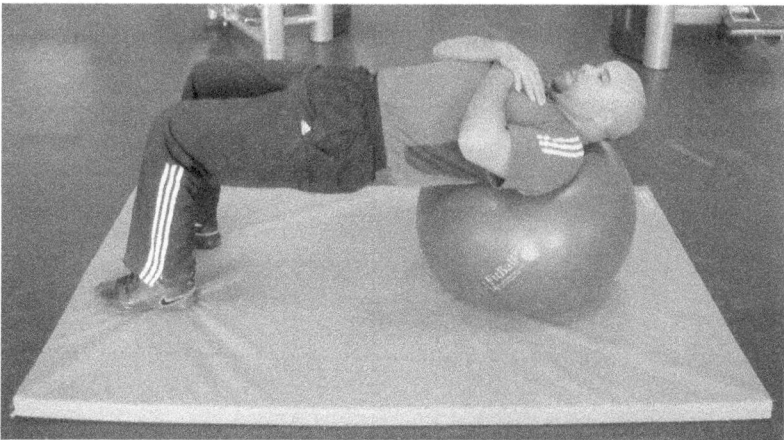

Abductor/Adductor

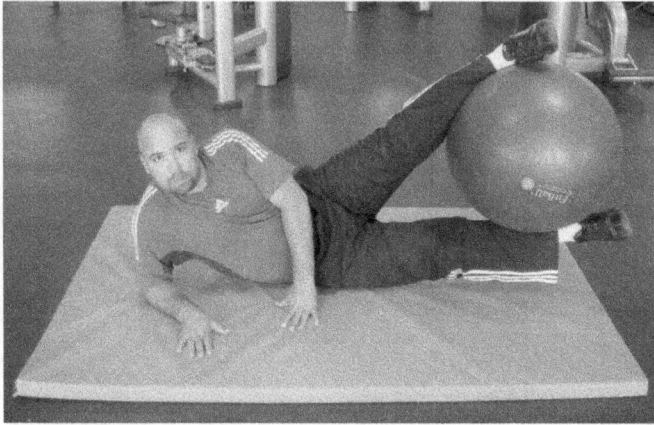

Lie on your side with your body as straight as possible, keeping the ball squeezed between your feet. Raise your legs as high off the ground as you can without twisting the body, whilst breathing out and return back to the start position whilst breathing in. Your aim should be to keep the legs from touching the floor and to apply a 3-5 second hold whilst keeping the legs as straight as possible. You must initiate the movement from the abdominals and try not to use your upper body too much, relax the shoulders at all times.

Wall Squat

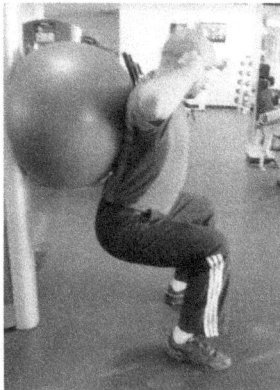

Place the ball behind you and position your feet shoulder width apart, relax the head and shoulders. Lower your body until your legs are at a 90 degree angle whilst breathing out. Return to the start position whilst breathing in ensuring that your legs are straight and the ball remains just above the small of the back. Your feet should be level and so use a line for guidance, your knees should also be behind your toes at all times.

Single Leg Squat

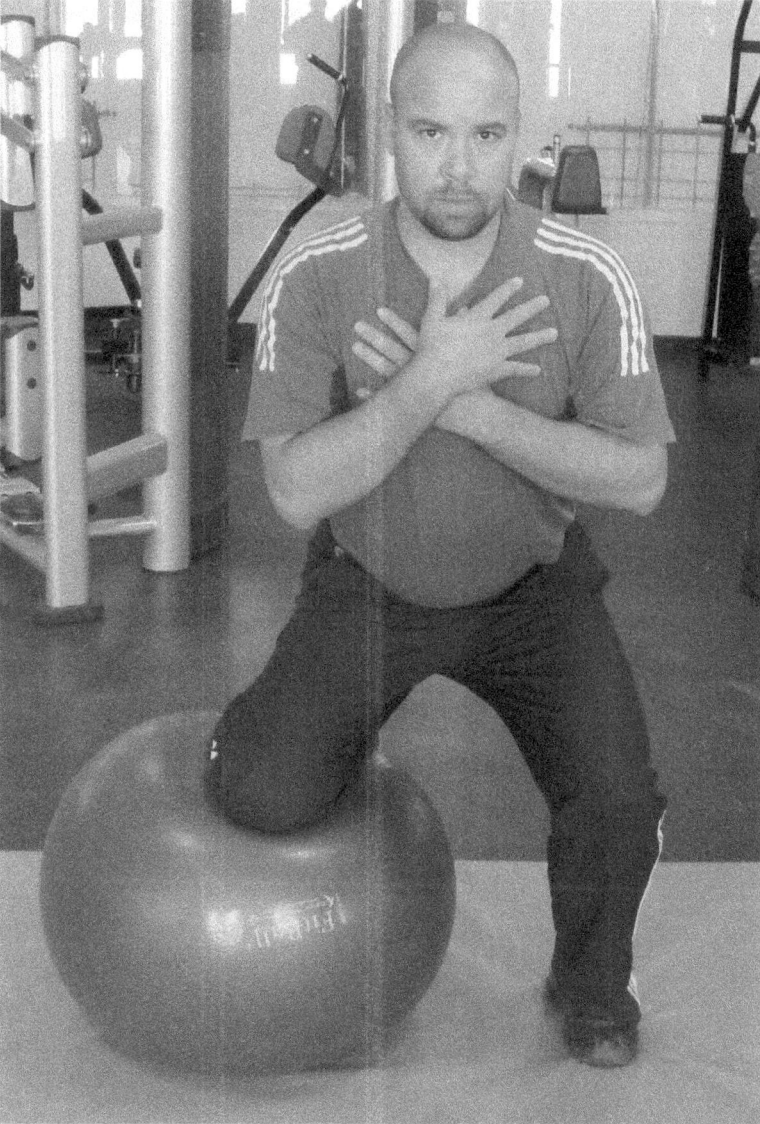

Place one knee on the ball with the other flat on the floor, relax the head and shoulders. Lower your body until your leg is at a 90 degree angle whilst breathing out. Return to the start position whilst breathing in ensuring that your leg is straight and the ball remains as still as possible. You should endeavour to keep your knee behind your toe at all times, change legs accordingly.

LEG EXERCISES USING MACHINES

Squat machines

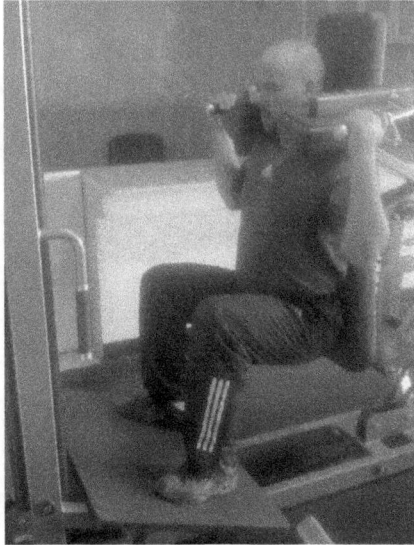

Select a weight that is low enough for you to master the technique first, stand with your feet flat and wide enough to maintain good balance. Lower your body down & backwards until your thighs are parallel to the ground, your hips, shoulders, head and eyes should be inline and facing forwards. Initiate the movement via the abdominals whilst keeping the back straight and breathing out, breathe in as you return to the start position and repeat. All movements should be under control and safe!!

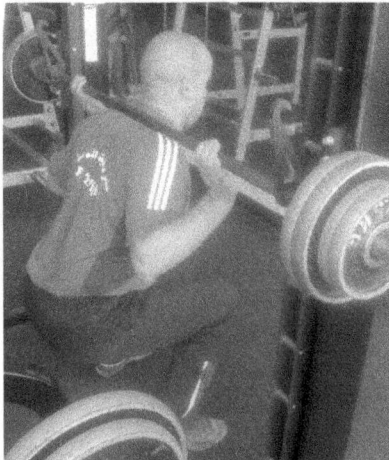

232

Leg extension

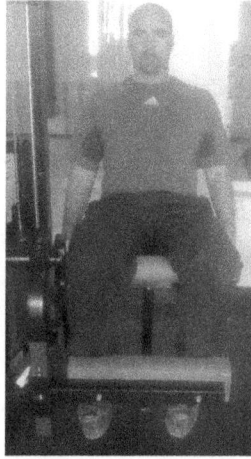

First of all, always select a safe weight that is achievable and this will generally be a lighter one until you have mastered the technique. Adjust the seat so that your lower legs hang comfortably down towards the foot pad which should also be comfortable and around shin height. The hand grips are optional but try not to use your upper body too much to assist, initiate the abdominals before raising the pad until it is level with your knees whilst breathing out. Breathe in as you lower the pad under control. Repeat accordingly.

Hamstring curl

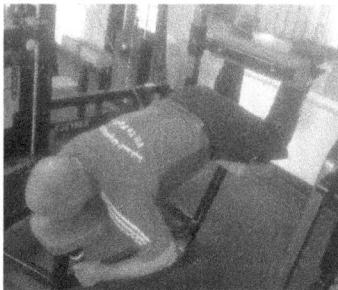

First of all, always select a safe weight that is achievable and this will generally be a lighter one until you have mastered the technique. Adjust the foot pad so that it is far enough back and just above the ankle. Ensure it is comfortable and your legs are straight. The hand grips are optional but try not to use your upper body too much to assist, initiate the abdominals before raising the pad until it is as close to your backside as possible whilst breathing out. Breathe in as you lower the pad under control. Repeat accordingly.

Calf machines

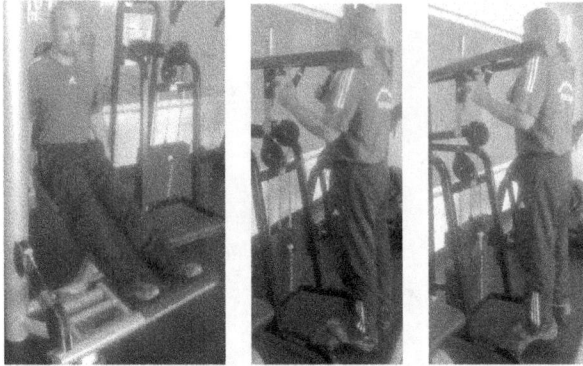

First of all, always select a safe weight that is achievable and this will generally be a lighter one until you have mastered the technique. Adjust the relevant machine so that your legs are straight but your heels are pointing towards the ground. Your position in the machine should be comfortable and the hand grips only as optional but try not to use your upper body too much to assist. Initiate the abdominals before raising the heels upwards whilst breathing out. Breathe in as you lower the heels under control. Repeat accordingly

Abductors / Adductors

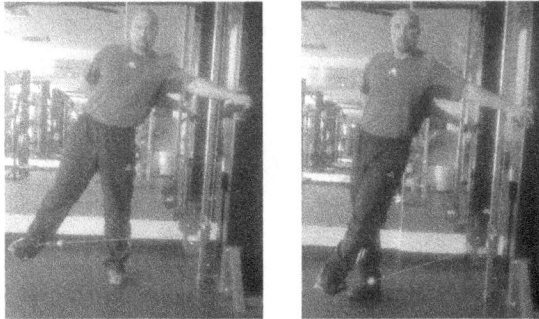

First of all, always select a safe weight that is achievable and this will generally be a lighter one until you have mastered the technique. Attach the cable to one of your feet whilst ensuring your other foot is firmly stable on the ground. Begin by holding onto something as you progress the exercise, although your aim should be to not do so and this will also work the stationary leg. Begin by standing as upright as possible, initiate your abdominals and pull the cable away from the midline of the body whilst breathing out. Breathe in as you return to the start position under control and repeat accordingly. Your leg should be as straight as possible. As you progress you can place your arms out to the side, by your side or across your chest.

234

Hip extension / Hip flexion

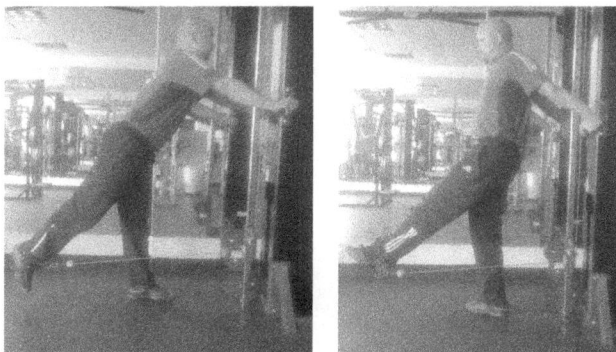

First of all, always select a safe weight that is achievable and this will generally be a lighter one until you have mastered the technique. Attach the cable to one of your feet whilst ensuring your other foot is firmly stable on the ground. Begin by holding onto something as you progress the exercise, although your aim should be to not do so and this will also work the stationary leg. Begin by standing as upright as possible, initiate your abdominals and pull the cable away from the midline of the body whilst breathing out. Breathe in as you return to the start position under control and repeat accordingly. Your leg should be as straight as possible. As you progress you can place your arms out to the side, by your side or across your chest.

Leg press

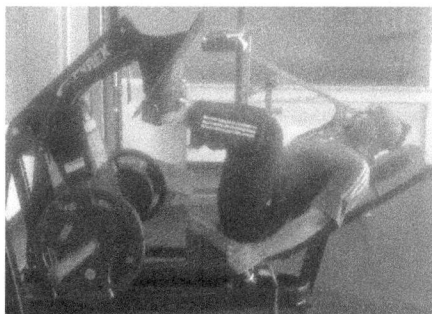

Select a weight that is low enough for you to master the technique first, sit with your feet flat and wide enough to maintain good balance. Release the weight using the handle at the left hand side of the machine and lower the plate towards you (under control) until your thighs are parallel to the ground, your hips, shoulders, head and eyes should be inline and facing forwards. Keep the back pressed into the seat and lower the weight whilst breathing in. Initiate the movement via the abdominals and breathe out as you push the weighted plate away from you whilst straightening the legs and repeat. All movements should be under control and safe!!

235

LEG EXERCISES USING A BARBELL

Barbell Squat

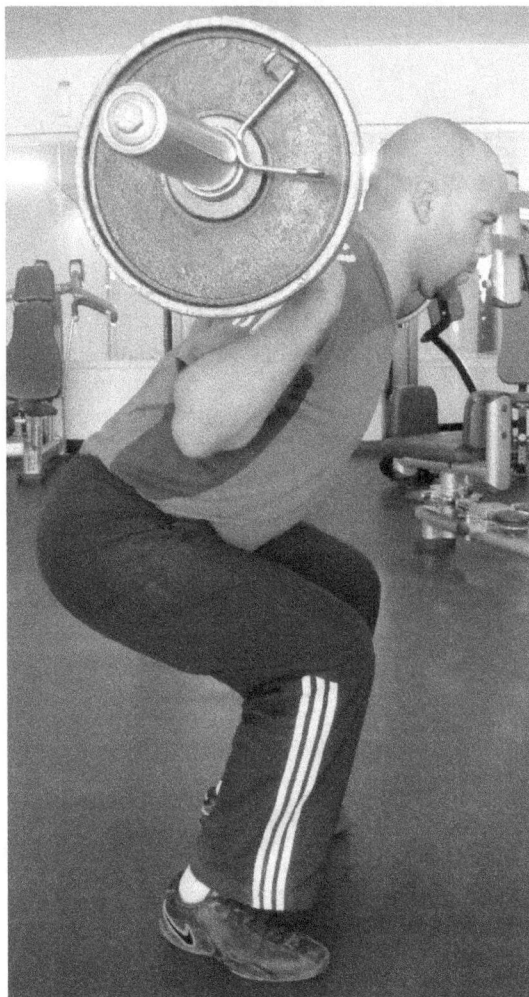

Select a weight that is low enough for you to master the technique first, stand with your feet flat on the floor and wide enough to maintain good balance. Lower your body down & backwards until your thighs are parallel to the ground, your hips, shoulders, head and eyes should be inline and facing forwards. Initiate the movement via the abdominals whilst keeping the back straight and breathing out, breathe in as you return to the start position and repeat. All movements should be under control and safe!

Barbell Lunge

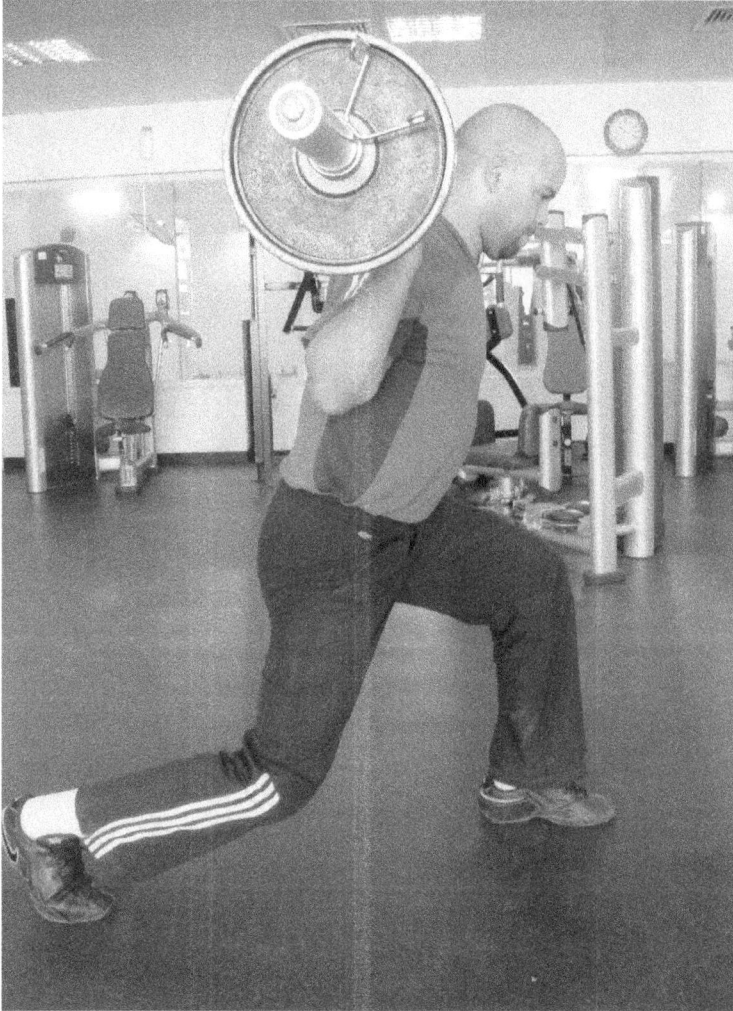

Select a weight that is low enough for you to master the technique first, stand with your feet flat on the floor and wide enough to maintain good balance. Step backwards with one leg until the thigh of the forward leg is parallel to the ground, your hips, shoulders, head and eyes should be inline and facing forwards. Initiate the movement via the abdominals whilst keeping the back straight and breathing out, breathe in as you return to the start position and repeat. All movements should be under control and safe!! This exercise can be changed so that you step forwards instead.

Dead lift

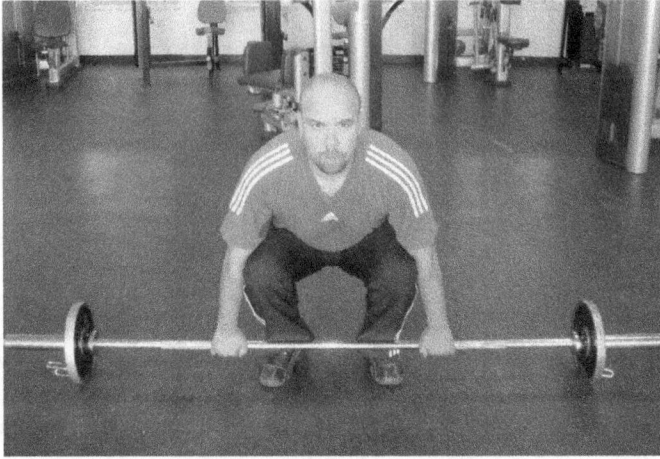

Select a weight that is low enough for you to master the technique first, stand with your feet flat on the floor and wide enough to maintain good balance. Lower your body down & backwards until your thighs are parallel to the ground, grip the bar so that your hands are outside of the legs. Your hips, shoulders, head and eyes should be inline and facing forwards. Initiate the movement via the abdominals and breathe out when you stand upright whilst keeping the back straight. Breathe in as you return to the start position and repeat. The shoulders should remain relaxed and all movements should be under control and safe!!

An alternative ex is the **clean pull exercise** – Hold the bar (as above) approx. shoulder width apart. The bar starts on the floor (approx. mid-shin height and close to touching your shin) your hips are down, feet flat and shoulders tall. Your back should not be rounded at all. Forcefully drive into the ground to pull the bar off the floor. You are pulling with your hips and not arms on this exercise, so ensure your arms stay extended throughout the movement. Try to keep the angle of your back constant as the bar comes off the ground. Your legs start to straighten to bring your body up. As the bar begins to cross the knees, you should be in the perfect power position. Pull and shrug as hard as you can in an attempt to make the bar move as fast as possible.

Barbell Step ups

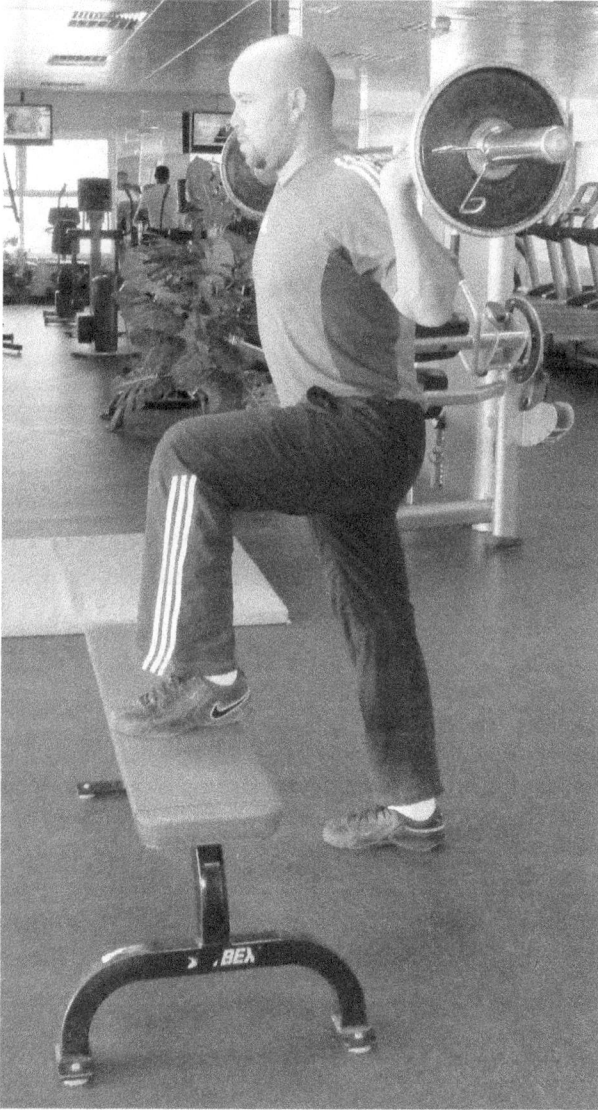

Select a weight that is low enough for you to master the technique first, stand with your feet flat on the floor and wide enough to maintain good balance. Choose a surface that is not too low or too high and your foot is flat on it before you step up. Your hips, shoulders, head and eyes should be inline and facing forwards. Initiate the movement via the abdominals and breathe out when you step up and attempt to stand upright. Your back should remain straight and the weight even on the shoulders. Breathe in as you return to the start position and repeat. All movements should be under control and safe!!

Barbell Split Squat

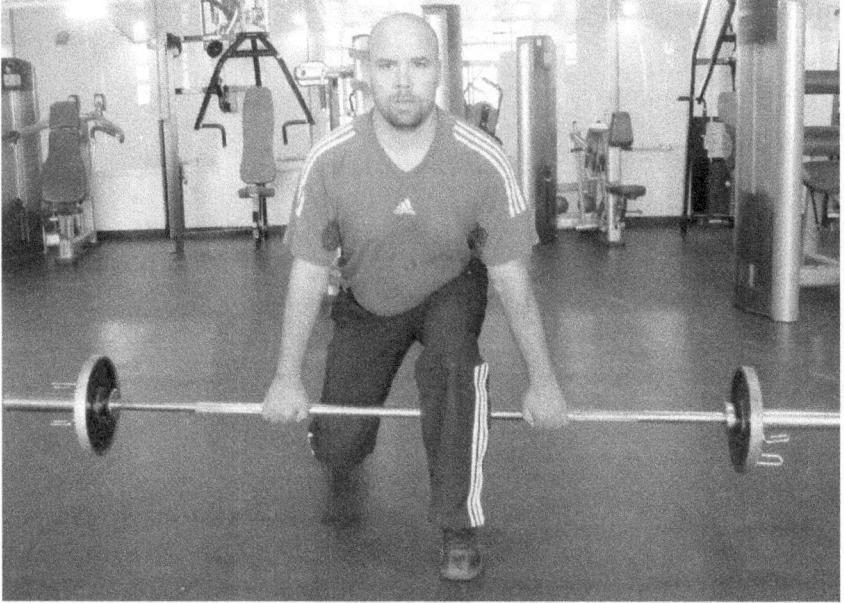

Select a weight that is low enough for you to master the technique first. Get in the position for the Lunge but with the bar in between your legs. Your front thigh should be parallel to the ground, grip the bar so that your hands are outside of the legs. Your hips, shoulders, head and eyes should be inline and facing forwards. Initiate the movement via the abdominals and breathe out when you stand upright whilst keeping the back straight. Breathe in as you return to the start position and repeat. The shoulders should remain relaxed and all movements should be under control and safe!!

LEG EXERCISES USING DUMBBELLS

Dumbbell Squat

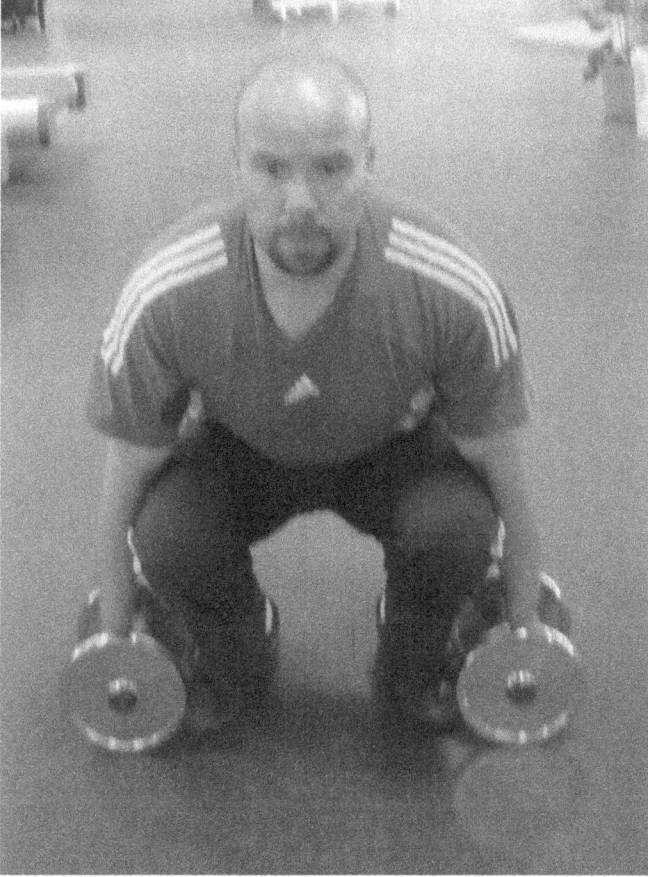

Select weights that are low enough for you to master the technique first, stand with your feet flat on the floor and wide enough to maintain good balance. Lower your body down & backwards until your thighs are parallel to the ground, your hips, shoulders, head and eyes should be inline and facing forwards. Initiate the movement via the abdominals whilst keeping the back straight and breathing out, breathe in as you return to the start position and repeat. All movements should be under control and safe!!

Dumbbell Lunge

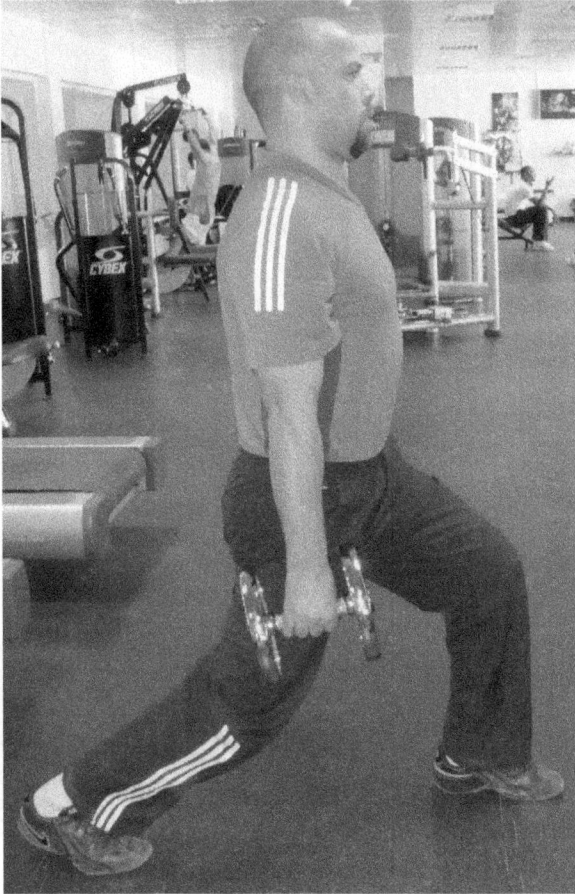

Select weights that are low enough for you to master the technique first, stand with your feet flat on the floor and wide enough to maintain good balance. Step backwards with one leg until the thigh of the forward leg is parallel to the ground, your hips, shoulders, head and eyes should be inline and facing forwards. Initiate the movement via the abdominals whilst keeping the back straight and breathing out, breathe in as you return to the start position and repeat. All movements should be under control and safe!! This exercise can be changed so that you step forwards instead.

Dumbbell Step Up

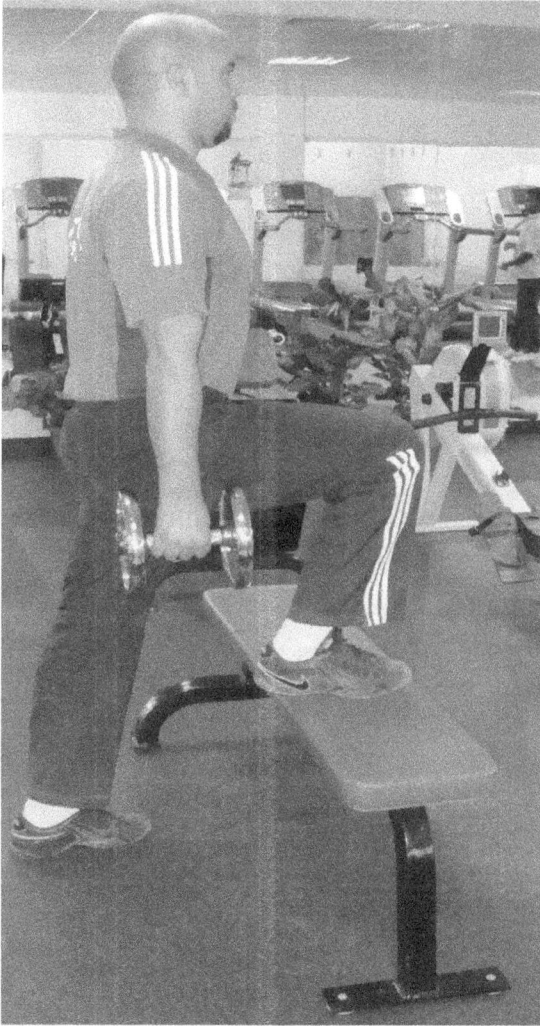

Select weights that are low enough for you to master the technique first, stand with your feet flat on the floor and wide enough to maintain good balance. Choose a surface that is not too low or too high and your foot is flat on it before you step up. Your hips, shoulders, head and eyes should be inline and facing forwards. Initiate the movement via the abdominals and breathe out when you step up and attempt to stand upright. Your back should remain straight and the weights secure in your hands at all times, with your shoulders relaxed. Breathe in as you return to the start position and repeat. All movements should be under control and safe!!

Dumbbell Dead lift

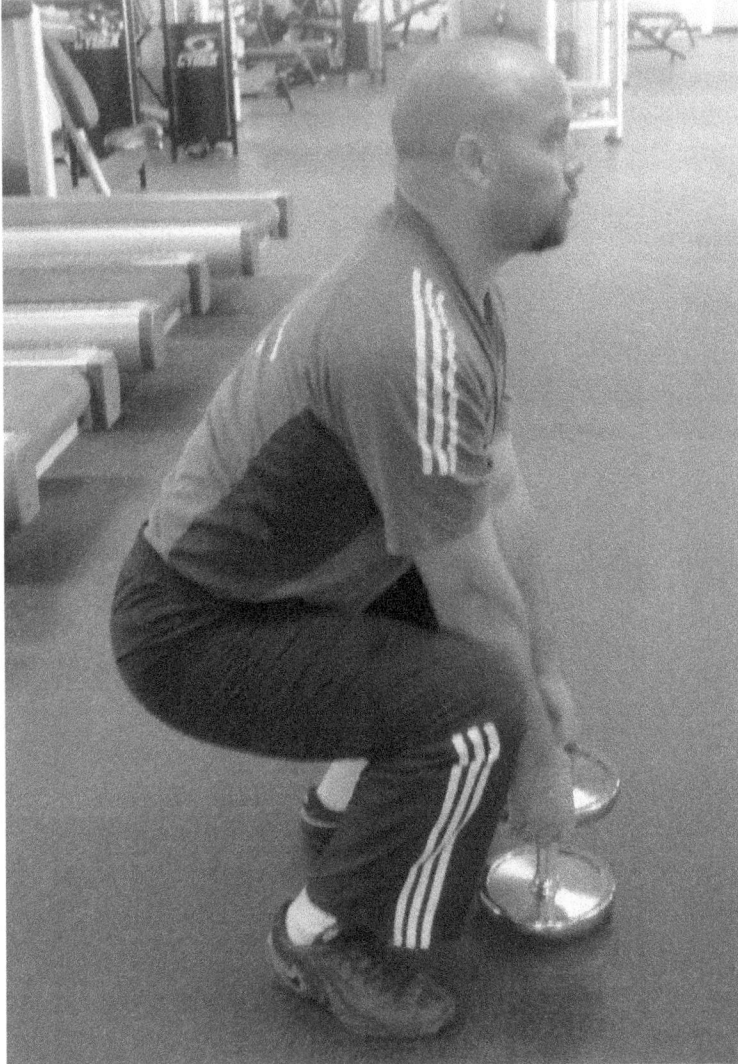

Select a weight that is low enough for you to master the technique first, stand with your feet flat on the floor and wide enough to maintain good balance. Lower your body down & backwards until your thighs are parallel to the ground, grip the weight so that your hands are inside of the legs. Your hips, shoulders, head and eyes should be inline and facing forwards. Initiate the movement via the abdominals and breathe out when you stand upright whilst keeping the back straight. Breathe in as you return to the start position and repeat. The shoulders should remain relaxed and all movements should be under control and safe!!

OPTIONAL EXERCISES

BODYWEIGHT EXERCISES		
Side plank	Tibialis anterior	Neck flex/extension (ISO)
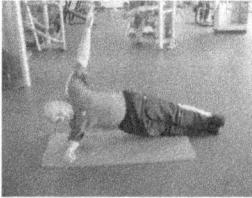	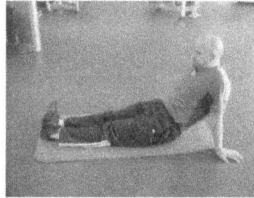	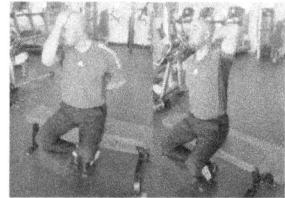
Brachioradialis	Calves (general)	Calves (soleus)
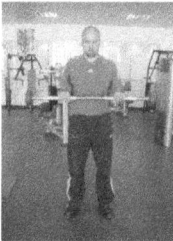	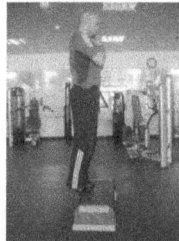	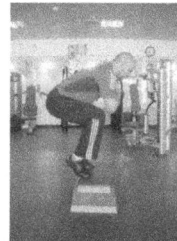
RESISTANCE BAND EXERCISES		BARBELL EX'S
Tibialis anterior	Shoulder shrugs	Wrist flexion
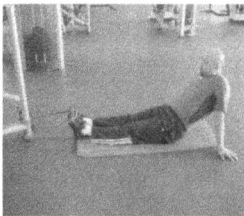	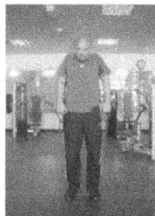	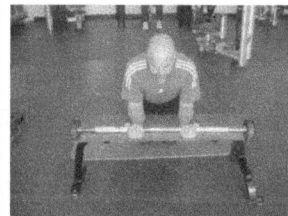
BARBELL EXERCISES		DUMBBELLS
Wrist extension	Shoulder shrugs	Shoulder shrugs
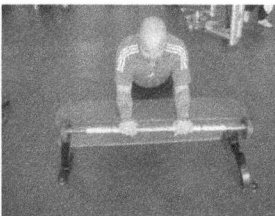	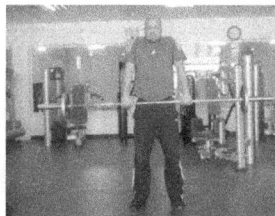	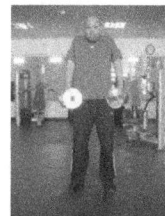

ISO - Isometric

AEROBIC & ANAEROBIC
RESISTANCE TRAINING

As you are already aware, there are many different types of training that will help you to build strength, but they each have their own unique twist. Some people prefer pyramid strength training, others prefer basic strength training. The best advice any professional can give you is to keep your body guessing, and change your program every 4-6 weeks. Use the different types of strength training to keep things interesting, especially if your current routine is going stale. Read all about the different types of strength training when you have the time, but for now just acknowledge what your training goals are, and put together your plan.

PYRAMID TRAINING

Pyramid training is very challenging due to the high intensity. Below is an example of an upper body pyramid workout, whilst alternating 1, 2 or 3 exercises per muscle group.

AIM	TARGET	EXAMPLE OF PYRAMID
Pyramid upper body workout	Chest, Back, Shoulders, Triceps and Biceps	For each exercise perform 12reps, increase the weight for 10reps, and again for 8 reps. Work your way back up for a total of 5 sets.

Breakdown of pyramid workout

BODY PARTS	1,2 OR 3 EXERCISES PER MUSCLE GROUP	REPS	REMARKS
CHEST	Alternating chest flies and chest press	12/10/8reps whilst adding weight each time	You may need different weights for each ex. Or just perform x1 ex per muscle group.
BACK	Lat pull downs and bent over row	**As above** - Work your way back up for a total of 5 sets.	**As above** - Work your way back up for a total of 5 sets.
SHOULDERS	Rear, lateral and front deltoid raises	**As above**	**As above** - A set of x3 ex's to target anterior, posterior and medial deltoid.
TRICEPS	Kickbacks and seated extensions		**As above** - 2 counts up, 2 counts down for each set
BICEPS	Normal curls and hammer curls		

247

Alternating 1, 2 or 3 exercises per muscle group is quite advanced, therefore for beginners you would just complete x1 exercise and progress accordingly. Below is an example of a lower body pyramid workout, whilst alternating 5 exercises per muscle group, it operates in the same way as the upper body workout. With this workout there aren't as many sets due there not being as many exercises. However, these particular leg exercises are mostly multi-joint compound exercises.

BODY PART	1,2 OR 3 EXERCISES PER MUSCLE GROUP	REPS	REMARKS
LEGS	Leg Press	12/10/8reps whilst adding weight each time	You may need different weights for each exercise. Work your way back up for a total of 5 sets.
	Lunges	**As above -** Work your way back up for a total of 5 sets.	
	Alternating Squat types	**As above**	2 counts up and 2 counts down for each set
	Dead-lifts		
	Calf Raises		

The main drawback of this workout will be the constant weight changes, especially if you choose to use a barbell i.e. constantly changing the weighted plates. A full body pyramid workout would challenge you more, especially if you chose more than x1 exercise per muscle group, and creating more sets etc. Overall, pyramid workouts and perfect when you want an intense training session. You can complete a pyramid workout by using any exercises, and also by using any equipment. Always remember that when you decrease your reps, to increase the resistance and add intensity by slowing down the movement, but mainly to progress safely.

SUPERSETS

By definition is one set of two different exercises completed back to back with no rest in between, and generally the exercises are for opposing muscle groups but can be completed for the same muscle group too. Supersets are a proven technique for increasing intensity and bringing up lagging body parts. They also allow you to gain muscle while working around injuries that might be aggravated with heavy weights. If your training program is getting stale, supersets can also help relieve your boredom. Supersetting is a legitimate way to get more results in a short period of time, and is thought to be the king of muscle building.

Below is a superset for opposing muscle groups:

BODY PART	OPPOSING MUSCLE GROUPS	EXAMPLE
LEGS	Quadriceps	Split squat
	Hamstring	Romanian dead lift

Another example would be:

BODY PARTS	OPPOSING MUSCLE GROUPS
BICEPS	Bicep curl
TRICEPS	Dips

Below is a superset for the same muscle group:

BODY PART	MUSCLE GROUP
CHEST	Chest press
	Chest flyes

If you've been training seriously for any length of time, super-setting is something you're probably already familiar with but haven't fully exploited to the maximum.

- Supersets are simply another method of increasing intensity;
- Shortening the rest between sets;
- More intensity equals more muscle;
- Supersets prevent injury, or allow you to work around an injury;
- A way to maintain your leg size without performing super heavy squats.

Super setting seems to work especially well in producing muscular hypertrophy when using a rep scheme of 6-10 reps to failure.

Pre exhaustion supersets

Pre-exhaustion is probably the best known and most effective type of superset of all, and performed by choosing two exercises for the same muscle group i.e. an isolation exercise first, followed by a basic, compound movement. The idea behind pre-exhaust supersets is to take a muscle group beyond the normal point of exhaustion and thereby achieve muscle fiber stimulation and growth that you normally could not achieve from a straight set.

An example of this is overleaf:

BODY PARTS	ISOLATION EXERCISE	COMPOUND EXERCISE
Back	DB pullovers	Lat pull downs
Chest	DB flyes	Bench press
Shoulder	DB lateral raise	Shoulder press
Triceps	Triceps pushdown	Close grip bench press
Biceps	BB curl	Under grasp pull ups
Legs	Leg extension	Squat
	Leg curl	Straight leg dead-lift

Complete a particular exercise until you can't do another rep, and you'll find that you are still able to do a compound exercise (albeit with a lighter poundage than usual). other muscles that are used in the compound exercise will still be fresh and strong. By "pre-exhausting" the target muscle with an isolated movement, you can then continue to blast the fatigued muscle even further with the help of the assisting muscles in the compound movement.

ISOLATION EXERCISES
By definition are exercises that work muscles at only one joint for example: a leg extension or a bicep curl. Isolation exercises are useful for rehabilitation purposes and strengthening weaker muscles but they don't offer as many benefits as compound exercises.

PULL/PUSH EXERCISES
By definition are a variation of exercises that can be worked on alternate days that involve pulling muscles i.e. rows, pull ups etc and pushing muscles i.e. push ups, presses etc. You can also perform Push/Pull exercises for the upper body on one day and then Push/Pull exercises for the lower body on another day, amongst other variations.

ALTERNATING SETS
By definition are, completing one set of one exercise, rest and then one set of another exercise resting for a prescribed amount of time and repeat, this is sometimes referred to as alternating supersets. For example: bicep curls (flexion), rest, followed by a triceps exercise (extension), bicep curls rest and repeat.

ASSISTED / FORCED REPS TRAINING
This type of training is quite simply, the performing of repetitions to fatigue (alone) and then being assisted for a few more repetitions by your workout partner. Good technique should still be your main priority throughout, irrespective of the fact that your partner will be assisting you with 10-15% of the weight load.

BACK OFF SETS / DROP SETS / DE-LOADING

All different names yet having similar meanings… by definition are completing a lighter set after one or more very heavy sets. This is a way of taking advantage of the central nervous system and its increased efficiency and this is down to completing the heavier set first than you would otherwise use with a higher amount of reps. To keep the muscles working hard these back off sets can also be completed with slightly less weight than was used on the previous set of heavy weight for example: around 10% less but of course ensuring that you don't over train them.

COMPOUND EXERCISES

By definition are exercises that work muscles over more than one joint such as squats etc. These exercises are the most effective as they work larger areas and therefore burn more calories than the one joint isolated exercise. They are of course more functional for example: they carry over better into everyday life and sport, offering more benefits to you. There are many benefits of compound exercises for strength training.

- They require more physical effort and output;
- They burn more calories;
- They involve multiple muscle groups;
- They require a certain level of balance and body coordination;
- They assist in developing core strength;
- They help build joint stability;
- They are the best exercises you can perform to build strength.

Generally, you can achieve an entire body workout using compound strength exercises, but the level of physical exertion required to perform compound exercises allows you to get a great cardio workout at the same time.

Some of the best compound exercises are listed below:

1. Bench press;
2. Dead-lifts;
3. Squats;
4. Front squats;
5. Military press;
6. Clean and press;
7. Pull ups.

Pure strength training - Use compound exercises to build raw strength

To develop a well rounded physique - Make combined use of both compound exercises and isolation exercises to stimulate the maximum amount of muscle fibres.

251

SUPER SLOW TRAINING

A popular version of this type of training is comprised of the following:

- A 10sec lifting phase i.e. concentric;
- A 5sec lowering phase i.e. eccentric.

This technique can also be reversed i.e. 5sec concentric / 10sec eccentric but generally you should be aiming for 4-6 reps in the slowest amount of time possible i.e. between 15-60secs. 15secs or less if strength and hypertrophy are your goal, remembering at all times that overload = intensity i.e. working harder for less time.

NEGATIVE TRAINING

By definition is the lowering portion of a lift for example: when you bring the bar down towards the ground on a bicep curl. Negatives should be used sparingly but they normally involve using heavier weights than you would normally during the positive aspect of an exercise i.e. the concentric or upward movement. Negatives only involve the slow lowering of the weight which builds strength, but can be accomplished by any one of the following:

1. Adding manual resistance on the lowering phase of any lift;
2. Adjusting the weight lifted / lowered when using a selectorized plate machine;
3. Have a partner assist you through the lifting phase with an amount heavier than you could lift alone, and lower unassisted.

Negative training allows for approx. 30% more muscle force production than concentric contraction.

The remainder of this sub-chapter, are added extras and should be used for your additional information purposes only, as they are words or phrases that you may have come across previously or will do in the future.

1RM training (1RM = one repetition maximum)

By definition is the heaviest weight you can lift for one repetition on any given exercise. The 1RM can be tested or even estimated based on what you know about your past exercise programs or what you know you can lift for other numbers of reps. Exercise programs occasionally require you to use a weight that is a certain percentage of your 1RM.

Plateau

By definition is a period in which your training progress stops. A plateau is normally reached due to a lack of variety in your workouts, or simply lifting too heavy weights for too long. Plateaus are normally a warning sign of overtraining.

Overtraining

By definition is the condition that results from training too intensely or too consistently for too long without a break or a change in the program.

The symptoms of overtraining are generally related to the following: Injuries, a lack of interest in training, lethargy and a decrease in performance. Overtraining can be avoided but it is very specific to each person but try the following examples: every 4-6 weeks change your workout, take adequate rest, de-load for a week, stretch regularly, sleep 8-10 hours per night and follow a good nutrition plan.

Tri-set

By definition is 1 set each of 3 exercises completed back to back, usually with little or no rest between each set.

Leave one in the tank

By definition is taking your set to one rep short of failure. This technique avoids the risk of injury or overtraining, yet the muscles are still worked sufficiently and it should be how most people train.

Failure

By definition is performing an exercise for a number of reps until you cannot continue. There are different types of failure for example: You can stop the set before beginning the rep or you can fail halfway through the rep, alternatively you can be assisted by someone to assist you going beyond failure where you would normally fail. These techniques should be used sparingly so as not to risk injury or overtraining and generally your sets should finish one or two reps before failure.

Workout split

By definition is the way in which you organise your training schedule over a period of time i.e. each week etc. The purpose of your program will be dictated around your overall aim and would depend on whether you want to split your body parts i.e. chest & triceps, legs & shoulders, back & biceps or simply do upper and lower body. There are of course many other options, most of which are enclosed within this book

COMMON CARDIOVASCULAR ACTIVITIES

DEVELOPING YOUR CARDIOVASCULAR PROGRAM

Given the wide range of cardiovascular activities that you can choose from, almost anyone who enjoys working up a sweat can find something he or she enjoys. If you can integrate working out into your lifestyle, then this will ultimately leave you feeling fit and healthy. Even walking, jogging, running, cycling or even blading / roller skating etc to and from your home to your workplace and back several times a week will help you immensely.

Some large muscle group cardiovascular activities are listed for you below:

- Walking;
- Jogging;
- Running;
- Non-sprint cycling (on-or off road);
- Swimming;
- In line skating;
- Hiking;
- Stair climbing;
- Cross country skiing;
- Any other…

Exercising wherever you can will keep your routine flexible with variation. Even if you have no genetic predisposition to endurance in a muscular body i.e. you are a fast twitch muscle fiber person, then long periods of aerobic activity will not be your idea of fun at all. However, once you are comfortably able to sustain 20-30mins of any cardiovascular activity, you should endeavour to extend your aerobic exercise session to 45mins, or at least by 5mins per week. At this duration, your body burns through its available glycogen energy and begins to burn stored fat.

Overload
Overload is defined as a rhythmic, continuous, large muscle activity that promotes a simultaneous increase in heart rate and blood return to the heart. It is recommended that before you decide how long, hard or often you are going to train your cardiovascular system, you plan to apply the correct overload. In order to gain continued improvements the overload must be progressive in nature i.e. you will need to work harder in order to keep seeing progress.

Frequency of your cardiovascular exercise

3-5 days per week for most cardiovascular exercise programs is recommended. Alternating days of more intense exercise with a day of rest or easy exercise such as walking and stretching or yoga will give your body time to build and repair muscles.

Duration of your cardiovascular exercise

For cardiovascular benefits, you should aim for 20-60mins in your target heart rate zone, apart from the time you spend in warm-up and cool down. As explained previously, at this duration, your body burns through its available glycogen energy and begins to burn stored fat. While you will still have the benefits of burning calories if you exercise for less than 20mins in your zone, the best fitness benefits still come from setting aside the 20-60mins to spend in your aerobic zone. When beginning any type of fitness program your main focus should be to concentrate on increasing your duration with good posture and good form before you work on increasing the intensity of your workout. If you are using walking for your workout, work on increasing the number of minutes walked in each session. It is ultimately safer to increase your time by 10% per week. Once you are walking comfortably and with good posture and good form for 60mins at a time, then work on increasing the intensity by adding speed, hills, or intervals which you have previously learnt about in the interval training chapter.

Intensity

Steady state is a level of cardiovascular effort that is easy for you to maintain, and if you want to train to your full potential it is important for you to recognize this particular level of intensity i.e. a pace that you can maintain for a very long period of time. This zone is quite simply your comfort zone, but you must know and understand how you feel whilst working in this zone. Knowing what this steady state of effort feels like is what you are attempting to discover and ultimately improve upon i.e. gradually push yourself beyond it or, whilst in your active rest phase you may need to work at or below this effort level, especially when you are working with intervals. In order to optimize your results start thinking about what easy steady state exercise feels like, then you can compare these feelings when you are performing hard exercise. You will need to gauge your effort level throughout your training, whether this is via HRT or the rating of perceived exertion (RPE) method of 1 being easy 10 being extremely difficult. Whichever method you choose, you need to understand that no training intensity recommendation is set in stone i.e. Ranges for VO2 max, Target Heart Rate (THR) etc, so when you record your results you will find what works best.

In this chapter there are many cardio choices for you, you can then begin to plan your training program once you know what you want to achieve from it.

OUTDOOR ACTIVITIES

Tips for walking on the treadmill

Technique
Same as walking on the treadmill (unless interval training)

Safety

1. Change your outdoor walking program to an indoor one if the weather is too hot/humid;

2. Always be aware of traffic, uneven surfaces and think safety at all times;

3. Always wear luminous or bright colored clothing especially if it is not completely bright;

4. You should always have all your senses on high alert and therefore headphones can be a dangerous accessory.

Walking gear
A pedometer is completely optional even though it measures the distance you cover by counting your steps; it must be calibrated to your stride length first.

TIPS FOR RUNNING OUTDOORS

Technique
As per indoor running

Transition from walking to running
In the beginning it is advisable to run at a steady pace for 1 minute at a time, alternating walking and running throughout your allocated training time. Mix walking with running and endeavour to run for longer periods each time until you can run continuously for the whole time period. Focus on technique and distance rather than speed, do not overdo it in the beginning, be realistic and listen to your body.

Safety
Before you begin to run you should at least be accustomed to walking first, especially if you have been inactive and/or have an injury. You may want to attempt an activity with less stress on your body which involves less weight bearing.

1. Attempt to use dirt paths rather than pavements where necessary and change your outdoor running program to an indoor one if the weather is too hot/humid;

2. Always be aware of traffic, unpopulated areas and uneven surfaces and think safety at all times;

3. Always wear luminous or bright colored clothing especially if it is not completely bright;

4. You should always have all your senses on high alert and therefore headphones can be a dangerous accessory.

Running gear
A pedometer is completely optional even though it measures the distance you cover by counting your steps; it must be calibrated to your stride length first. Using a watch in the beginning is important to keep track of your performance.

TIPS FOR ROPE SKIPPING

Introduction

Skipping has many health and fitness benefits, and once you learn how to skip properly and you manage to maintain coordination, it will enable you to continue skipping for longer periods.

Skipping can be utilised in several ways:

1. Used as a warm up, either on its own or with body weight exercises;

2. Used as a conditioning tool for intervals i.e. 30secs of work / 30secs rest (active or complete);

3. Used whilst on your vacation because they are cheap and easy to carry;

4. Used as a CV workout when the weather doesn't allow you to go outdoors.

Skipping is an ideal exercise for a great cardio workout to help develop higher fitness levels. Skipping also assists you in losing weight, and if done correctly can burn many calories, and because skipping is a fairly energetic exercise, lots of calories can be burned in as little as a twenty minute session.

Skipping is generally considered an anaerobic type of exercise and therefore as mentioned it burns a great deal of energy.

Skipping has the following benefits:

- It is simple to learn;
- Inexpensive;
- Strengthens your bones;
- Assists in improving your strength and endurance;
- Increases your fitness levels;
- Improves your coordination and agility;
- Can be fun;

All exercises have their benefits and it is sometimes best to use a variation of exercises if you are attempting to lose weight. Variation in general helps you to maintain your motivation levels because you're never doing the same exercises day in day out.

TIPS FOR OUTDOOR CYCLING

Technique: As per indoor cycling

Safety:
Change your outdoor cycling program to an alternative indoor one if the weather is hot or humid. Prior to cycling you should plan your route according to your ability and observe traffic, uneven surfaces and use the proper hand signals whilst remaining alert at all times. If cycling at night you should use a head light and at the rear of the bike use a red light that flashes, combined with this it is wise to choose a well lit route. Your anticipation of other road users is very important as is using your gears effectively to slow down and/or your brakes to stop therefore to avoid any dangerous situations your speed should be controlled at all times. In order for you to be alert and have use of all your senses headphones should not be worn.

Cycling gear

Bike - The bike that you choose, whether it is a mountain bike or a racer should fit your body perfectly.

Clothes - It is of the utmost importance that you wear visibly bright and reflective clothing that is not baggy. For comfort wear padded shorts and gloves and ensure your glasses keep insects out of your eyes by wearing wraparound ones.

Shoes - A well fitted shoe is advised that is not only lightweight, thin and rigid but also low –cut so not to restrict your ankle.

Helmet - Do not ride outdoors if you have no helmet, as a helmet can and will prevent injuries or may save your life should you have an accident. The helmet should fit correctly on your head without pinching.

Getting started
You would ensure that the frame size is adequate for your height by straddling the top tube of the bike and making sure you clear it by 2-5 cm. You would also ensure that the brakes and gears are of a good standard by practicing shifting gears and braking in a quiet location prior to going into traffic. Once you actually sit on the bike you should adjust the height of the seat to ensure that you have a slight bend at the knee when you extend the leg downwards. The saddle should be parallel to the ground and the handlebars comfortable with reference to your reach and general posture. Toe straps should not be used if you are a beginner to cycling.

TIPS FOR SWIMMING

Technique
Body position – because of the horizontal position of the body in the water, you should avoid heart rate training as it is not a very good indicator of intensity.

Breathing – exhale fully under the water and endeavour to control the speed over time, patience is the key. If tired switch to a less strenuous stroke or take a break and

Arm and leg stroke can be concentrated on individually by using a float/kick board.

Safety
Generally - whether you are swimming in a pool or in the sea, always endeavour to swim with someone else and in case of extreme weather always avoid swimming in the sea. Apply sunscreen on sunny days and never chew gum to avoid choking.

In a pool – ensure there is a lifeguard present where possible or swim with a friend in case of emergency, avoid running at all times due to slippery surfaces

In the sea – familiarize yourself with the location and be aware of shallow/deep water, low/hide tides, rips and any possible hazard that may be under the surface.

Swimming gear
Goggles – endeavour to wear ones that fit the contours of your face to avoid problems on turns or dives. Whether you are swimming in the sea or in the pool, goggles will protect your eyes so long as they fit tightly and comfortably.

Costume – to minimize water resistance it should be tight fitting but comfortable.

Warm up & cool down
Mobility exercises and stretching can be followed by an easy paced swim for 5-10 minutes, use a variation of strokes to warm up all muscle groups to avoid injuries.

Variations
Break the swimming down into sets i.e. so many lengths of one stroke and then another etc and even using kickboards and floats to alternate arm work and leg work. Water aerobics and walking/running in water drills are also excellent forms of cardiovascular fitness.

INDOOR ACTIVITIES

Tips for walking on the treadmill

Technique
To prevent injuries good posture should be used at all times for e.g.

- Shoulders relaxed, (back and down)
- Chest up;
- Abdominals tight, with pelvis slightly tilted forwards;
- Walk tall;
- Avoid looking down.

Bend your arms to a 90 degree angle and as you swing your arms grasp your hands slightly. Roll as you step, form your heels to the balls of the feet and onto your toes and keep an even stride (unless interval training), breathe naturally and keep a record of your performance.

Safety
Whether you are using it anywhere or in the gym you should familiarize yourself with the treadmill first and know how it works before you attempt to use it. The most important button on the control is the emergency button, so be aware of its location. If you are unsure about anything you should ask the sales person or a gym instructor.

Before you turn the treadmill on you should stand on the step rails which are either side of the treadmill and depending on the type of treadmill that you are using you will have to program it first i.e. set your age, weight, time you want to workout etc but it is best advised to use the manual setting first because that way you will be in full control of your workout.

You should start the running belt with a slow speed first, ensure your feet are flat on the belt and hold onto the hand rails whilst slowly increasing the speed. Concentrate on your walking technique (explained above) and once you have cooled down you should finish by gradually decreasing the speed until it comes to a complete stop.

Try not to get into the habit of leaving the treadmill running when you are not on it and likewise getting on it when it is running.

Position yourself central on the treadmill i.e. not slipping off the backend or kicking the front panel.

TIPS FOR RUNNING ON THE TREADMILL

Technique
To prevent injuries good posture should be used at all times for e.g.

- Shoulders relaxed (back and down)
- Chest up;
- Abdominals tight, with pelvis slightly tilted forwards;
- Walk tall;
- Avoid looking down.

Bend your arms to a 90 degree angle and as you swing your arms grasp your hands slightly. Land softly on the heel and roll forward to the toes, try to avoid running on your toes and bouncing, keep an even stride (unless interval training) and maintain a steady pace, breathe naturally and keep a record of your performance.

Safety
Before you begin to run you should at least be accustomed to walking first, especially if you have been inactive and/or have an injury. You may want to attempt an activity with less stress on your body which involves less weight bearing. Whether you are using it anywhere or in the gym you should familiarize yourself with the treadmill first and know how it works before you attempt to use it. The most important button on the control is the emergency button, so be aware of its location. If you are unsure about anything you should ask the sales person or a gym instructor.

Before you turn the treadmill on you should stand on the step rails which are either side of the treadmill and depending on the type of treadmill that you are using you will have to program it first i.e. set your age, weight, time you want to workout etc but it is best advised to use the manual setting first because that way you will be in full control of your workout. You should start the running belt with a slow speed first, ensure your feet are flat on the belt and hold onto the hand rails whilst slowly increasing the speed. Concentrate on your running technique (explained above) and once you have cooled down you should finish by gradually decreasing the speed to a slow walk until it comes to a complete stop.

Try not to get into the habit of leaving the treadmill running when you are not on it and likewise getting on it when it is running. Position yourself central on the treadmill i.e. not slipping off the backend or kicking the front panel.

TIPS FOR INDOOR CYCLING

Technique

To avoid injuries use good posture at all times, keep the abdominals tight, a slight bend at the elbows and move your knees straight up and down, also:

1. Ensure the ball of the foot is on the pedals at all times;

2. Push forward at the top and bring your foot up and over;

3. Imagine scraping mud from the bottom of your shoes and relax to bring your foot back up;

4. Breathe naturally.

Your progress should be monitored regularly to ensure your intensity level is maintained and/or improved. To add variety and to work more muscle groups you should alternate between sitting and standing.

Safety

Adjust the height of the seat to ensure you have a slight bend at the knee when you sit on the bike and extend the leg downwards. Progress at a steady state which will reduce the risk of fatiguing quickly, you should adjust the resistance according to your fitness levels. Whether you use a manual setting or a set program on the machine the (RPM) rotations per minute should be maintained at a medium to high intensity level.

Cycling gear

Bike - If you are taking part in a spinning class, always ask a member of staff for a thorough brief before you begin. Attempt to buy a comfortable seat should you take cycling seriously and/or ride for long periods of time. For the best results your session should be progressive and challenging.

Shoes - Always try to ensure that your laces are tucked away at all times and purchase low cut (lightweight) shoes to avoid restricting any ankle movement.

Clothes - Avoid baggy clothes

TIPS FOR INDOOR ROWING

Technique

If you get your technique right you'll be efficient, produce better scores/results and avoid potential injuries.

1. Lean back slightly with the legs flat, the handle drawn to the body with the forearms horizontal;
2. The arms are relaxed and extended fully with the body rocking forward from the hips;
3. AFTER the arms have fully extended and the body rocked forward, slide forward maintaining arm and body position;
4. Shins vertical with body pressed up to the legs, the arms are straight and relaxed this position should not feel uncomfortable;
5. The legs push down and the body begins to lever back;
6. The legs continue to push as the body levers back, the arms remain straight;
7. The arms draw the handle past the knees and then strongly to the body, returning to the Finish position, the legs remain flat with the forearms horizontal;
8. Lean back slightly, legs flat, handle drawn to the body with the forearms horizontal. You are now ready to take the next stroke.

Safety

Always have the frame lock in the locked position when the flywheel and monorail sections are connected. To avoid possible injury, use caution while attaching the monorail section to the flywheel section and while operating the frame lock. Always ensure that you leave adequate free space around the rower clear of obstacles, walls, furniture etc to avoid contact or injury whilst rowing.

Rowing gear

Generally, any type of athletic wear that you would normally wear providing it is not loose fitting is a good choice. Shorts that fit tightly are encouraged and tops such as athletic bra tops or other tightly fitting tops are recommended. If you wear anything loose you take the chance of it getting caught in the rowing machine. Adequate footwear should be worn, preferably with rubber soles, and you have to strap your foot in. Do not wear sandals or attempt to use a rowing machine in bare feet ever.

If you have long hair and are using an indoor rowing machine you should always make sure that you tie it up and out of the way. Not only will this be cooler for you, but also it will prevent you from getting your hair caught in any part of the rowing machine.

TIPS FOR THE STAIR CLIMBER

Advantages of the stair climber – A non-weight bearing cross trainer ideal for working different muscle groups and supplementing other activities.

Technique

- Your posture should be perfect at all times with tight abs;
- Keep your knees over your toes at all times;
- Ensure your feet are flat on the platforms;
- Breathe naturally and pace yourself;
- Progress from holding handrails to not holding them;
- Monitor your intensity regularly;
- Avoid bouncing movements at the top/bottom of range;

Safety

Progress slowly and be patient as you build up the endurance of your leg muscles, keep the resistance low and speed high i.e. stairs climbed per minute. Avoid the following:

- Your heels hanging over the platforms;
- Standing on the balls of your feet;
- Your toes tingling or becoming numb (occasionally lift your forefoot off the platform).

Stepping gear

Adapt our program to suit your stair climber or if in a gymnasium ask an instructor to brief you fully on its use prior to using it.

Clothes

Wear baggy shorts and a comfortable loose fitting t-shirt.

TIPS FOR THE ELLIPTICAL TRAINER

The elliptical trainer is sometimes still referred to as a cross trainer, and it combines the fluidity of running with the low impact motion of cycling. The elliptical trainer puts a minimal amount of strain on your joints, yet provides one of the best workouts available today. Most elliptical trainers have a pair of handles connected to your foot pedals i.e. as your feet move, so do the arm handles. Moving your arms is optional, so you can choose to lightly grasp the stationary handlebar found in between the two swinging handles or you can choose not to hold onto anything at all. Below is the technique you use should you choose to use your arms.

Technique

1. Leg Movement

As you get on the machine for the first time pay attention to your foot placement, as each foot needs to be securely placed on its pedal, ideally on the center of each pedal; Your stride length should feel natural i.e. a stride length that is too long and wide makes for an uncomfortable workout. Also, a stride length that is too short is apt to create an unpleasant jerky movement. Some newer elliptical trainers now offer an adjustable stride length. This is great news for gym owners and others who need to share their equipment with people of different stature.

2. Arm Movement

Moving your arms in a manner similar to that of a runner or speed walker is the best option for increasing the intensity of your workout. Not holding onto anything causes the stabilising muscles of your midsection to work harder, thus maximizing your calories burned. However, leaning with your bodyweight on the handles will only decrease the intensity of your lower body workout.

Safety

If you choose to hold onto the handles of the elliptical trainer, whether they are movable or stationary, take care to do so with great care.

Digital Readout

The digital readout on any fitness machine is certainly a motivator for many exercisers. Readouts are usually programmed using a preset model exerciser so be aware of the accuracy i.e. use the digital readout as a guide. Gradually work your way up to at least a 20min workout, also increase the resistance gradually but maintain good posture at all times i.e. back straight, neck neutral, and shoulders down and relaxed.

CORE STRENGTH TRAINING

WHAT IS CORE TRAINING

By definition is working groups of muscles of the abdomen, including the obliques and lower back. Working this group of muscles assists in providing stability for the entire body (see the specific sections within the book i.e. the injury prevention & rehabilitation section and the section on abdominal exercises). Thousands if not millions of gym users often wonder why it is so difficult to get a six pack. The actual processes of getting a six pack are quite straight forward. When it comes to your abs it requires only that you decrease your intake of Fatty foods and of course specific exercises performed correctly. Everything that you do fitness wise should be initiated by the power of your abdominals, from standing up straight, walking, or any exercise (especially with weights).

Aim

The aim of this section is to give you a large selection (library) of exercises so that you can select ones that work best for you. Your core region consists of far more than just the abdominal muscles in fact core strength training aims to target all the muscle groups that stabilise your spine and pelvis. It is these muscle groups that are critical for the transfer of energy from large to small body parts during many sporting activities. Core conditioning and abdominal conditioning have become synonymous in recent years but the abdominal muscles alone are overrated when it comes to real core strength or conditioning. In reality, the abdominal muscles have a very limited and specific action, and your core actually consists of many different muscles that stabilise the spine and pelvis and run the entire length of the torso. These muscles stabilise the spine, pelvis and shoulder and provide a solid foundation for movement in the extremities, and core conditioning exercise programs need to target all these muscle groups to be effective. The muscles of the core make it possible to stand upright and move on two feet, these muscles help control movements, transfer energy, shift body weight and move in any direction. A strong core distributes the stresses of weight bearing and protects the back it also acts as a shock absorber for jumps and rebounds etc.

The main benefits of core strength training are:

1. Greater efficiency of movement, and improved body control and balance;
2. Increased power output from both the core musculature and peripheral muscles such as the shoulders, arms and legs;
3. Reduced risk of injury and improved balance and stability;
4. Improved athletic performance.

Core strength training and performance

Because the muscles of the trunk and torso stabilise the spine from the pelvis to the neck and shoulder, they allow the transfer of powerful movements of the arms and legs. All powerful movements originate from the centre of the body out, and never from the limbs alone. Before any powerful rapid muscle contractions can occur in the limbs, the spine must be solid and stable, and the more stable the core the more powerful the extremities can contract. Training the muscles of the core also corrects postural imbalances that can lead to injuries. The biggest benefit of core training is to develop functional fitness i.e. fitness that is essential to both daily living and regular activities. Core strengthening exercises are most effective when the torso works as a solid unit and both front and back muscles contract at the same time, multi joint movements are performed and stabilization of the spine is monitored.

What makes up your core muscles?

The list of muscles that make up your core is somewhat arbitrary and different experts include different muscles. In general, the muscles of your core run the length of your trunk and torso, and when they contract they stabilise your spine, pelvis and shoulder girdle and create a solid base of support. You are then able to generate powerful movements of the extremities. The goal of core stability is to maintain a solid foundation and transfer energy from the centre of your body out to the limbs. The following list includes the most commonly identified core muscles as well as the lesser known groups:

1. Rectus Abdominis - located along the front of your abdomen, this is the most well known abdominal muscle and is often referred to as the six pack;

2. Erector Spinae - This group of 3 muscles runs along your neck to lower back;

3. Multifidus - located under your erector spinae along the vertebral column, these muscles extend and rotate the spine;

4. External Obliques - located on the side and front of your abdomen;

5. Internal Obliques - located under your external obliques, running in the opposite direction

6. Transverse Abdominis (TVA) - located under your obliques, it is the deepest of your abdominal muscles and wraps around your spine for protection and stability;

7. Hip Flexors - located in front of your pelvis and upper thigh;

8. Gluteus medius and minimus - located at the side of your hip;

9. Gluteus maximus, hamstring group, piriformis - located at rear of your hip and upper thigh leg;

10. Hip adductors - located at medial thigh.

Strengthening your core muscles

There are many exercises that will strengthen your core, as well as exercise equipment that will aid this training. Some of the best products for developing core strength include:

- Medicine balls;
- Stability balls;
- Balance products such as the bosu ball, balance boards, wobble boards etc
- Dumbbells, Kettle-bells to name but a few.

Using no equipment

Body weight exercises are very effective for developing core strength, they are also the type of exercises many athletes and coaches rely on for regular core training, and they include:

➤ Abdominal Bracing

Abdominal bracing is the main technique used during core exercise training, and it refers to the contraction of the abdominal muscles. To correctly brace, you should attempt to pull your navel back in toward your spine, and this action primarily recruits transverse abdominus. Be careful not to hold your breath as you should be able to breathe evenly while bracing.

Some other general exercises can be used such as:

- Plank exercise;
- Side plank exercise;
- The basic push up;
- V-sits;
- Push ups;
- Squats;
- Back bridge;
- Hip lift;
- Russian twists;
- Lunges;
- Side lunges
- Back Extensions, to name only a few.

Yoga is also an excellent way for you to build core strength, and for a simple core strength program you can begin with push ups and crunches, but try to work with a trainer to find the exercises that work best for you.

Core Tests

These tests determine the strength of your abdominal muscles and the muscles around your lumbar spine. Since core muscles should be activated and used in almost every activity you do, doing well on theses specific core tests will prove that you are more than capable on the other tests. The plank is explained within the back exercise sub-chapter, just simply hold this good form for as long as you can, record and repeat.

Intensity levels

High intensity interval training (H.I.I.T) should accompany the exercises in this work-book. As with all exercises you should aim to control all movements i.e. whatever the exercise, it should be completed slowly during the concentric and eccentric aspects (up & down). The abdominals should be initiated prior & during every exercise and this way you will work them 100%. As mentioned previously, the position of your feet & arms whilst on the fit-ball is also very vital to your results i.e. hands out to the side takes less control of your abdominals than your hands across your chest. The closer together your feet are, the more balance is required; try this out as you master the technique on the fit-ball for each exercise.

How much is enough

As always, use a journal to write down what you can achieve in the time you have, you can start off by doing each exercise to a certain amount of reps or to a set time, so long as you control each movement. Stay out of your comfort zone and don't just do the exercises you find easy i.e. always test your body and keep it thinking about what is coming next. The more difficult you find a certain exercise you can guarantee that it is that exercise that will get you the better results.

Posture & Breathing

You should retain good posture throughout any exercise i.e. your head, shoulders and hips should be inline & facing forwards at all times. This should not change irrespec-tive of which position you are in, whether it is standing, sitting, on your back or on your front. It is advised that you breathe out during any exertion to avoid any health issues. It is extremely important that the abdominals are initiated first, before all movements.

Important notes

Some people believe that you have to do 1000's of sit ups to get results, but with a healthy diet and a reduction in body fat, alongside controlled exercises that require you to focus, you will achieve the results you require. Before attempting any exercise you must always see your doctor before exercising, especially if you have any existing inju-ries or conditions.

FIT-BALL EXERCISES

In order to reap the benefits of a total workout, most people prefer to purchase home fitness equipment that is not only effective for them, but also something they can do during their own flexible timings. If you prefer to workout at home then one of the best options you should consider is buying a fitness ball. There are various other names given to a fitness ball and they include: exercise ball, Pilate's ball, gym ball, therapy ball, balance ball, body ball, yoga ball, sports ball, and Swiss ball, to name but a few. Fitness balls come in different sizes, an example being one with a diameter of 55-85 cm's and they are generally made of elastic rubber. To establish the correct size for you, when you sit on the ball there should be a 90 degree angle at your knees.

The main benefit of a fitness ball exercise is enabling your body to respond to the ball's instability while keeping your balance and engaging more muscles simultaneously. Compared to normal sit up exercises, your core muscles, back muscles, hip muscles, abdominal and pelvic muscles are the main target of fitness ball exercises in helping you stay on the ball. The exercises can be made easier to give you more stability on the fitness ball, and progressed in order to be made more difficult for e.g. if you are performing a sit up on the fitness ball and your feet are spread apart, this makes it easier and can be made more difficult when the feet are closer together. The same principles apply for placing your arms out to the side for more balance, and across your chest when you want to progress and make it more difficult. Closing your eyes is another way although this is very advanced, but your muscles are strengthened upon struggling to maintain your balance whilst performing specific exercises on the fitness ball. Each exercise requires you to maintain correct posture and support from your stomach muscles and back to help in keeping the trunk muscles firm, and even though the fitness ball is still prescribed by some therapists in treating patients with back pain, the fitness ball can also cause injury if not used correctly. Workout templates specific to fitness ball exercises can be found at the rear of the book.

ABDOMINAL EXERCISES (Beginner to advanced)

Beginner exercises

Bent knee Sit Up (arms across chest)

Start Position:

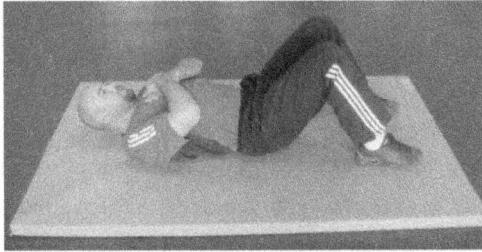

Variation of exercises:

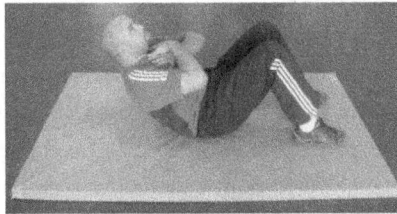

A: Raise your shoulders off the ground using the abdominals only

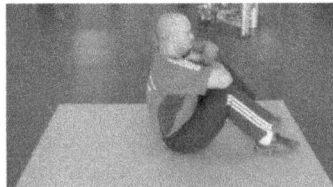

B: Raise your back off the ground using the abdominals only

Leg Raises (arms by side)

Start Position: Endeavour to keep your feet off the ground

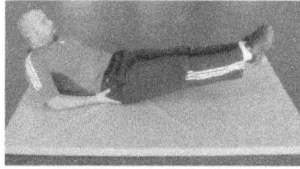

Choice of Exercises:

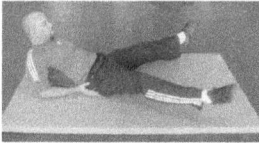

A: open/close your legs to the side   **B:** up and down

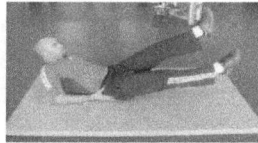

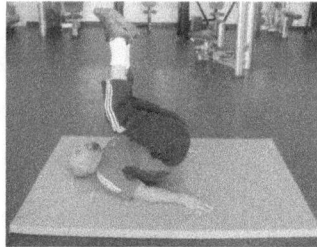

C: Raise your hips off the ground using the abdominals only

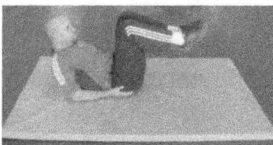

D: Raise your knees to your chest   **E:** Add a weight

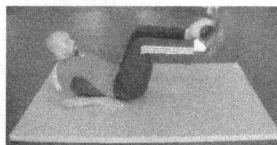

Sit Ups (arms above head)

Start Position:

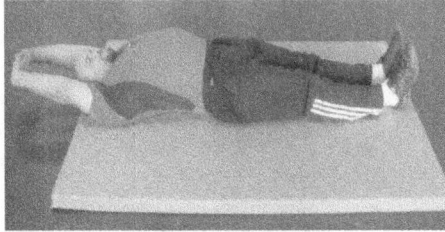

Choice of Exercises:

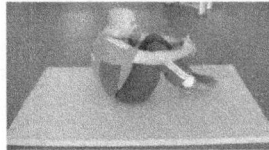

A: Sit up to grasp your bent knees

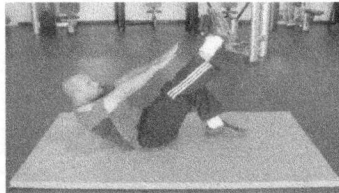

B: Sit up to touch the ankle of one straight leg

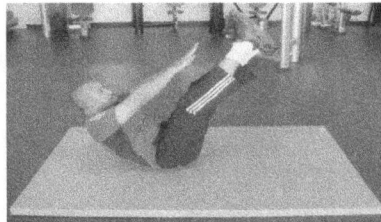

C: Sit up and hold with 2 straight legs

Sit Ups (hands on head)

Start Position: On your back or on your side

Choice of Exercises:

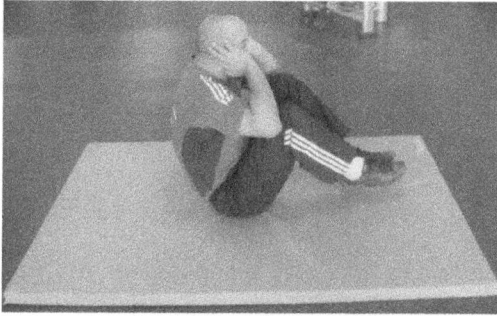

A: Sit up to touch the knees with your elbows

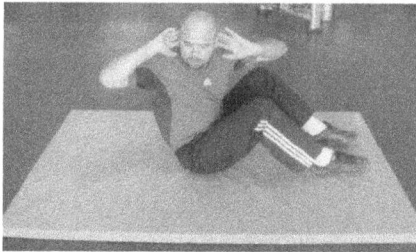

B: Sit up to touch the knee with the opposing elbow

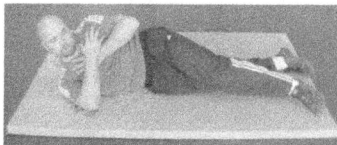

C: Sit up to the side and hold (hands across chest)

Beginner Sit Ups (utilising a fit-ball)

Start Position: Sat on the ball, legs on the ball or between your feet

Choice of Exercises:

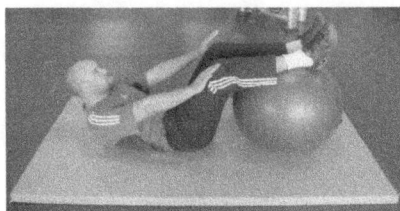

A: Sit up to touch the knees with your finger tips

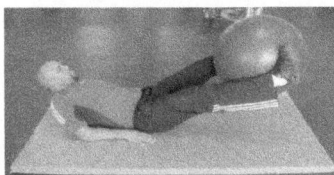

B: Raise the ball towards your hips with legs bent

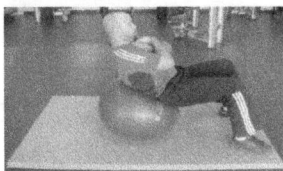

C: Sit up slowly and hold

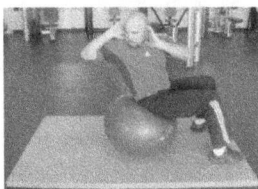

D: Sit up slowly and twist

Beginner Machines

Starting out: Always consult a personal trainer or gym   instructor first

Choice of Exercises:

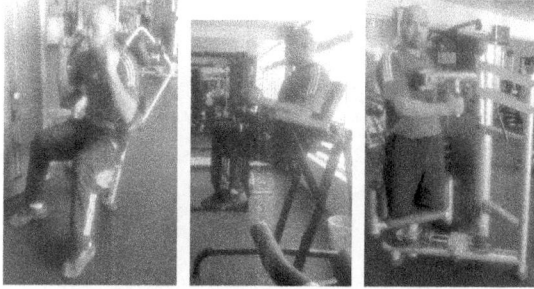

A: Crunch, twist and raise the knees to chest height

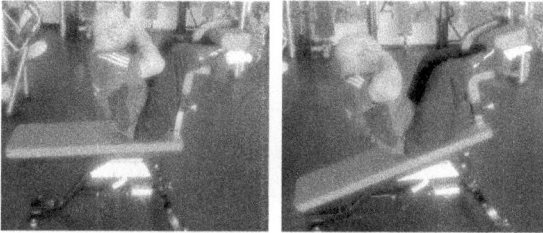

B: Fix the legs and curl up and down slowly

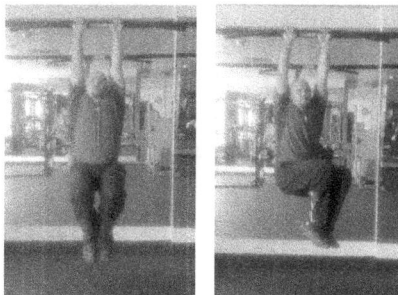

C: Ensure your grip is tight; raise the knees to waist height and / or twist to work your obliques.

Intermediate Abdominal Exercises

Weighted ball in hands

Start positions: Ball in your outstretched arms

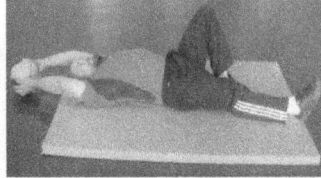

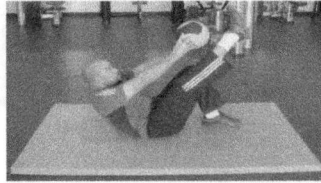

A: With 1 leg bent curl up, touch your other leg with the ball

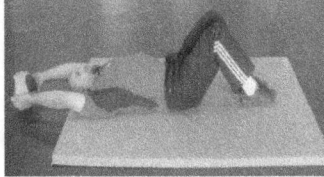

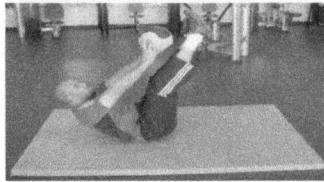

B: With both legs bent curl up, touch both your legs with the ball

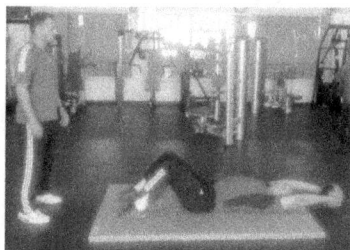

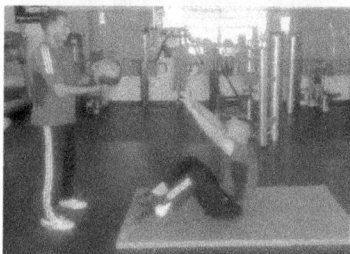

C: With both legs bent, keep ball above head as long as possible with arms straight, curl up, breathe out and throw at the wall - or to someone.

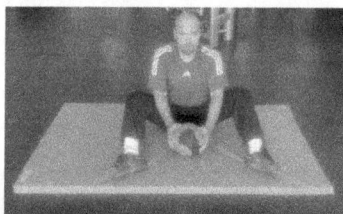

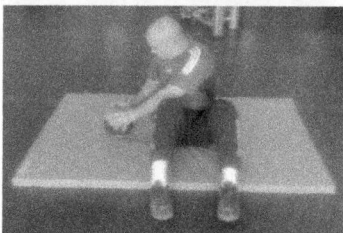

D: Twist at the waist and touch the ball down behind you, repeat to opposite side.

Weighted ball in feet

Starting out: Keep your feet off the ground at all times

Choice of Exercises:

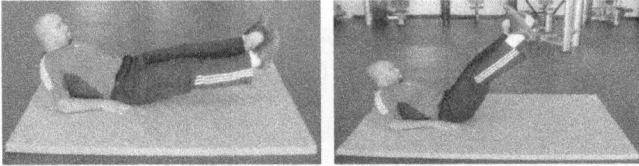

A: Raise your legs from the floor, hold, lower and raise.

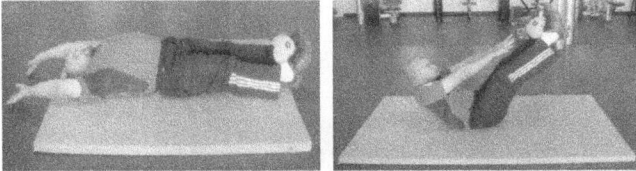

B: With both legs straight, curl up, touch the ball with both hands & slowly lower

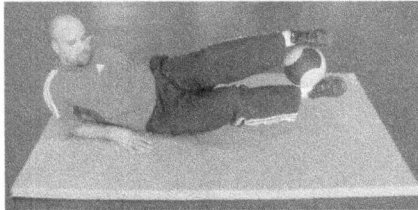

C: Twist at the waist; touch your knees down to each side, repeat to other side

Partner Exercises

Choice of Exercises:

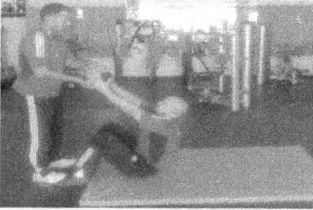

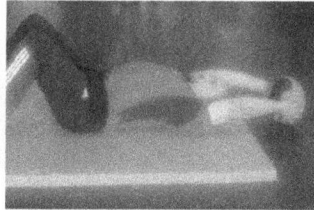

A: With both legs bent, keep ball above head for as long as possible with arms straight, curl up, breathe out and pass the ball to your partner

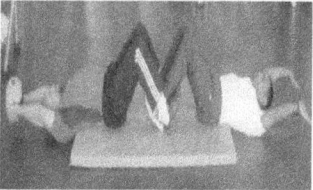

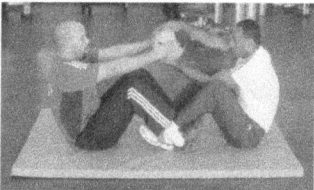

B: With both legs bent, curl up & pass the ball to your partner

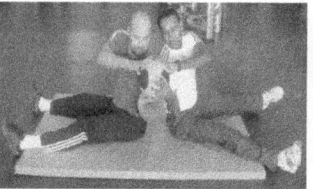

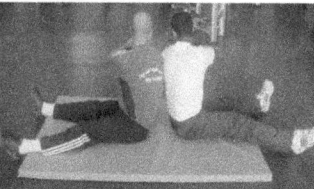

C: Twist at the waist; pass the ball to your partner, repeat to other side

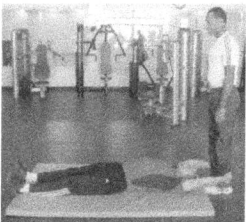

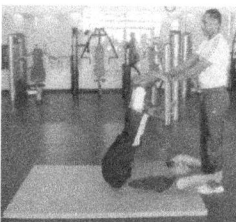

D: Contract your abs, raise your legs towards your partner and breathe out

Intermediate Abs (utilising a fit-ball)

Choice of Exercises:

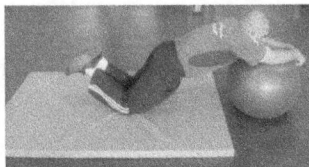

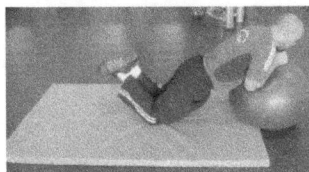

A: With both knees resting, lean on the ball with your arms outstretched, pull the ball towards you as you breathe out and without moving at the waist

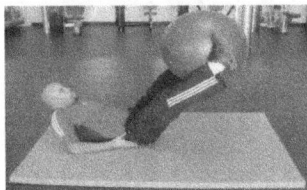

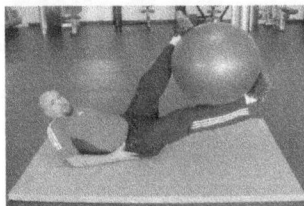

B: With both legs straight, keep the ball in between your feet & twist at the waist

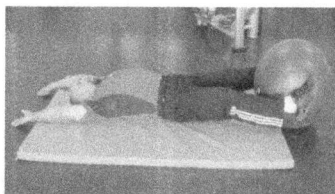

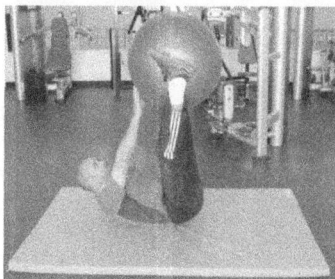

C: Raise both your upper & lower body whilst breathing out, touch the ball

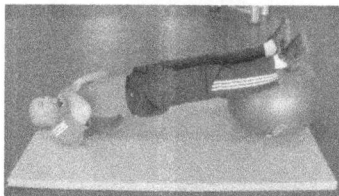

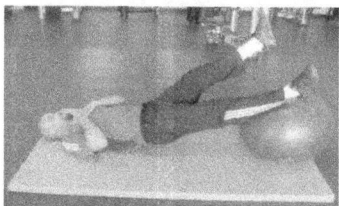

D: With just your shoulders on the floor, press down on the ball with one leg, whilst raising the other, trying to keep your hips high at all times

Advanced Abdominal Exercises

Bodyweight with minimum equipment

Choice of Exercises:

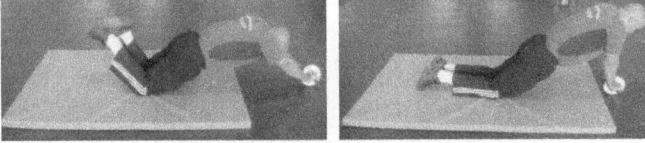

A: With both knees resting, lean on the wheel with your arms outstretched, push & pull the wheel without moving at the waist, Progress to feet on floor

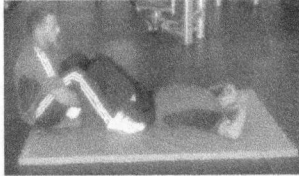

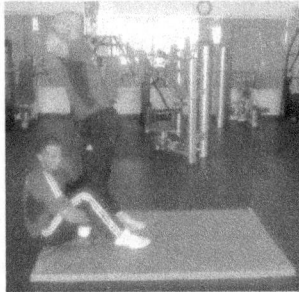

B: Stand up from lying on your back, with or without a partner

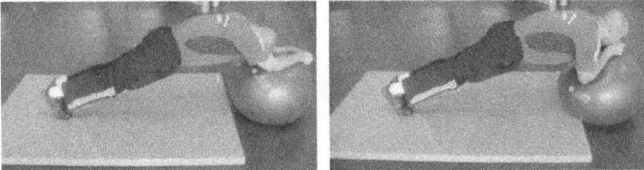

C: With both feet on the floor with your arms outstretched, pull the ball towards you as you breathe out and without moving at the waist

Advanced Abs (utilising machines)

Choice of Exercises:

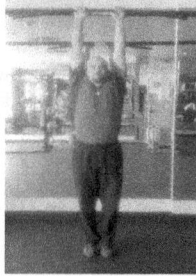

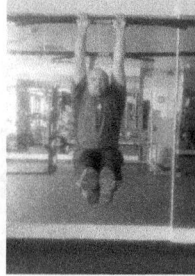

A: Ensure your grip is tight; raise the legs to waist whilst breathing out

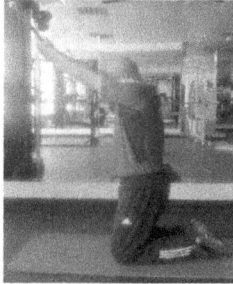

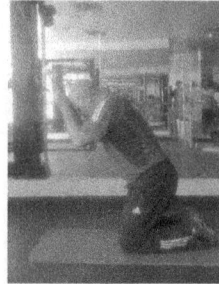

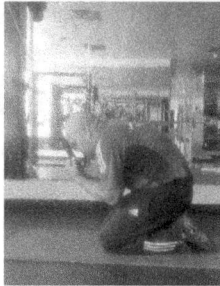

B: Pull cable or rope whilst contracting your abdominals & breathing out

Cable rotating extension

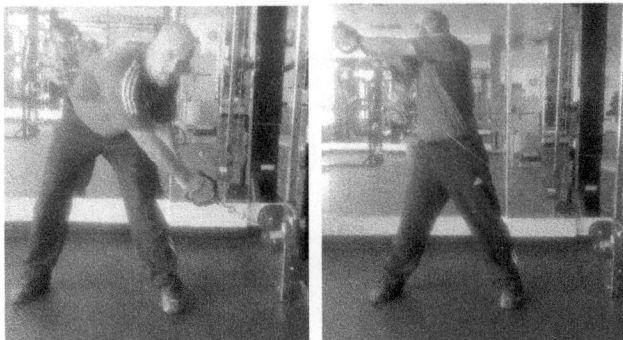

Cable rotation

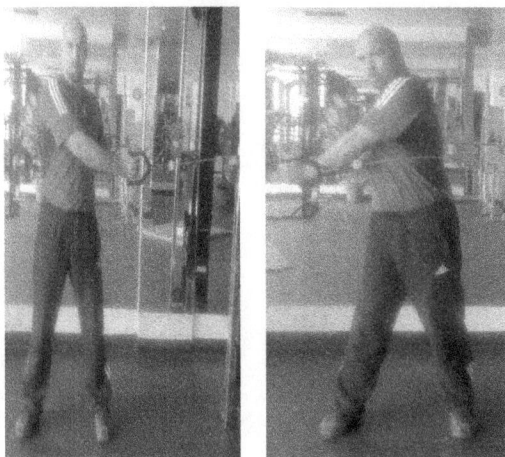

C: Pull the cable up or down dependant on setting, also pull from the side & twist, initiate the abdominals/obliques in order to pull the cable, not the arms.

Advanced Abs (utilising barbell)

Choice of Exercises:

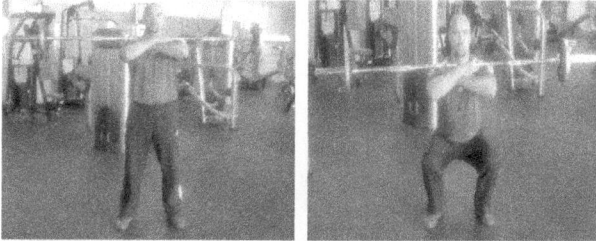

A: Squat down & up under the sole control of your abdominals, control breathing

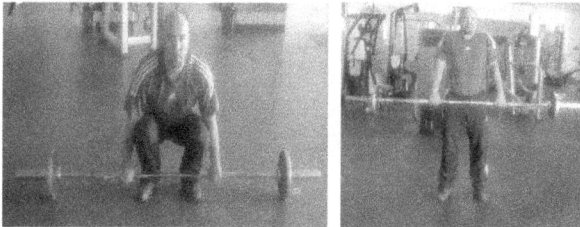

B: Stand up & raise your shoulders utilising your abdominals, whilst breathing out

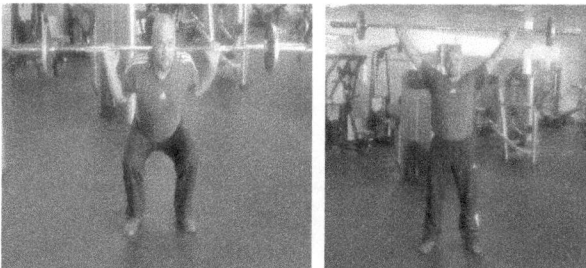

C: Stand up & raise the bar up above your head, utilising your abdominals, whilst breathing out.

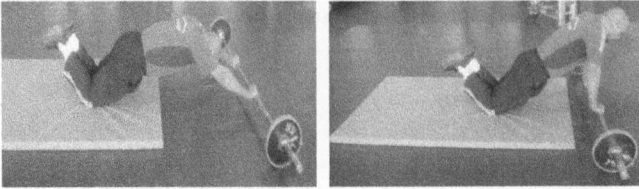

D: With both knees on the floor with your arms outstretched, pull the ball towards you as you breathe out, without moving at the waist. Progress to feet on the floor

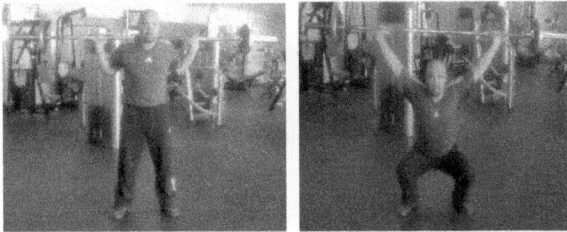

E: Squat down under the sole control of your abdominals, raise the bar up above your head whilst breathing out. Breathe in as you stand up and lower the bar

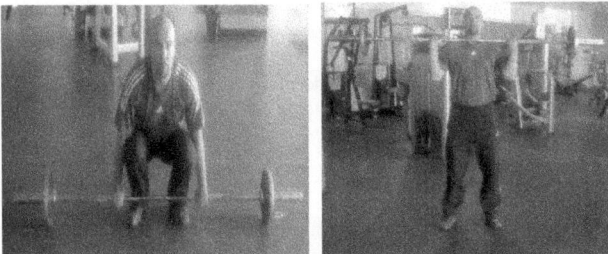

(1)   (2)

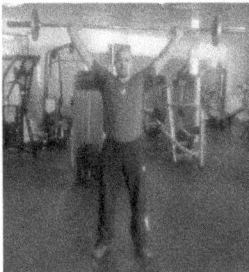

(3)

F: Stand up & raise the bar to your shoulders & then above your head whilst breathing out. Attempt to do this at speed whilst using your abdominals.

Advanced Abs (utilising dumbbells)

Choice of Exercises:

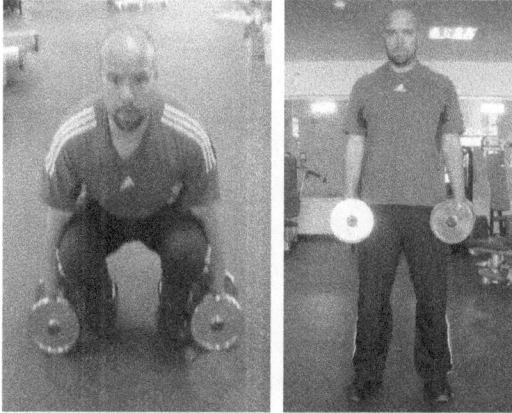

A: Stand up utilising your abdominals, whilst breathing out

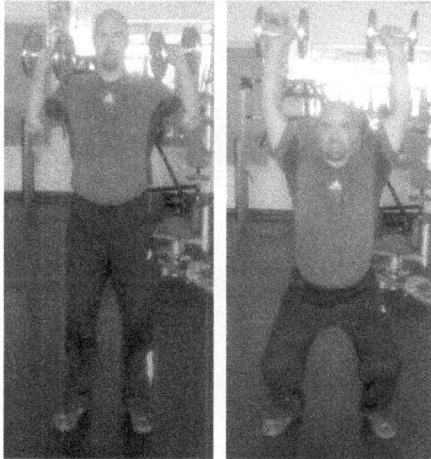

B: Squat down under control of your abs, raise the dumbbells above your head whilst breathing out. Breathe in as you stand up & lower them

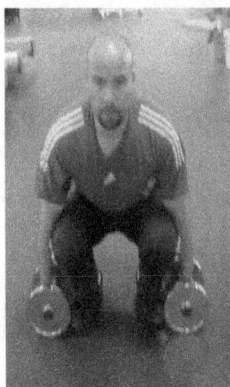

(1)

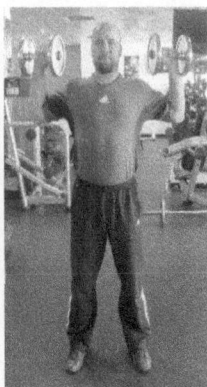

(2)

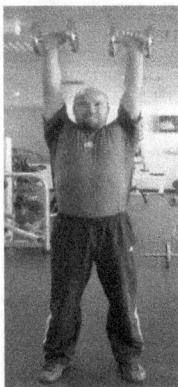

(3)

C: Stand up & raise the dumbbells to your shoulders & then above your head whilst breathing out. Attempt to do this at speed whilst using your abs

Stretching your abdominals

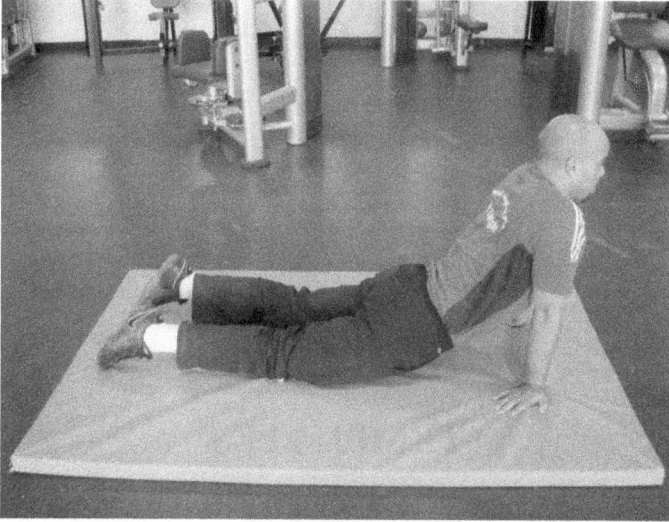

Lie on your front with your hips as close to the floor as possible, lift your upper body from the floor using your arms and push your hips into the floor. Breathe normally throughout the stretch without holding your breath.

To stretch your obliques, quite simply lie on a fit-ball (on your side) and lower your upper body below the height of your hips to ensure you get a good stretch, obviously ensure you are stable and your bottom leg is firmly on the ground.

TEMPLATES

The following templates consist of all the exercises included within this book. They provide you with all that you need to construct programs which you can tailor to your own specific needs.

SPORTS SPECIFIC TEMPLATE

In order to improve your level of performance within your chosen sport many considerations need to be taken into account. You need to increase your working capacity, your skill effectiveness and your psychological qualities. Most training programs tend to neglect the physical training component and focus on the technical and tactical training. Physical training must be the foundation of your training program with physical efficiency being provided by technical proficiency. The number one rule for different types of sports is as follows:

SPEED & POWER SPORTS	ENDURANCE SPORTS
Emphasize intensity	Volume

For sports requiring more intricate skills, training complexity is paramount.

The chart below shows you the basics of what is required related to training objectives for specific sports, however the technical elements are not included.

SPORT	GENERAL PREPERATION	SPECIFIC PREPERATION
Rowing	Aerobic endurance, general and Maximum strength	Aerobic endurance and Muscular endurance
Physical team sports	As above	Anaerobic endurance and Power
(100m) **Swimming**	As above	Anaerobic & aerobic endurance, Maximum strength and power
(800m)		Aerobic & anaerobic endurance, Muscular endurance

In simple terms, if a particular workout template hits the zone for your sport then use it.

CIRCUIT TRAINING TEMPLATES

Overview of the different circuit types

There are many different types of circuits but we have summarized the main types for you i.e. general circuits, which can involve alternating arm, trunk, leg body parts in order to work your whole body. Or specific circuits that can overload certain muscle groups or focus on certain skills and drills. But generally it will depend on your goals.

EXERCISE	INTENSITY	LOAD	REST
Upper body	Dictated by time or reps and by the amount of rest	Bodyweight only	Generally 30-60secs rest in between
Abdominals			
Lower body			
Upper body			
Abdominals			
Lower body			

Setting your own level of fitness

You can develop your own circuit utilising whatever exercises you want i.e. body-weight, fit-ball, resistance band, BB, DB or exercises using fitness machines. Test yourself by performing the maximum amount of reps in a set time for e.g. a minute, and record your results within the chart below. In this way you are rating your own level of fitness in order to see your improvements over time. Controlling the exercise order, amount of sets etc will dictate your intensity. You can also perform each exercise to failure, and share it with others to challenge their level of fitness.

EXERCISES	LEVEL										
	1	2	3	4	5	6	7	8	9	10	REMARKS (Max effort)
Squat thrusts	12	14	16	18	22	*24	26	28	30	32	Did 24 in 1min

Create your own sports specific circuits

Sports specific circuits can include many agility type drills (lateral hopping, sliding, stepping etc) also balance, coordination and of course resistance type exercises. A circuit may be performed once or repeated several times. You can fit any exercises you choose into a circuit template, and your choice of exercises will depend on your sport and specific goals. Additionally a circuit can be performed once or twice per week or less frequently depending on your training needs. Your imagination will be the deciding factor related to the results you require

For footballers, boxers, wrestlers, gymnasts, martial artists and certain other team sports personnel who require acyclic muscular endurance.

TYPE	INTENSITY	% of LOAD	RHYTHM	REST
Acyclic muscular endurance	Intensive n.o of reps: (10-30 reps)	Dynamic loads of 50-80%	Slow	2-3 x more than work-out time

EXERCISE	REPS (10-30)	LOAD	REST	REMARKS
			2-3 times more than it takes to execute the exercise	
		50-80%		

Generally 6, 9 or 12 stations are used

For distance runners, swimmers, cross country runners, skiers and rowers who require cyclic muscular endurance.

TYPE	INTENSITY	% of LOAD	RHYTHM	REST
Cyclic muscular endurance	Extensive n.o: (30-50 reps per min)	Low loads of 20-50%	Med-slow	Shorter rest intervals

EXERCISE	REPS (extensive number)	LOAD	REST	REMARKS
		20-50%	Shorter rest intervals	

Generally 6, 9 or 12 stations are used

AEROBIC ENDURANCE TRAINING TEMPLATES
(Beginner to Intermediate for 20-40mins)

OUTDOOR WALKING

Week	Times per week	Choose the time or distance option	
		Time option (minutes)	Distance option (kilometers)
1	3	25	2.5
2	3	25	2.5
3	3	25	2.5
4	3	25	2.5
5	3	30	3.0
6	3	30	3.0
7	3	30	3.0
8	3	30	3.0
9	3	35	3.5
10	3	35	3.5
11	3	35	3.5
12	3	35	3.5
13	3	40	4.0
14	3	40	4.0

TREADMILL WALKING

Week	Times per week	Time goal (minutes)	Speed (km/hr)	Alternate (flat / incline)	
				Flat	5%
1	3	20	5.5	-	
2	3	20	5.5	-	
3	3	20	5.5	5mins	3mins
4	3	20	5.5	5mins	5mins
5	3	25	5.5	-	
6	3	25	6.0	5mins	5mins
7	3	25	6.0	-	
8	3	25	6.0	-	
9	3	30	6.0	-	
10	3	30	6.0	5mins	3mins
11	3	30	6.5	-	
12	3	30	6.5	-	
13	3	35	6.5	-	
14	3	35	6.5	-	
15	3	35	6.5	5mins	3mins
16	3	35	6.5	5mins	5mins

Whether or not you are an experienced walker, feel free to increase or decrease the time/speed/incline guides according to your current fitness level.

AEROBIC THRESHOLD TRAINING TEMPLATES

OUTDOOR RUNNING (70-80% MHR)

Week	Times per week	Activity	Choose the time or distance option	
			Time option (min)	Distance option (km)
1	3	Walk/Run	20	2.5
2	3	Walk/Run	20	2.5
3	3	Walk/Run	20	2.5
4	3	Run	20	2.5
5	3	Run	20	2.5
6	3	Run	20	3.0
7	3	Run	20	3.0
8	3	Walk/Run	25	3.5
9	3	Walk/Run	25	3.5
10	3	Run	25	3.5
11	3	Run	25	3.5
12	3	Run	25	3.5
13	3	Run	25	4.0
14	3	Run	25	4.0

TREADMILL RUNNING (70-80% MHR)

Week	Times per week	Time goal (minutes)	Alternate			
			Walking (km/hr)		Running (km/hr)	
			Minutes	Speed	Minutes	Speed
1	3	20	3	6.8	2	11
2	3	20	2	6.8	3	11
3	3	20	2	6.8	5	11
4	3	20	2	6.8	5	11
5	3	20	-	-	20	11
6	3	25	2	6.8	5	11
7	3	25	2	6.8	5	11
8	3	25	-	-	25	11
9	3	30	2	6.8	5	11
10	3	30	2	6.8	5	11
11	3	30	-	-	30	11
12	3	30	-	-	30	11
13	3	35	2	6.8	5	11
14	3	35	2	6.8	5	11
15	3	35	-	-	35	11
16	3	35	-	-	35	11

Whether or not you are an experienced runner, feel free to increase or decrease the time/speed guides according to your current fitness level.

ANAEROBIC THRESHOLD TRAINING TEMPLATES
(Above 20mins)

OUTDOOR CYCLING (80%+ MHR)

Week	Times per week	Choose the time or distance option	
		Time option (min)	Distance option (km)
1	3	20	6
2	3	20	6
3	3	20	6
4	3	20	6
5	3	25	8
6	3	25	8
7	3	25	8
8	3	25	8
9	3	30	10
10	3	30	10
11	3	30	10
12	3	30	10
13	3	35	12
14	3	35	12

INDOOR CYCLING (80% MHR)

Week	Times per week	Time goal in minutes	Cycling speed (rotations per minute)	Resistance
1	3	20	50+	Low
2	3	20	50+	Low
3	3	20	60+	Low
4	3	20	60+	Low/Medium
5	3	25	60+	Low/Medium
6	3	25	60+	Low/Medium
7	3	25	70+	Low/Medium
8	3	25	70+	Medium
9	3	30	70+	Medium
10	3	30	70+	Medium
11	3	30	80+	Medium
12	3	30	80+	Medium/Hard
13	3	35	80+	Medium/Hard
14	3	35	80+	Medium/Hard
15	3	35	80+	Medium/Hard
16	3	35	80+	Medium/Hard

Whether or not you are an experienced cyclist, feel free to increase or decrease the time/speed/resistance guides according to your current fitness level.

INDOOR ROWING (80% MHR)

Day	Workout	Heart rate range	Total time	Average pace	Total distance (m)
Monday		-	:	:	
Tuesday		-	:	:	
Wednesday		-	:	:	
Thursday		-	:	:	
Friday		-	:	:	
Saturday		-	:	:	
Sunday		-	:	:	

Weekly combined time/distance

:	

STAIR CLIMBING & ELLIPTICAL (80%-90% MHR)

Week	Times per week	Time goal in minutes	Exercise intensity
1	3	10	Low
2	3	10	Low
3	3	15	Low
4	3	15	Low/Medium
5	3	20	Low/Medium
6	3	20	Low/Medium
7	3	20	Low/Medium
8	3	20	Medium
9	3	25	Medium
10	3	25	Medium
11	3	25	Medium
12	3	25	Medium/Hard
13	3	30	Medium/Hard
14	3	30	Medium/Hard
15	4	30	Medium/Hard
16	4	30	Medium/Hard

Feel free to increase or decrease the time/intensity guides according to your current fitness level.

2-6 DAY TRAINING PROGRAM TEMPLATES
(Beginner to Advanced)

MUSCULAR ENDURANCE TEMPLATES
(For field sports, rowers and martial artists etc)

Full bodyweight program template – (2 times per week + cardio)

Back exercises	20-30 Reps	2-5 Sets	Remarks
Back extensions			
Alt arm/leg raise 1&2			
Straight leg hold			
Plank progressions			
Hip raises			
Chest exercises	**Reps**	**Sets**	**Remarks**
Isometric hold			
Incline Push Ups			
Normal Push Ups			
Decline Push Ups			
Bodyweight Dips			
Shoulder exercises	**Reps**	**Sets**	**Remarks**
Isometric holds 1-4			
Advanced Hold			
Partner Resisted Ex's			
Caterpillar			
Additional Holds			
Bicep exercises	**Reps**	**Sets**	**Remarks**
Isometric hold			
Partner Res Holds			
Under-grasp pull ups			
Behind neck pull ups			
Triceps exercises	**Reps**	**Sets**	**Remarks**
Bench Dips			
Incline Press Ups			
Advanced press ups			
Partner walk			
Body raises			
Leg exercises	**Reps**	**Sets**	**Remarks**
Static Hold			
Bridge			
Squat			
Lunge			
Step Up			
Squat Jump			

*Choose 3-5 ex's per muscle group, and either overload or alternate each muscle group

RESISTANCE BAND PROGRAM TEMPLATE - (2 times per week + cardio)

Each band has a different strength and colour e.g. Yellow = light, green = Medium and red = heavy etc. Colour band used (_____)

Back exercises	20-30 Reps	2-5 Sets	Remarks
Single arm row			
Bent over row			
Seated row			
Lat pull down			
Reverse flyes			
Chest exercises	Reps	Sets	Remarks
Chest Press			
Flyes 1			
Flyes 2 & 3			
Pullovers			
Shoulder exercises	Reps	Sets	Remarks
Isometric Holds			
Shoulder Press			
Frontal Raise			
Rear Deltoid			
Lateral Raise			
Upright Row			
Bicep exercises	Reps	Sets	Remarks
Isometric Hold			
Standing Curls			
Overhead Pull			
Bent over curl			
Triceps exercises	Reps	Sets	Remarks
Overhead press			
Kickbacks			
Overhead push			
Forward press			
Leg exercises	Reps	Sets	Remarks
Squats			
Hip extension			
Hip flexion			
Abd/Adduction			

*Choose 3-5 ex's per muscle group, and either overload or alternate each muscle group

FITNESS MACHINE PROGRAM TEMPLATE – (2 times per week + cardio)
(30-50% 1RM)

Back exercises	20-30 Reps	2-5 Sets	Remarks
Lat pull down (wide arm)			
Standing pull downs 1			
Standing pull downs 2			
Pull ups (assisted)			
Standing row			
Back Extension			
Chest exercises	**Reps**	**Sets**	**Remarks**
Seated press & smiths machine			
Seated fly machine			
Cable Pullover			
Cable Flyes 1 & 2			
Cable Flyes 3,4 & 5			
Shoulder exercises	**Reps**	**Sets**	**Remarks**
Shoulder Press machines			
Forward raise (cable)			
Rear Deltoid (cable)			
Lateral Raise (cable)			
Medial Deltoid –Single Arm (cable)			
Bicep exercises	**Reps**	**Sets**	**Remarks**
Seated Curls			
Standing Cable Curls			
Alternative overhead curls			
Assisted under-grasp pull ups			
Triceps exercises	**Reps**	**Sets**	**Remarks**
Seated tricep push			
Overhead press			
Pull downs			
Close arm press			
Dips			
Leg exercises	**Reps**	**Sets**	**Remarks**
Squat machines			
Leg extension			
Hamstring curl			
Calf machines			
Abductors / Adductors			
Hip extension / Hip flexion			
Leg press			

*Choose 3-5 ex's per muscle group, and either overload or alternate each muscle group

BARBELL EXERCISE PROGRAM TEMPLATE - (2 times per week + cardio)
(30-50% 1RM)

Back exercises	20-30 Reps	3-5 Sets	Remarks
Back extension			
Dead lift			
Bar Pull with knees bent			
Bent over row 1			
Bent over row 2			
Chest exercises	Reps	Sets	Remarks
Barbell Pull Over			
Bench Press			
Incline Press			
Decline Press			
Barbell Fly			
Shoulder exercises	Reps	Sets	Remarks
Isometric holds			
Frontal Raise			
Rear Deltoid			
Shoulder Press			
Lateral Raise			
Upright Row			
Bicep exercises	Reps	Sets	Remarks
Isometric holds			
Standing Curls			
Preacher Curls			
Triceps exercises	Reps	Sets	Remarks
Lying overhead push			
Seated press			
Close arm press			
Tricep press (fixed bar)			
Leg exercises	Reps	Sets	Remarks
Barbell Squat			
Barbell Lunge			
Dead lift			
Barbell Step ups			
Barbell Split Squat			

*Choose 3-5 ex's per muscle group, and either overload or alternate each muscle group

DUMBBELL EXERCISE PROGRAM TEMPLATE - (2 times per week + HIIT)
(30-50% 1RM)

Back exercises	20-30 Reps	3-5 Sets	Remarks
Bent over row 1			
Bent over row 2			
Straight leg dead lift			
Reverse flyes			
Dumbbell pull			
Chest exercises	**Reps**	**Sets**	**Remarks**
Dumbbell Press			
Incline Press			
Decline Press			
Pull Overs			
Flyes			
Shoulder exercises	**Reps**	**Sets**	**Remarks**
Shoulder Press			
Forward Raise			
Rear Deltoid			
Bent Over Flyes			
Lateral Raise			
Upright Row			
Bicep exercises	**Reps**	**Sets**	**Remarks**
Isometric Hold			
Normal & Hammer Curls (standing)			
Preacher normal/hammer curls			
Normal & Hammer Curls (seated)			
Seated or bent over curl			
Triceps exercises	**Reps**	**Sets**	**Remarks**
Seated overhead push			
Kick Backs			
Lying overhead press			
Double arm seated push			
Leg exercises	**Reps**	**Sets**	**Remarks**
Dumbbell Squat			
Dumbbell Lunge			
Dumbbell Step Up			
Dumbbell Dead Lift			

*Choose 3-5 ex's per muscle group, and either overload or alternate each muscle group

CORE STRENGTH TRAINING TEMPLATES
Beginner to Advanced - (2 times per week + HIIT + Cardio)

Abdominal exercise program template - (Pages 274-292)

BEGINNER EXERCISES (30secs rest intervals)	20-30 REPS	2-3 SETS	REMARKS
Bent knee Sit Up			
(Exercise A)			
(Exercise B)			
Leg Raises			
(Exercise A)			
(Exercise B)			
(Exercise C)			
(Exercise D)			
(Exercise E)			
Sit Ups (arms above head)			
(Exercise A)			
(Exercise B)			
(Exercise C)			
Sit Ups (hands on head)			
(Exercise A)			
(Exercise B)			
(Exercise C)			
Utilising a fit-ball			
(Exercise A)			
(Exercise B)			
(Exercise C)			
(Exercise D)			
Beginner Machines			
(Exercise A)			MUSCLE ENDURANCE (Below 67% 1RM)
(Exercise B)			
(Exercise C)			
INTERMEDIATE EXERCISES (30-90secs rest intervals)	**6-12 REPS**	**3-6 SETS**	**REMARKS**
Weighted ball in hands			
(Exercise A)			
(Exercise B)			
(Exercise C)			
(Exercise D)			

Weighted ball in feet			
(Exercise A)			
(Exercise B)			
(Exercise C)			
Partner Exercises			
(Exercise A)			
(Exercise B)			
(Exercise C)			
(Exercise D)			
Utilising a fit-ball			
(Exercise A)			
(Exercise B)			
(Exercise C)			
(Exercise D)			
ADVANCED EXERCISES (2-5mins rest intervals)	**1-8 REPS**	**3-5 SETS**	**POWER** (70-85% 1RM)
B/wt & minimum equipment			
(Exercise A)			
(Exercise B)			
(Exercise C)			
Utilising machines			
(Exercise A)			
(Exercise B)			
(Exercise C)			
Utilising barbell			
(Exercise A)			
(Exercise B)			
(Exercise C)			
(Exercise D)			
(Exercise A)			
(Exercise F)			
Utilising dumbbells			
(Exercise A)			
(Exercise B)			
(Exercise C)			

*Choose 3-5 ex's per muscle group, and either overload or alternate each muscle group

CORE STRENGTH TRAINING
Power & maximum strength - (3 times per week + HIIT)

FIT-BALL EXERCISE PROGRAM TEMPLATE

Back exercises	6-10 Reps	4-6 Sets	Remarks
Alt arm & leg raise			
Ball Pull bent & straight legs			
Res-band rev flyes			
Db reverse flyes			
Single arm Db row			
Chest exercises	**Reps**	**Sets**	**Remarks**
Chest Press			
Flyes			
Pull Over			
Push Up			
Shoulder exercises	**Reps**	**Sets**	**Remarks**
Isometric Holds			
Shoulder Press			
Frontal Raise			
Prone lying raises			
Fit-ball Caterpillar			
Bicep exercises	**Reps**	**Sets**	**Remarks**
Isometric Holds			
Resistance band curls			
Hammer Curls			
Variation of Curls			
Triceps exercises	**Reps**	**Sets**	**Remarks**
Dumbbell overhead press (Back lying)			
B-bell overhead press			
Kickbacks			
Close arm press			
Other variations			
Leg exercises	**Reps**	**Sets**	**Remarks**
Hip Flexors			
Leg Bridge			
Abductor/Adductor			
Wall Squat			
Single Leg Squat			

*Choose 3-5 ex's per muscle group, and either overload or alternate each muscle group

OPTIONAL EXERCISES – (Page 245)

BODYWEIGHT EXERCISES	20-30 Reps	3-5 Sets	Remarks
Side plank			
Tibialis anterior			
Neck flexion (ISO)	MUSCULAR ENDURANCE		
Neck extension (ISO)	(Below 67% 1RM)		
Brachioradialis			
Calves (general)			
Calves (soleus)			
RESISTANCE BAND EXERCISES	**6-12 Reps**	**3-6 Sets**	**Remarks**
Tibialis anterior	MUSCLE SIZE		
Shoulder shrugs	(67-85% 1RM)		
BARBELL EXERCISES			
Wrist flexion	Muscle endurance		
Wrist extension	20-30 Reps / 3-5 Sets		
Shoulder shrugs (70-85% 1RM)	1-5 Reps	3-5 Sets	Power
DUMBBELL EXERCISES			
Shoulder shrugs (70-85% 1RM)	1-5 Reps	3-5 Sets	Power

MUSCLE SIZE TRAINING TEMPLATES
(3 times per week, alternated with Cardio, Flexibility + HIIT)

EXAMPLE 1

 # 1: Pushing exercises

Muscle groups	Weight (67-85% 1RM)	6-12 Reps	3-6 Sets	Remarks (30-90s rest)
Chest (General)				
Quadriceps				
Chest (Upper)				
Deltoid (Front)				
Calves (General)				
Optional exercises				
Quadriceps, Hip Adductors, Triceps and Obliques				

 # 2: Pulling exercises

Muscle groups	Weight (67-85% 1RM)	6-12 Reps	3-6 Sets	Remarks (30-90s rest)
Back (Lats)				
Hamstrings				
Back (General)				
Deltoid (Side)				
Biceps				
Optional exercises				
Hip Abductors, Hip Flexors, Trapezius (Upper) Abdominals and Obliques				

 # 3: Legs and arms

Muscle groups	Weight (67-85% 1RM)	6-12 Reps	3-6 Sets	Remarks (30-90s rest)
Quadriceps				
Hamstrings				
Calves (General)				
Triceps				
Biceps				
Optional exercises				
Hip Flexors, Abdominals and Obliques				

EXAMPLE 2

 # 1: Upper Body

Muscle groups	Weight (67-85% 1RM)	6-12 Reps	3-6 Sets	Remarks (30-90s rest)
Chest (General)				
Back (General)				
Deltoid (Side)				
Triceps				
Biceps				
Optional exercises				
Chest (Upper), Back (Lats), Deltoid (Front) and Trapezius (Upper)				

 # 2: Lower Body

Muscle groups	Weight (67-85% 1RM)	6-12 Reps	3-6 Sets	Remarks (30-90s rest)
Quadriceps				
Hamstrings				
Calves (General)				
Optional exercises				
Hip Abductors / Adductors / Flexors, Abdominals and Obliques				

 # 3: Torso exercises

Muscle groups	Weight (67-85% 1RM)	6-12 Reps	3-6 Sets	Remarks (30-90s rest)
Chest (General)				
Back (Lats)				
Chest (Upper)				
Back (General)				
Deltoid (Front)				
Deltoid (Side)				
Optional exercises	**Weight**	**Reps**	**Sets**	**Remarks**
Deltoid (Rear) and Trapezius (Upper)				

MUSCLE POWER TRAINING TEMPLATES
(3-4 times per week, alternated with CV, Flexibility + HIIT)

EXAMPLE 1 – Explosive, Bilateral, Unilateral and rotational exercises

1

Muscle groups	Weight (70-85% 1RM)	1-8 Reps	3-5 Sets	Remarks (2-5mins rest)
BB Bent over row				
Hang power clean				BB Adv ex
Cable rotating ext'n				P288
B/W Pull ups				

2

Muscle groups	Weight (70-85% 1RM)	1-8 Reps	3-5 Sets	Remarks (2-5mins rest)
BB Split squat				P240
Cable push/pull				P138
DB Shoulder press				Alternate
BB Bench press				Close grip

3

Muscle groups	Weight (70-85% 1RM)	1-8 Reps	3-5 Sets	Remarks (2-5mins rest)
BB Clean pull				P238
Lat pull downs				Dble or S-arm
Back ext'n				+W.T
Cable rotation				P288

4

Muscle groups	Weight (70-85% 1RM)	1-8 Reps	3-5 Sets	Remarks (2-5mins rest)
BB Squat				Front/rear sh.
DB Inc B/Press				
BB Push press				P171
Jump squats				+W.T

EXAMPLE 2 – Less functional type exercises

 # 1: Chest and back

Muscle groups	Weight (70-85% 1RM)	1-8 Reps	3-5 Sets	Remarks (2-5mins rest)
Chest (General 1)				Chess Press
Back (Lats 1)				Lat pull down
Chest (Upper)				Incline Press
Back (General)				Bent over row
Optional exercises				
Chest (General 2)				DB Flyes
Back (General or Lats)				Pull ups
Trapezius (Upper)				Shoulder shrug

 # 2: Legs

Muscle groups	Weight (70-85% 1RM)	1-8 Reps	3-5 Sets	Remarks (2-5mins rest)
Quadriceps 1				BB Squat
Hamstrings 1				S-L Dead lift
Calves (General)				S-L Heel raise
Optional exercises				
Quadriceps 2, Hamstrings 2, Hip Add/Abductors & Flexors, Calves (Soleus), Tibialis Anterior, Abdominal & Obliques.				

#3: Shoulders and arms

Muscle groups	Weight (70-85% 1RM)	1-8 Reps	3-5 Sets	Remarks (2-5mins rest)
Deltoid (Front)				D/B Fr raise
Deltoid (Side)				D/B Lat raise
Deltoid (Rear)				Rear delt row
Triceps				BB O-H Press
Biceps				DB Curls
Optional exercises				
Brachialis (Preacher curls), Brachioradialis, Wrist Flexors/Extensors & Neck Extensors & Flexors.				

MAXIMUM STRENGTH TRAINING TEMPLATES
(4 times per week, alternated with CV & Flexibility)

EXAMPLE 1

 # 1: Back and biceps

Muscle groups	Weight (85%+ 1RM)	Below 6 Reps	2-6 Sets	Remarks (2-5mins rest)
Back (Lats 1)				
Back (General)				
Back (Gen2 / Lats2)				
Biceps				
Optional exercises				
Brachialis (Preacher curls), Brachioradialis & Wrist Flexors				

 # 2: Chest and triceps

Muscle groups	Weight (85%+ 1RM)	Below 6 Reps	2-6 Sets	Remarks (2-5mins rest)
Chest (Upper 1)				
Chest (General 1)				
Triceps				
Optional exercises				
Chest (Gen 2 / upper2), Wrist Extensors				

 # 3: Thighs

Muscle groups	Weight (85%+ 1RM)	Below 6 Reps	2-6 Sets	Remarks (2-5mins rest)
Quadriceps 1				Target a specific glute exercise instead of hamstrings & quadriceps if required.
Hamstrings 1				
Quadriceps 2				
Hamstrings 2				
Optional exercises				
Hip Abductors & Adductors				

 # 4: Shoulders, calves and abdominals

Muscle groups	Weight (85%+ 1RM)	Below 6 Reps	2-6 Sets	Remarks (2-5mins rest)
Deltoid (Front 1)				
Calves (General 1)				
Deltoid (Side 1)				
Deltoid (Rear)				
Calves (Soleus)				
Trapezius (Upper)				
Abdominal				Can be exercised elsewhere
Optional exercises	**Weight**	**Reps**	**Sets**	**Remarks**
Calves (General 2)				Hip flexors, obliques, neck extensors & flexors can be exercised with another workout if required.
Deltoid (Front 2 or Side 2)				
Tibialis Anterior				
Hip Flexors				
Neck Extensors				
Neck Flexors				
Obliques				

EXAMPLE 2

 # 1: Torso pulling exercises

Muscle groups	Weight (85%+ 1RM)	Below 6 Reps	2-6 Sets	Remarks (2-5mins rest)
Back (Lats 1)				Neck Flexors may be exercised with the back if desired.
Deltoid (Sid 1)				
Back (General 1)				
Trapezius (Upper)				
Back (Gen 2 / Lats2)				
Deltoid (Rear)				
Optional exercises	**Weight**	**Reps**	**Sets**	**Remarks**
Deltoid (Side 2)				

#2: Torso pushing exercises

Muscle groups	Weight (85%+ 1RM)	Below 6 Reps	2-6 Sets	Remarks (2-5mins rest)
Chest (General 1)				
Chest (Upper 1)				
Chest (General 2)				
Deltoid (Front)				
Optional exercises	**Weight**	**Reps**	**Sets**	**Remarks**
Chest (Gen 3/Upper 2)				
Neck Extensors				
Neck Flexors				
Deltoid (Front)				

 # 3: Leg and arm pulling exercises

Muscle groups	Weight (85%+ 1RM)	Below 6 Reps	2-6 Sets	Remarks (2-5mins rest)
Hamstrings				
Biceps				
Abdominal				
Optional exercises	**Weight**	**Reps**	**Sets**	**Remarks**
Hip Abductors				Hip flexor, abdominal and oblique exercises may be exercised with another workout, and wrist extensors may be exercised with triceps.
Brachialis				
Hip Flexors				
Brachioradialis				
Wrist Flexors				
Obliques				
Wrist Extensors				

 # 4: Leg and arm pushing exercises

Muscle groups	Weight (85%+ 1RM)	Below 6 Reps	2-6 Sets	Remarks (2-5mins rest)
Quadriceps 1				
Triceps				
Calves (General 1)				
Calves (Soleus)				
Optional exercises	**Weight**	**Reps**	**Sets**	**Remarks**
Quadriceps 2				
Hip Adductors				
Calves (General 2)				
Tibialis Anterior				May be exercised with the hamstrings

319

6 DAY MIXED STRENGTH & CV TRAINING TEMPLATE

Day 1: Chest and biceps

Specific exercises	Weight	Reps	Sets	Remarks
BB Bench press	45% 1RM	15	1	
Incline DB press	60% 1RM	8	2	
Weighted dips (M)	Bodyweight	10-12	1	
" pull ups (M)	Bodyweight	10	1	
BB bicep curl	60% 1RM	8	1	

Day 2: High intensity interval training (HIIT)

Sprint	Recovery	Time for 1 set	Sprints per workout	Remarks
30secs	90secs	120secs	10-15 sprints	
20secs	60secs	80secs	15-22 sprints	
15secs	45secs	60secs	20-30 sprints	
10secs	30secs	40secs	30-45 sprints	

Day 3: Legs and lower back

Muscle groups	Weight	Reps	Sets	Remarks
BB Squat	45% 1RM	15	1	
Leg press (M)	60% 1RM	15	2	
BB S-leg dead-lift	45% 1RM	15	1	
BB Good mornings	60% 1RM	1	2	

Day 4: Off

Day 5: Shoulders and abdominals

Muscle groups	Weight	Reps	Sets	Remarks
BB Clean & Jerk	45% 1RM	10	1	
DB Lateral raises	60% 1RM	12	1	
DB B-O Lat raises	60% 1RM	12	1	B-O = bent over
Weighted sit ups	60% 1RM	12	1	Disc across chest
Weighted leg raises	60% 1RM	10	2	Weight in feet

Day 6

Aerobic endurance

Activity	Time	Intensity	Remarks
Steady state run	40-60mins	Moderate to hard	

Day 7: Back and triceps

Muscle groups	Weight	Reps	Sets	Remarks
OG pull ups (M)	45% 1RM	15	1	
BB bent over row	60% 1RM	8	2	
BB Bench press	45% 1RM	15	1	Close grip
Weighted dips (M)	Bodyweight	10	1	
Cable tri pull downs	60% 1RM	8	1	

Progressions

Strength
Depending on the exercise, increase the % of 1RM, whilst decreasing the repetitions. The number of sets should be dictated by the time you have, continuous maintenance of perfect form and ultimately how you are feeling.

High intensity interval training (HIIT)
If you are a beginner progress from 1:3+ ratio i.e. same as the example on Day 2, progress to 1:2 i.e. 30s / 60s or 1:1 30s / 30s. The timings can be adjusted accordingly for example instead of 30s use 1m etc.

MIXED STRENGTH TRAINING TEMPLATE

MUSCLE GROUPS & EXERCISES	MUSCLE ENDURANCE (30-50% 1RM)		POWER (70-85% 1RM)		MAXIMUM STRENGTH (85%+ 1RM)	
Back	Weight	20–30 reps	Weight	6 – 10 reps	Weight	1 – 5 reps
Chest						
Shoulder						
Biceps						
Triceps						
Legs						

FLEXIBILITY PROGRAM TEMPLATE (Page 33-52)

Timings will depend on whether it's a warm up (6-12secs for 6-10 sets) or cool down i.e. hold for longer.

Back stretches	Time	Sets	Remarks
Forward bends			
Tree hug			
Twist & hold			
Pelvic tilt			
Knees to chest			
Chest stretches	Time	Sets	Remarks
Hands to rear			
Wall Stretch 1			
Wall Stretches 2 & 3			
Arms above head			
Arm out to side-floor			
Shoulder stretches	Time	Sets	Remarks
Most Common			
Anterior Deltoid			
Posterior Deltoid			
Additional			
Bicep stretches	Time	Sets	Remarks
Common stretch			
Kneeling (all fours)			
Arm out to side-floor			
Seated (arms to rear)			
Triceps stretches	Time	Sets	Remarks
Common stretch			
Using a towel			
Using a bench			
Using a partner			
Variations			
Leg stretches	Time	Sets	Remarks
Hip flexors			
Glutes			
Hamstrings			
Quadriceps			
ITB			
Inner thigh			
Calf			

EXTRAS

During recovery, your muscle glycogen stores are replenished and muscle tissue repaired. The time it takes to replenish muscle glycogen depends on the severity of depletion and the amount and timing of carbohydrate intake in your diet. On average, this takes between 24 hours and three days. You need to ensure that you consume enough protein to provide the raw material for new muscle growth. An inadequate intake will result in slower repair and growth and therefore your strength gains will be compromised. On the other hand, an excessive intake will not further enhance muscle growth or strength.

BALANCED DIET

FOOD TYPE	IMPORTANCE	AMOUNT
Bread and other cereals	These foods are the main energy source for the body.	You should eat 6-11 portions a day
Fruit and vegetables	These foods are important to provide the vitamins and minerals your body needs to stay healthy and are an important source of fibre.	You should eat 5 portions of fruit and vegetables a day
Dairy foods	These foods are important for healthy bones and teeth.	You should eat 3-4 portions a day.
Meat, fish and alternatives (proteins)	Often called muscle foods, as they help build your muscles.	You should eat 2-3 portions a day.
Foods with added fat and sugar	These should only be eaten in small amounts and are not essential for a healthy balanced diet.	

Here are some more specific choices:

Carbohydrates - Oatmeal, rice, breads, yams beans, potatoes, fruits and veggies.

Proteins - Steak, chicken, lean beef, cottage cheese, whole milk, eggs and salmon

Fats - Olive oil, flax oil, avocados, nuts and peanut butter

Extras (high calorie cheat food)
Ice cream, raisins, dried fruit and trail mix.

Hydration
When the climate is hot and humid or when you are participating in exercise, you will need more water than what is considered a normal intake i.e. 6-8 glasses or 1.5 -2L per day.

EATING FOR EXERCISE - (before, during & after)

Before exercise - Never Train Hungry

Choices:

- 3 meals in your body prior to training;
- Or eat the biggest meal of your day immediately after your workout.

During exercise
Drinking carbohydrate and Protein drinks
Mix up a 2:1 ratio of carbohydrate to protein as described below, for 100-200 extra calories per day.

After exercise
Same as the workout drink as above, which is easily an extra one pound per week. You should only really use this strategy if you are weight training at a very high intensity.

BULKING UP
Consuming more of the following than normal is by far the easiest and fastest method that you should aim for:

- Protein i.e. replacing 1 chicken breast for 2
- Nuts;
- Protein powder;
- Carbohydrates i.e. more high fibre bread, whole-wheat pasta etc.

You body will have no other option but to start gaining weight if this is your aim.

Super-healthy protein drink
Drink at least 5 times a week and several times a day during peak training cycles

x1 scoop of egg white protein adjusted to your body weight i.e. 1.5g per b/wt and x1g per b/wt when doing two shakes a day.

Ingredients

x1 raw egg	1 to 1.5 cups of pure water	5g of powdered L-glutamine	Raw almonds	Handful of fresh or frozen berries
Sweetner - stevia	Ice	5g of creatine monohydrate	Small amount of pumpkin seeds	

Eat every 2-3 hours, and ensure you are eating your first meal within 15-30mins of waking up. Your 1st meal of the day should always consist of nutritious food to flood your body with quality nutrients. Spend more of your time preparing food, more time eating food and more time shopping for food. Focus on caloric-rich foods that are loaded with nutrients, avoid foods with empty calories i.e. no fat and sugar eat a high caloric meal loaded with slow releasing carbohydrates, proteins, fats, vitamins, minerals and fibre. Push your body's threshold regarding food and eating, your body requires more food as you gain more muscle on your body and your metabolism increases. So, if you are not eating, then you are not growing.

SUMMARY

As with every exercise workout, you can make it as easy or as difficult as you choose and this book was put together in such a way that the exercises shown are progressive according to your present fitness level. You can of course begin where you feel more comfortable, so long as you are safe. Of course there are many more exercises you can perform to exercise your whole body but this selection contains specific groups of exercises which utilise your own bodyweight, the fit-ball and other equipment to further ensure that your whole body is worked thoroughly. The selected exercises compliment each other and with the respective progressions you can definitely challenge yourself accordingly and get enormous benefit from using them in a correct and safe manner. Ensure as always that you warm up and stretch accordingly prior to any exercise and more importantly cool down and stretch for longer periods on completion of your workout in order to prevent injuries and reduce muscle soreness.

Utilising equipment such as the fit-ball and weighted balls etc prevent you from repetition of the same bodyweight exercises and will ultimately add variety to your training. If you use the fit-ball to compliment your normal routine then it is advised that you complete these type of exercises towards the latter part of your workout. Focus is the key factor with core strength training which in turn ensures that your body remains balanced, not just on the fit-ball but with reference to its musculature and respective supporting structures. Training with weights is the most beneficial and most underrated way to work your whole body, especially with regards to weight loss. So many people think that you need to do just sit ups to work the abs, but the exercises with weights if performed correctly and safely require a large amount of strength from your abdominals and this is due to the majority of your power coming from this area.

Safety is the key factor, so long as you master the technique with minimum resistance/weight initially and progress accordingly. Muscle imbalances can and will cause problems in other areas of your body, especially later in life. These imbalances should be targeted immediately by tightening and/or stretching the relevant muscles involved (explained in more detail within the rehabilitation book on the website below). Maintaining good posture at all times will undoubtedly help too. The amount of repetitions and sets you complete will depend on your current level of fitness, try out all of the exercises and create a program for yourself using the templates provided. Depending on your aim and how you plan your time and workout program, your personal success will only be dictated by you. Whole body workshop can only provide you with the information, you must provide the mind and body to compliment the content.

'Maximise Your Fitness Potential' is for all levels, but especially those of you who have reached a plateau and the time is right for you to advance on the knowledge you learned from 'Exercise your whole body at home'

More related article can be found on our websites:

www.wholebodyworkshop.com / info@wholebodyworkshop.com
www.weightlossdubai.com / info@weightlossdubai.com

BIBLIOGRAPHY

Bompa, Tudor O. Periodization: Theory and methodology of training, 4th Ed, 1999.

Brooks, D. your personal trainer. 1999.

Chuen Hui S. Yuen P Y. Validity of the modified sit and reach test: a comparison with other protocols, Medicine & Science in sports & exercise, Official journal of the american college of sports medicine Volume 32, Number 9, Lippincott Williams, Hagerstown, U.S.A, 2000.

Durstine, L J. King, A C. Painter, P L. Roitman, J L. Zwiren, L D. Kenney, L W. ACSM'S Resource manual for guidelines for exercise testing and prescription, second edition. American college of sports medicine,Williams & Wilkins, U.S.A, 1993.

Egger G. Champion N. The fitness leaders handbook, third edition, Kangaroo press, Australia, 1991.

Harre, D. (Ed.) 1982. Trainingslehre. Berlin: Sportverlag.

MacDougall D J. Wenger H A. Green H J. Physiological testing of the high performance athlete. Published for the Canadian association of sport sciences, second edition, Human Kinetics, U.S.A.

Mahler D A. Froelicher V F. Houston Miller N. York T D. ACSM'S Guidelines for exercise testing and prescription, 5th edition, Williams & Wilkins U.S.A, 1995.

Nadori, L. 1989. Theoretical and methodological basis of training planning with special considerations within a microcycle. Lincoln, NE: National strength and conditioning association.

Nikiforov, I. 1974. About the structure of training in scientific work.

Piehl, 1974; Recovery times for muscular endurance, Fox et al, 1989.

Scholich, M. 1974. Kreistraining. Berlin: Bartels and weritz.

Schroeder, W. 1969. The correlation between force and the other motor abilities.

Thomas D G. Swimming steps to success, second edition, Leisure press, U.S.A, 1989.

An excellent source for fitness information: - www.exrx.net

www.ingramcontent.com/pod-product-compliance
Lightning Source LLC
Chambersburg PA
CBHW020335270326
41926CB00007B/189